To Raffaele and Cettina,
my father and mother
with deep gratitude
for their life's teachings

Springer-Verlag Italia Srl.

New Advances in Heart Failure and Atrial Fibrillation

Edited by
Michele Gulizia

Proceedings of the
Mediterranean Cardiology Meeting

(Taormina, April 10-12, 2003)

Springer

MICHELE GULIZIA, MD
Chief of Cardiology Division
S. Luigi - S. Currò Hospital
Viale A. Fleming, 24
95126 - Catania, Italy

Originally published by Springer-Verlag Italia, Milan in 2003
Softcover reprint of the hardcover 1st edition 2003

ISBN 978-88-470-2169-3 ISBN 978-88-470-2087-0 (eBook)
DOI 10.1007/978-88-470-2087-0

Library of Congress Cataloging-in-Publication Data: Applied for

Cover design: Simona Colombo, Milan
Typesetting: Graphostudio, Milan

SPIN: 10917053

Preface

Clinical practice is evolving at a rapid pace. In no place more so than in the field of cardiology, has this change been so evident.

Heart Failure and Atrial Fibrillation are two emerging pathologies where many investigators are addressing their researches. Less than 10 years ago, Heart Failure was considered only of relevance to internists and Atrial Fibrillation as a common benign arrhythmia. Today, the diffusion of Heart Failure and Atrial Fibrillation amongst the population represents one of the major public health problems at the beginning of the third millennium.

The need to have a *state of the art* about the epidemiology, physiopathological and electrogenetic mechanisms, diagnosis, pharmacological or electrical treatment, prognosis, in- and outhospital management, organizational and economical implications of Heart Failure and Atrial Fibrillation inspired us to organize a biannual international meeting.

This book contains the Proceedings of the Mediterranean Cardiology Meeting held in Taormina - Italy, at Villa Diodoro on 10th–12th April 2003. Even though this is the first meeting, it boasts the participation of many nationally and internationally renowned speakers in the field of Heart Failure and Atrial Fibrillation who will interact actively with the delegates.

The book is divided into seven sections, each dedicated to a different topic: atrial fibrillation and heart failure: the chicken-egg dilemma; in- and outhospital management of heart failure patients; current trends and treatments of atrial fibrillation and flutter; 10 years of biventricular pacing in congestive heart failure; atrial arrhythmias: drugs, devices or ablation for the prevention and treatment of the recurrences; new approaches in electrical treatment and management of heart failure patients and, last but not least, the role of ICD in the prevention of sudden death in heart failure, the brilliant lecture of my best friend Antonio Raviele who inspired and incited me in the field of arrhythmology.

This book is aimed at providing the latest information about the most recent and modern aspects concerning the above mentioned pathologies. It is intended not only for cardiologists, but also for those who are actively interested in the evidence-based approach to clinical care, such as internists, first aid clinicians, fellows, students, nurses and technicians. It may also be helpful for those engaged in the development and coordination of research strategies in biological engineering, industry and regulatory affairs, who have a high interest in the whole management of these cardiac pathologies.

A Faculty, selected among the Italian and foreign leading experts in the field, provided the highest quality of this volume. In these last years, the publications of many of them contributed to my scientific development and influenced many of my professional considerations and decisions. I am really most indebted to all these Authors who have dedicated invaluable time and efforts without which this book would not have been completed.

I also wish to thank the Springer-Verlag staff and in particular Donatella Rizza, Executive Editor, who has facilitated the publication of this book at the start of the Mediterranean Cardiology Meeting and who has kindly assisted me throughout. Special and deep words of thanks are addressed to Rita Reggiani, professional, tireless and very kind Project Leader of Adria Congrex, who has helped and supported me in the optimal organization of this International Meeting, together with her staff members Sara and Silvana.

I cannot forget to acknowledge the role of my two teachers Antonio Circo and Salvatore Mangiameli who encouraged my passion for cardiology and particularly for arrhythmology and cardiostimulation.

Also, I would like to thank my colleagues Cacia, Francese, Raciti, Rubino and all the nursing staff of my Division at the "S. Luigi-S. Currò" Hospital of Catania for their active collaboration and support during these years of work and for the organization of this Meeting.

Finally, a special mention for my wife Luisa and my daughters Alice and Raffaella. I am especially and deeply grateful to them. Without their love and patience I could not have spent so many nights and weekends preparing the Meeting and this volume.

Michele Gulizia

Table of Contents

CURRENT TRENDS AND TREATMENTS OF ATRIAL FIBRILLATION AND FLUTTER

List of Contributors

LECTURE

Sudden Death Prevention in Heart Failure: What Role for ICD?

A. Rossillo, A. Raviele

Heart failure is one of the most frequent cardiovascular diseases, with a high cost to health care; in Italy about 1 million people are estimated to suffer from heart failure. The annual mortality due to heart failure ranges from 16% to 30%, increasing to 70% when patients with severe symptoms are considered. The relative rates of sudden death decrease with increase in NYHA class [1]. In 70%-80% of patients sudden death is due to an arrhythmia such as monomorphic ventricular tachycardia, polymorphic ventricular tachycardia, ventricular fibrillation, or in 15%-20%, bradyarrhythmias.

In recent years an effort has been made to improve the treatment of heart failure. Prevention of sudden death has been considered using many drugs, classically divided in two groups: therapeutic agents commonly used in heart failure and antiarrhythmic treatment. A meta-analysis of randomized clinical trials showed that ACE inhibitor treatment reduces total mortality by 17% and the sudden cardiac death rate by 20% [2]. In a digoxin study, treatment with digoxin caused a slight increase in deaths from arrhythmia, and a recent analysis of the data showed an increase of mortality in female patients [3, 4]. Use of diuretic agents theoretically increases the risk of sudden death due to hypokalemia, hypomagnesemia, and activation of the renin-angiotensin system, but the RALES trial showed a significant reduction in sudden deaths during spironolactone treatment. Second-generation calcium channel blockers improve survival in patients with nonischemic cardiomyopathy; amlodipine reduced the mortality rate by 16% in severe heart failure patients, but its efficacy in preventing sudden death is unknown [5].

There are other types of drugs that are able to reduce the mortality and the risk of sudden death, such as statin and N3-polyunsaturated fatty acids; we are waiting for more data on the real efficacy of omega- 3 [6, 7].

As for antiarrhythmic drugs, it has been well known since the end of the 1980s that class I drugs have no effect or a deleterious effect on mortality [8,

Division of Cardiology, Umberto I Hospital, Mestre-Venice, Italy

9]. Studies like CIBIS-II and MERIT HF have shown the role of the "old" β-blockers in the treatment of heart failure and the significant reduction of the risk of sudden cardiac death; recently, these results have also been confirmed for noncardioselective β-blockers with ancillary vasodilatatory properties, such as carvedilol [10-12]. An important meta-analysis on amiodarone concludes that this drug is also effective in the prevention of sudden death [13]. Other antiarrhythmic drugs have been tested in recent years, but none was able to reduce the risk of sudden death: D-sotalol in the SWORD trial increased mortality, while in other studies dofetilide and azimilide showed a neutral effect [14-16].

Another possible therapy for sudden cardiac death is the implantable cardioverter-defibrillator (ICD); the first studies have evaluated the efficacy of the ICD in secondary prevention of sudden death. The Dutch, CIDS, CASH and AVID studies have confirmed that the ICD is superior to the best medical therapy in patients with ventricular fibrillation, syncopal ventricular tachycardia, and ventricular tachycardia associated with left ventricular dysfunction [17-20]. Domanski et al. in a post-hoc analysis have demonstrated that the patients with best outcome for ICD therapy are those that have the worst left ventricular ejection fraction [21].

In recent years all the trials have been trying to establish the efficacy of the ICD in primary prevention of sudden death: the MADIT, MUSTT, and CABG Patch trials have been performed in patients with coronary artery disease with left ventricular dysfunction and a high risk of sudden death. The first two studies have shown that ICD significantly reduces mortality during a long-term follow-up, while the last concluded that ICD is not the best therapy to prevent sudden death [22-27]. Recently other two important papers have been published on the SCD-HEFT and MADIT II trials.

These trials have been trying to demonstrate how fundamental ICD therapy is in the battle against sudden cardiac death, and for this purpose simple criteria for enrolment were selected.

In the ICD arm of the MADIT II study mortality was about 30% lower than in the control group. The results of this study have enlarged the population who need an ICD [25, 26].

On the basis of these data we can conclude that the ICD is the basic therapy in combination with conventional drug therapy to prevent sudden cardiac death. We must hope for a reduction in the device costs so that this treatment can become more widely spread among heart failure patients.

References

1. Uretsky BF, Sheahan RG (1997) Primary prevention of sudden cardiac death in heart failure: will the solution be shocking? J Am Coll Cardiol 30(7):1589-1597
2. Domanski MJ, Exner DV, Borkowf CB et al (1999) Effect of angiotensin converting enzyme inhibition on sudden cardiac death in patients following acute myocardial

infarction. A meta-analysis of randomized clinical trials. J Am Coll Cardiol 33:598-604

3. The Digitalis Investigation Group (1997) The effect of digoxin on mortality and morbidity in patients with heart failure. N Engl J Med 336:525-533
4. Rathore SS, Wang Y, Krumholz HM (2002) Sex based differences in the effect of digoxin for the treatment of heart failure. N Engl J Med 347:1403-1411
5. Packer M, O'Connor CM, Ghali JK et al (1996) Effect of amlodipine on morbidity and mortality in severe chronic heart failure. N Engl J Med 335:1107-1114
6. The long term intervention with pravastatin in ischaemic disease (LIPID) study group (1998). Prevention of cardiovascular events and death with pravastatin in patients with coronary heart disease and a broad range of initial cholesterol levels. N Engl J Med 339:1349-1357
7. GISSI Prevenzione Investigators (1999) Dietary supplementation with n-3 polyunsaturated fatty acids and vitamin E after myocardial infarction: results of the GISSI-Prevenzione trial. Lancet 354:447-455
8. CAST I investigators (1989) Preliminary report: effect of encainide and flecainide on mortality in a randomized trial of arrhythmia suppression after myocardial infarction. N Engl J Med 321:406-412
9. The CAST II investigators (1989) Effect of the antiarrhythmic agent morozine on survival after myocardial infarction. N Engl J Med 321:406-412
10. Packer M, Bristow MR, Cohn JN et al, for the US Carvedilol Heart Failure Study Group (1996) The effect of carvedilol on morbidity and mortality in patients with chronic heart failure. N Engl J Med 334:1349-1355
11. CIBIS-II Investigators and Committees (1999) The Cardiac Insufficiency Bisoprolol Study II (CIBIS-II): a randomised trial. Lancet 353:9-13
12. The International Steering Committee on behalf of the MERIT-HF Study Group (1997) Rationale, design, and organization of the metoprolol CR/XL randomized intervention trial in heart failure (MERIT-HF). Am J Cardiol 80:54J-58J
13. Amiodarone Trials Meta-Anlysis Investigators (1997) Effect of prophylactic amiodarone on mortality after acute myocardial infarction and in congestive heart failure: meta-analysis of individual data from 6500 patients in randomized trials. Lancet 350:1417-1424
14. Waldo AL, Camm AJ, deRuyter H et al, for the SWORD investigators (1996) Effect of D-sotalol on mortality in patients with left ventricular dysfunction after recent and remote myocardial infarction. 348:7-12
15. Torp-Pedersen C, Moller M, Bloch-Thomsen PE et al, for the Danish Investigations of Arrhythmia and Mortality on Dofetilide Study Group (1999) Dofetilide in patients with congestive heart failure and left ventricular dysfunction. N Engl J Med 341:857-865
16. Køber L, Bloch-Thomsen PE, Møller M et al, on behalf of the Danish Investigations of Arrhythmia and Mortality on Dofetilide (DIAMOND) Study Group (2000) Effect of dofetilide in patients with recent myocardial infarction and left-ventricular dysfunction: a randomised trial. Lancet 356:2052-2058
17. The Antiarrhythmics versus Implantable Defibrillator (AVID) Investigators (1997) A comparison of antiarhythmic-drug therapy with implantable defibrillators in patients resuscitated from near-fatal ventricular arrhythmias. N Engl J Med 337:176-1583
18. Connoly SJ, Gent M, Roberts RS et al, for the CIDS investigators (2000) Canadian Implantable Defibrillator Study (CIDS). A randomized trial of the implantable cardioverter defibrillator against amiodarone. Circulation 101:1297-1302

19. Kuck KH, Cappato R, Siebels J, Ruppel R, for the CASH investigators (2000) Randomized comparison of antiarrhythmic drug therapy with implantable defibrillators in patients resuscitated from cardiac arrest. The Cardiac Arrest Study Hamburg (CASH). Circulation 102:748-754
20. Cappato R (1999) Secondary prevention of sudden death: the Dutch Study, the Antiarrhythmics Versus Implantable Defibrillator Trial, the Cardiac Arrest Study Hamburg, and the Canadian Implantable Defibrillator Study. Am J Cardiol 83:68D-73D
21. Domanski MJ, Sakseena S, Epstein AE et al, for the AVID investigators (1999) Relative effectiveness of the implantable cardioverter-defibrillator and antiarrhythmic drugs in patients with varying degrees of left ventricular dysfunction who have survived malignant ventricular arrhythmias. J Am Coll Cardiol 34:1090-1095
22. Moss AJ, Hall WJ, Cannom DS et al, for the MADIT investigators (1996) Improved survival with an implanted defibrillator in patients with coronary disease at high risk for ventricular arrhythmia. N Engl J Med 335:1933-1940
23. Buxton AE, Lee KL, Fisher JD et al, for the MUSTT (1999) A randomized study of the prevention of sudden death in patients with coronary artery disease. N Engl J Med 341:1882-1890
24. Bigger JT for the CABG Patch trial investigators (1997) Prophylactic use of implanted cardiac defibrillators in patients at high risk for ventricular arrhythmias after coronary artery bypass graft surgery. N Engl J Med 337:1569-1575
25. Klein H, Auricchio A, Reek S, Geller C (1999) New primary prevention trials of sudden cardiac death in patients with left ventricular dysfunction: SCD-HEFT and MADIT-II. Am J Cardiol 83:91D-97D
26. Moss AJ, Zareba W, Hall WJ et al, for the MADIT II Investigators (2001) Prophylactic implantation of a defibrillator in patients with myocardial infarction and reduced ejection fraction. N Engl J Med 346:877-883

ATRIAL FIBRILLATION AND HEART FAILURE: THE CHICKEN-EGG DILEMMA

Incidence and Diagnosis of Atrial Fibrillation in Patients with Heart Failure

A. Curnis, G. Mascioli, L. Bontempi, M. Metra, L. Dei Cas

Atrial fibrillation (AF) and congestive heart failure (CHF) can have common symptoms and are often coexistent. It is likely that they are the most common cardiac diseases and they undoubtedly constitute major sources of health expenditure.

It is often impossible to establish if, in a patient with AF and CHF symptoms, the "primum movens" was AF or CHF, because it is well known that AF, especially if ventricular rate is not optimally controlled, can lead to a disturbance of left ventricular function, just as CHF, by causing an enlargement of the atria, can promote CHF. Furthermore, both AF and CHF are common diseases among older people: the prevalence of CHF is 1-3% among older people [1], and AF affects almost 10% of octogenarians [2]. This increased prevalence is commonly attributed mainly to improved medical treatment of patients with acute cardiac diseases, especially coronary artery disease.

The prevalence of AF is even higher in patients with CHF: in fact, this arrhythmia is present in 40-50% of patients in NYHA functional classes III and IV, whereas its prevalence drops to 10% in patients in class II. Overall, AF affects approximately 15-30% of patients with clinically overt CHF [3], and CHF itself is one of the most powerful independent predictors of AF (sixfold increased risk) [2].

Nevertheless, as already stated, AF can be a cause of CHF: loss of atrial contraction and irregular ventricular rhythm decrease cardiac output [4], just as restoration of sinus rhythm (SR) improves it [5]. Moreover, it must not be forgotten that antiarrhythmic drugs used to mantain SR can also have negative effects on hemodynamic function, both in terms of a direct negative inotropic effect and in terms of possible proarrhythmic effects.

Despite this tight relationship, the prognostic impact of AF in patients with CHF is still unclear. Whereas V-HeFT [3] and two other small studies [6, 7] were not able to find an AF-related increase in mortality, other, more recent,

Department of Cardiology, Spedali Civili di Brescia, Italy

larger trials showed an increase in mortality directly due to AF [8, 9]. Recently, a prospective international multicenter AF-CHF trial has begun patient enrollment in order to evaluate the effect on mortality of two different strategies: rhythm control with electrical cardioversion and drugs, and rate control with drugs or the ablate-and-pace procedure. This study will, it is hoped, give physicians dealing with CHF patients a more detailed idea of which is the better strategy for patients with CHF who develop AF. At present, which of these two strategies would be best to follow is still unknown. Although it is true that the presence of a stable SR could be extremely important in maintaining active atrial contraction, thus increasing the cardiac output, it is also true that controlling the ventricular rate - especially if mainteinance of SR is impossible - can help physicians to avoid derangement of the ejection fraction.

Ablate-and-pace has shown to be an extremely useful approach in 10-15% of patients in whom rate control cannot be obtained with drugs [10]. In a meta-analysis of 21 studies that enrolled a total of 1181 patients, ablate-and-pace significantly improved quality of life, functional status, left ventricular function, and exercise capacity, and reduced hospitalisations [11]. It is extremely interesting that the patients who benefited most from this treatment were those with the worst basal left ventricular function.

Recently, pacing has also been proposed as a treatment to prevent AF recurrences. New pacing algorithms, dual-site atrial pacing, and biatrial pacing have all been proposed for this pathology, with the aim of reducing the post-extrasystolic interval, improving interatrial and intra-atrial conduction delays, and homogenizing refractory periods. Although, some studies have shown effectivity in reducing the AF burden [12], others have failed to find positive effects [13]. Nevertheless, the availability of devices that can monitor patients' rhythm and offer specifically designed algorithms to prevent and treat atrial tachyarrhythmias could be extremely useful in CHF.

It should not be forgotten that other pacing modalities, such as biventricular pacing, that could significantly improve hemodynamic function in patients with AF might have positive effects for the reduction of AF in this population.

References

1. Cleland J, Clark A (1999) Has the survival of the heart failure population changed? Lessons from trials. Am J Cardiol 83:112D-119D
2. Kannel WB, Abbott RD, Savage DD, McNamara PM (1982) Epidemiologic features of chronic atrial fibrillation: the Framingham study. N Engl J Med 306:1018-1022
3. Carson PE, Johnson GR, Dunkman WB et al (1993) The influence of atrial fibrillation on prognosis in mild to moderate heart failure. The V-HeFT studies. Circulation 87:102-110
4. Pozzoli M, Cioffi G, Traversi E et al (1998) Predictors of primary atrial fibrillation and concomitant clinical and hemodynamical changes in patients with chronic heart failure: a prospective study in 344 patients with baseline sinus rhythm. J Am Coll Cardiol 32:197-204

5. Gosselink AM, Crijns HJ, Van den Berg MP et al (1994) Functional capacity before and after cardioversion of atrial fibrillation: a controlled study. Br Heart J 72:161-166
6. Crijns HJ, Van den Berg MP, Van Gelder IC, Van Veldhuisen DJ (1997) Management of atrial fibrillation in the setting of heart failure. Eur Heart J 18:C45-C49
7. Mahoney P, Kimmel S, De Nofrio D, Wahl P, Loh E (1999) Prognostic significance of atrial fibrillation in patients at a tertiary medical center referred for heart transplantation because of severe heart failure. Am J Cardiol 83:1544-1547
8. Dries DL, Exner DV, Gersh BJ et al (1998) Atrial fibrillation is associated with an increased risk for mortality and heart failure progression in patients with asymptomatic and symptomatic left ventricular dysfunction: a retrospective analysis of the SOLVD trial. J Am Coll Cardiol 32:695-703
9. Mathew J, Hunsberger S, Fleg J et al (2000) Incidence, predictive factors and prognostic significance of supraventricular tachyarrhythmias in congestive heart failure. Chest 118:914-922
10. Crijns HJ, Van Gelder IC, Van Gilst WH et al (1991) Serial antiarrhythmic drug treatment to maintain sinus rhythm after electrical cardioversion for chronic atrial fibrillation or atrial flutter. Am J Cardiol 68:335-341
11. Wood MA, Brown-Mahoney C, Kay GN, Ellenbogen KA (2000) Clinical outcome after ablation and pacing therapy for atrial fibrillation. A meta-analysis. Circulation 101:1138-1144
12. Saksena S, Prakash A, Hill M, Krol RB et al (1996) Prevention of recurrent atrial fibrillation with chronic dual-site right atrial pacing. J Am Coll Cardiol 26:687-694
13. Mabo P, Daubert J, Bouhour A (1999) Biatrial synchronous pacing for atrial arrhythmias prevention: the SYNBIAPACE study. Pacing Clin Eelectrophysiol 22:755

Ablation of Atrial Fibrillation in Chronic Heart Failure Patients: Facts or Fancy?

F. Gaita, S. Grossi, R. Riccardi, C. Giustetto, E. Caruzzo, F. Bianchi, L. Vivalda, E. Richiardi, G. Pistis

Heart failure (HF) represents the natural evolution of many cardiovascular diseases. The prevalence of HF varies between 1% and 3% in the general population, being even more frequent in the elderly [1]. Atrial fibrillation (AF) on the other hand, is the most frequent arrhythmia, with a prevalence of 0.5%-1% in the general population and up to 10% in octogenarians [2]. These two diseases often have common causes and they are frequently associated. HF predisposes to AF, which is present in from 10% of patients in NYHA class II and up to 40%-50% of patients in NYHA class IV, with an average of 15%-30% in the whole group of patients with HF [3-6]. AF worsens the outcome of patients with HF. A rapid and irregular ventricular response and the lack of the atrial kick during AF may further reduce cardiac output [7].

In a prospective study, the onset of AF has been related to an increase in functional class and a decrease of the maximum O_2 consumption [7]. The prognostic impact, however, is controversial: some authors have shown a negative effect of AF on mortality, whereas in others studies AF fails to appear as an independent risk factor. However, none of these trials had the impact of AF on mortality as an end-point. Furthermore, the usefulness of maintaining sinus rhythm with respect to rate control in the treatment of AF is far from adequately assessed. In the AFFIRM study, in patients with HF a trend has been shown in favor of rhythm control. By contrast, the use of antiarrhythmic drugs may be harmful because of their proarrhythmic effect, particularly in patients with depressed left ventricular function and electrolytic imbalance due to diuretic therapy.

In this context, the role of ablation in the therapy of AF has not been clearly established. When the therapeutic choice is rate control, atrioventricular junction ablation with implantation of a pace maker may be considered in patients in whom this goal cannot be reached with drugs (about 10%). In 21 studies in 1181 patients, such an approach improved quality of life, functional status, and

Divisione di Cardiologia, Ospedale Mauriziano Umberto I, Turin, Italy hospitalization rate [8]. In about 1% of patients a risk of ventricular arrhythmias must be taken into account after nodal ablation: this risk can be lowered by increasing the pacing rate to 80-90 bpm during the first week after ablation [9]. This approach is linked to permanent pacing and is therefore suitable for older patients.

The attempt to maintain sinus rhythm may be necessary in patients with HF in whom the arrhythmia may be considered the cause of the cardiomyopathy, when the onset of AF significantly affects the hemodynamic state, or in cases of thromboembolism during appropriate anticoagulation therapy.

When pharmacological therapy is ineffective or not recommended, or even harmful, transcatheter ablation of AF can be considered.

Electrical disconnection of the pulmonary veins represents the main option and can be carried out with different techniques: radiofrequency is the most widespread, and its results are the best known. Alternative forms of energy are cryoenergy and ultrasound. The effectiveness of pulmonary vein isolation is around 70%; it increases up to 85% in association with antiarrhythmic drugs [10, 11]. However, these results have been achieved in patients without structural heart disease with paroxysmal AF and atria of normal dimensions. In HF, AF tends to be persistent or permanent with the atria dilated: in this setting, the effectiveness of pulmonary vein ablation is lower than 50% even when combined with antiarrhythmic drugs. In these cases the role of the trigger, the target of pulmonary vein ablation, is less important than the substrate. On the other hand, the results of transcatheter linear ablation of the substrate by means of atrial compartmentalization are less than completely satisfactory: if limited to the right atrium the treatment is hardly effective, and if it is extended to the left atrium the linear lesions are incomplete and not transmural because of the technological limitations of the catheter [12].

With a surgical approach an atrial linear lesion can be achieved with radiofrequency, cryoenergy, or microwave energy, allowing complete transmural linear lesions and pulmonary vein isolation in a high percentage of patients. In the majority of cases the surgical approach involves the posterior wall of left atrium connecting the pulmonary vein ostia. In 1996 our group was the first to propose a "7" lesion connecting the two pulmonary veins of each side, the two superior pulmonary veins and the left inferior to the mitral annulus [13]. If the "7" lesion is achieved by the surgeon and its completeness is confirmed by the electrophysiological study, the success rate in maintening sinus rhythm is greater than 90% without drugs even in patients with persistent AF, dilated atria, and associated valvulopathy. The surgical approach can be taken into account in patients with HF of ischemic or valvular origin with an indication to surgery and coexistent AF.

Sometimes AF may be the cause of the HF. Several cases have been reported of tachycardiomyopathy in the setting of AF. It is more frequent in young patients scarcely symptomatic with a rapid ventricular response. In these cases, slowing the ventricular rate and/or recovery of sinus rhythm may definitively cure the cardiomyopathy with normalization of left ventricular function and NYHA class [14, 15]. In these cases the stable maintenance of sinus rhythm may have a beneficial impact on prognosis. The effectiveness of pharmacological therapy in maintaining sinus rhythm does not exceed 50%. An ablative approach should be considered in order to improve the maintenance of sinus rhythm, which in these kind of patients without structural primitive heart disease can reach 70%.

Conclusions

Transcatheter ablation is an evolving approach in the treatment of AF. The aim of the electrophysiologist in future will be the elimination of AF even in patients with HF. However, the technology available at present does not allow the desired results to be achieved except in selected patients.

References

1. Cleland JG, Clark A (1999) Has the survival of the heart failure population changed? Lessons from trials. Am J Cardiol 83:112D-119D
2. Kannel WB, Abbott RD, Savage DD, McNamara PM (1982) Epidemiologic features of chronic atrial fibrillation: the Framingham study. N Engl J Med 306:1018-1022
3. Carson PE, Johnson GR, Dunkman WB et al, for the V-HeFT VA Cooperative Studies Group (1993) The influence of atrial fibrillation on prognosis in mild to moderate heart failure. The V-HeFT studies. Circulation 87:VI-102-VI-110
4. Deedwania PC, Singh BN, Ellenbogen KA et al (1998) Spontaneous conversion and maintenance of sinus rhythm by amiodarone in patients with heart failure and atrial fibrillation. Observation from the Veterans Affairs Congestive Heart Failure Trial on Antiarrhythmic Therapy (CHF-STAT). Circulation 98:2574-2579
5. Middlekauff HR, Stevenson WG, Stevenson LW (1991) Prognostic significance of atrial fibrillation in advanced heart failure. A study of 390 patients. Circulation 84:40-48
6. The CONSENSUS Trial Study Group (1987) Effect of enalapril on mortality in severe congestive heart failure. Results of Cooperative North Scandinavian Enalapril Survival Study (CONSENSUS). N Eng J Med 316:1429-1435
7. Pozzoli M, Cioffi G, Traversi E et al (1998) Predictors of primary atrial fibrillation and concomitant clinical and hemodynamic changes in patients with chronic heart failure: a prospective study in 344 patients with baseline sinus rhythm. J Am Coll Cardiol 32:197-204
8. Wood MA, Brown-Mahoney C, Kay GN et al (2000) Clinical outcome after ablation and pacing therapy for atrial fibrillation. A meta analysis. Circulation 101:1138-1144
9. Ozcan C, Jahangir A, Friedman A et al (2000) Sudden death after RF ablation of the atrioventricular node in patients with atrial fibrillation. J Am Coll cardiol 40:105-110
10. Haissaguerre M, Jais P, Shah DC et al (2000) Electrophysiological end point for catheter ablation of atrial fibrillation initiated from multiple pulmonary venous foci. Circulation 101:1409-1417
11. Pappone C , Rosanio S, Oreto G et al (2000) Circumferential radiofrequency ablation of pulmonary vein ostia. A new anatomic approach for curing atrial fibrillation. Circulation 102:2619-2628

12. Ernst S, Schluter M, Ouyang F et al (1999) Modification of the substrate for maintenance of idiopathic human atrial fibrillation: efficacy of radiofrequency ablation using non fluoroscopic catheter guidance. Circulation 100:2085-2092
13. Gaita F, Gallotti R, Calò L, Manasse E, Riccardi R, Garberoglio L, Nicolini M, Scaglione M, Di Donna P, Caponi M, Franciosi G (2000) Limited posterior left atrial cryoablation in patients with chronic atrial fibrillation undergoing valvular heart surgery. J Am Coll Cardiol 36:159-166
14. Grogan M, Smith HC, Gersh BJ, Wood DL (1992) Left ventricular dysfunction due to atrial fibrillation in patients initially believed to have idiopathic dilated cardiomyopathy. Am J Cardiol 69:1570-1573
15. Iga K, Takahashi S, Yamashita M, Hori K et al (1993) Reversible left ventricular dysfunction secondary to rapid atrial fibrillation. Int J Cardiol 41:59-64

Drugs and Ablation in Patients with Atrial Fibrillation and Heart Failure

A. Bonso, A. Rossillo, R. Valente, A. Raviele

Introduction

Atrial fibrillation (AF) is the most common cardiac arrhythmia in the general population. Its prevalence ranges from 0.5% to 9 % between the ages of 50 and 80 years. It may occur in the clinical history of any patient with cardiopathy and even in apparently healthy people or those with minor structural anomalies of the heart [1]. Its presence causes a rise in morbidity and mortality due to the loss of atrial function and the consequent decrease in heart performance and increase in embolic risk. Very often AF is associated with disabling symptoms such as palpitations, which alone can significantly influence quality of life. Moreover, literature data [2] suggest that the incidence of this arrhythmia increases dramatically in patients with heart failure. In those with asymptomatic or symptomatic left ventricular systolic dysfunction it is independently associated with an increased risk of all-cause mortality. Persistently elevated ventricular rate during AF can produce dilated ventricular cardiomyopathy. Heart failure may thus be a consequence of rather than the cause of AF in clinical practice. For this reason, recovery and maintenance of sinus rhythm is one of the main objectives of treatment. However, antiarrhythmic drug therapy of AF is often unsatisfactory because recurrences frequently occur. Only 60% of patients remain in sinus rhythm after 6 months [2]. Moreover, antiarrhythmic therapy with class I drugs in patients with heart failure leads to an increase in mortality, so that the only efficient and safe drug therapy is amiodarone.

Due to the low efficacy of drug therapy for AF, some alternative nondrug techniques have recently come out, such as pacing, atrial defibrillator placement, surgery, and radiofrequency catheter ablation. The results of nonpharmacological procedures - sometimes unsatisfactory - suggest the hypothesis that a combined pharmacological and nonpharmacological approach, a so-called "hybrid therapy" [3], could be more successful in controlling AF recur-

Department of Cardiology, Umberto I Hospital, Mestre-Venice, Italy

rences. The logic behind this therapeutic strategy is to obtain synergy of action between pharmacological and nonpharmacological therapy in order to improve efficacy in controlling AF recurrences while at the same time reducing complications and improving tolerability.

Hybrid Pharmacological and Ablative Therapy of AF

More data have been presented on the effect on the combination of radiofrequency ablation with drug therapy, particularly in those patients with AF in whom atrial flutter develops after administration of class IC or class III drugs [3-9]. It is well known that during treatment of AF with class IC or class III antiarrhythmic drugs, the arrhythmias can spontaneously convert into typical atrial flutter. The percentages in different reports vary from 5% to 22% for class IC drugs [10]. The reported variability is probably due to the fact that in some studies only atrial flutter episodes with high ventricular response were recorded. With amiodarone a rate of 18.5% is reported [11]. The mechanism of drug-related atrial flutter seems to involve depression of intra-atrial conduction velocity, followed by the transformation of conduction delay into conduction block. This prevents simultaneous occurrence of the multiple reentrant circuits necessary for the perpetuation of AF. However, in some cases the conduction slowdown can start the development of macrocircuits and thus the start of atrial flutter around of the tricuspid valve [12-14].

Recent studies [3-11] have shown that in patients undergoing treatment for recurrent episodes of AF with class IC drugs or amiodarone, the onset of atrial flutter is not a reason to consider the treatment ineffective; on the contrary, the elimination of atrial flutter through radiofrequency ablation combined with antiarrhythmic therapy is able to prevent both arrhythmias in the follow-up. Success rates in preventing AF recurrences in this type of hybrid therapy range from 40% to 90 % with class IC drugs [3, 7-10, 15, 16] and 80% with amiodarone [4, 9, 16]. These data are usually based on small case reports with a follow-up shorter than 1 year. Hybrid pharmacological and ablative therapy has shown a higher efficacy than the added effects of drug therapy alone and of ablative therapy of atrial flutter alone [15]. Therefore this therapy has shown synergetic action between the two therapies. In our experience in a multicenter trial of more than 100 patients [17], we documented efficacy of hybrid therapy maintained in time in almost 50% of patients. Patients who have recurrences show the first episode within 6 months after ablation. Usually at least 30% of patients, even if they have AF recurrences, have a dramatic decrease in the number of episodes and admissions to the emergency department, and on the whole an increase in quality of life [7]. In our experience, amiodarone was effective in 70% of cases compared to 40% for class IC drugs in a mean of 22 months follow-up from the date of onset of the first AF recurrence.

A randomized and controlled study to establish the real role of combined drug treatment and linear or focal ablation of AF has never been performed.

Antiarrhythmic drug therapy is usually resumed after failure of the ablation procedure. In these cases a certain number of patients, 10%- 20%, seem to benefit from antiarrhythmic drugs which were ineffective before ablation [18]. This is probably due to greater efficacy of the antiarrhythmic drugs on areas of arrhythmogenic substrate that are partially electrically disconnected. Complex flow charts of combined antiarrhythmic drug therapy, ablation, and atrial stimulation have been suggested to improve upon the results of single therapy [19].

Ablation applied to other organized arrhythmias such as atrial tachycardia and atypical atrial flutter that appear during treatment of AF with antiarrhythmic drugs at the moment can only be hypothetical, since no cases have yet been treated systematically.

Hybrid Pharmacological and Ablative Therapy of AF and Heart Failure

The results of AF radiofrequency ablation during open heart surgery [20] and using minimally invasive surgical techniques [21] or the results of endocardial electrical disconnection of pulmonary veins [22] show how important a role is played by the posterior left atrium and pulmonary veins in the genesis and maintenance of AF. However, despite a good percentages of success reported so far, AF ablation has still some unsolved problems. It has not yet been established what the best technique may be. Follow-ups are not yet adequate, and complications are still significant. The treatment is mainly suited to patients refractory to drug therapy with paroxysmal and persistent mild or moderate structural cardiopathy. It has not yet been extensively used in patients with structural heart disease with persistent or chronic AF and patients with heart failure. However, some data are encouraging [23]. At all events, amiodarone is still the best as being the only safe antiarrhythmic drug for patients with heart failure. At the moment hybrid pharmacological and ablative therapy depends on amiodarone in these patients. In our experience hybrid therapy of amiodarone atrial flutter in patients with structural heart disease and low ejection fraction prevents recurrences of AF in 70% during a mean follow-up of 22 months.

References

1. Kannel W, Wolff P, Benjamin E, Levy D (1998) Prevalence, incidence, prognosis, and predisposing conditions for atrial fibrillation: population-based estimates. Am J Cardiol 82:2N-9N
2. Fuster V, Gibbonns RJJ, Klein WW (2001) ACC/AHA/ESC guidelines for the management of patients with atrial fibrillation. Eur Heart J 22:1852-1923
3. Huang DT, Monaham KM, Zimetbaum P et al (1998) Hybrid pharmacological and ablative therapy: a novel and effective approach for the management of atrial fibrillation. J Cardiovasc Electrophysiol 9:462-469

4. Natale A, Tomassoni G, Fanelli R et al (1997) Occurrence of atrial flutter after initiation of amiodarone therapy of paroxysmal atrial fibrillation. Circulation 96:I-385, abstr 2156
5. Nabar A, Rodriguez LM, Timmermans C et al (1999) Effect of right atrial isthmus ablation on the occurrence of atrial fibrillation. Circulation 99:1441-1445
6. Nabar A, Rodriguez LM, Timmermans et al (2001) Class IC antiarrhythmic drug induced atrial flutter: electrocardiographic and electrophysiological findings and their importance for long term outcome after right atrial isthmus ablation. Heart 85:424-429
7. Schumacher B, Jung W, Lewalter T et al (1999) Radiofrequency ablation of atrial flutter due to administration of class IC antiarrhythmic drugs for atrial fibrillation. Am J Cardiol 83:710-713
8. Bonso A, Themistoclakis S, Gasparini G et al (1999) Class IC drug induced atrial flutter during treatment of atrial fibrillation: usefulness of a combined pharmacological and ablative therapy. Eur Heart J 20: abstr P 634,98
9. Reithmann E, Hoffmann G, Spitzlberger U et al (2000) Catheter ablation of atrial flutter due to amiodarone therapy for paroxysmal atrial fibrillation. Eur Heart J 21:565-572
10. Bianconi L, Mennuni M, Lukic V et al (1996) Effects of oral propafenone administration before electrical cardioversion of chronic atrial fibrillation: a placebo-controlled study. J Am Coll Cardiol 28:700-706
11. Riva S, Tondo C, Carbucicchio C et al (1999) Incidence and clinical significance of transformation of atrial fibrillation to atrial flutter in patients undergoing long-term antiarrhythmic drug treatment. Europace 1:242-247
12. Waldo A, Cooper TB (1996) Spontaneous onset of type I atrial flutter in patients. J Am Coll Cardiol 28:700-706
13. Kalman J, Olgin J, Saxon L et al (1996) Activation and entrainment mapping defines the tricuspid annulus as the anterior barrier in typical atrial flutter. Circulation 94:398-406
14. Lesh M (1997) What is the relationship between atrial fibrillation and flutter in man? In: Raviele A (ed) Cardiac arrhythmias . Springer, Milan, pp 144-151
15. Stabile G, De Simone A, Turco P et al (2001) Response to flecainide infusion predicts long-term success of hybrid pharmacologic and ablation therapy in patients with atrial fibrillation. J Am Coll Cardiol 37:1639-1644
16. Tai CT, Chiang CE, Lee SH et al (1999) Persistent atrial flutter in patients treated for atrial fibrillation with amiodarone and propafenone: electrophysiologic characteristics, radiofrequency catheter ablation, and risk prediction. J Cardiovasc Electrophysiol 10:1180-1187
17. Bonso A, Rossillo A, Zoppo F et al (2002) Class IC or amiodarone induced atrial flutter during chronic treatment of atrial fibrillation: long-term follow-up of hybrid pharmacological and ablative therapy (abs). Pacing Clin Electrophysiol 25:(4/PartII):523-750
18. Garg A, Finneran W, Mollerus M et al (1999) Right atrial compartmentalization using radiofrequency catheter ablation for management of patients with refractory atrial fibrillation. J Clin Electrophysiol 10:763-77
19. Krol RB, Saksena S, Prakash A (2000) New devices and hybrid therapies for the treatment of atrial fibrillation. J Intervent Card Electrophysiol 12:900-908
20. Deneke T, Khargi K, Grewe PH et al (2002) Left atrial versus bi-atrial maze operation using intraoperatively cooled-tip radiofrequency ablation in patients undergoing open-heart surgery. J Am Coll Cardiol 39:1644-1650

21. Kottkamp H, Hindricks G, Autschbach R et al (2002) Specific linear left atrial lesions in atrial fibrillation. J Am Coll Cardiol 40:475-480
22. Marrouche N, Dresing T, Cole C et al (2002) Circular mapping and ablation of the pulmonary vein for treatment of atrial fibrillation. J Am Coll Cardiol 40:464-474
23. Pappone C, Rosanio S, Tocchi M et al (2002) Outcome of circumferential pulmonary vein ablation in patients with atrial fibrillation and associated heart failure (abstract). Pacing Clin Electrophysiol 25:(4/PartII):523-750

Drugs and Pacemakers in Patients with Atrial Fibrillation and Heart Failure

R.M. Polimeni, G. Meduri, A. Amato

Atrial fibrillation (AF) is a common arrhythmia: its incidence increases markedly with age and it is frequently associated with heart failure (HF) [1]. In patients with HF the incidence of AF is estimated at between 20% and 40%.

HF gives rise to electrophysiologic and hemodynamic changes in atrial tissue that favor the onset and maintenance of atrial fibrillation: sympathetic tone, increased pressure, wall-stretching, and mitral regurgitation. On the other hand, the onset of AF in patients with HF often leads to a marked worsening of the clinical condition of these patients: loss of atrial systole, high and irregular ventricular rate, mitral regurgitation, low coronary and cerebral flow, and so on.

The common approaches to management are rate control plus anticoagulation and rhythm control with antiarrhythmic drugs. Neither of these two approaches is ideal, because anticoagulation reduces but does not eliminate the risk of stroke, and the antiarrhythmic drugs often do not maintain sinus rhythm. Thus, in recent years, a new therapeutic option using electrical devices has been introduced in the management of AF.

Drug Therapy

The best way to prevent arrhythmias in the HF patient is to optimize HF therapy. Where acute AF does occur, excluding cases where rapid electric cardioversion is needed, the therapeutic options are two: rate control and sinus rhythm restoration. In the first case, digitalis and diltiazem may be used in HF patients after a clinical assessment [2]. In the second case, amiodarone is the elective drug for rhythm control (it is also used for rate control): this drug can result in cardioversion of AF in 50%-90% of cases [3]. If AF is chronic, rate control (digitalis, β-blockers) and anticoagulation is the usual approach in patients with HF.

U.O. di Cardiologia, UTIC Ospedale S. Maria degli Ungheresi, Polistena (RC), Italy

If sinus rhythm is restored, rhythm control can be obtained using amiodarone with a good rate of success [4]. A recent analysis of the US Carvedilol Heart Failure Trials Program documented that, in patients with HF and AF, carvedilol significantly improves left ventricular ejection fraction and demonstrates effects on combined end-points (mortality and hospitalization for HF).

Prevention of AF by Atrial Pacing

In patients with HF, amiodarone represents the first choice to prevent recurrences of AF. The first evidence that permanent pacing affects atrial pathophysiology was derived from retrospective studies of patients who had pacemakers implanted for sick sinus syndrome. Patients with atrial or dual-chamber pacemakers had fewer episodes of AF than those with a ventricular pacemaker alone [5].

In an effort to promote more synchronized atrial activation in patients with AF, many studies were conducted to evaluate the effects of pacing in the atria at novel sites. Among patients with paroxysmal AF who required a pacemaker, those in whom the atrial lead was placed on the interatrial septum [6] or at Bachmann's bundle had a lower incidence of paroxysmal and chronic AF than those in whom the lead was positioned more traditionally in the right atrial appendage. Furthermore, biatrial stimulation (right atrium and left atrium through the coronary sinus) resulted in greater synchronization of the atrial tissue during depolarization and a lower incidence of AF recurrences [7]. These results, however, cannot be extrapolated to patients with HF.

In patients with sick sinus syndrome, special AF-suppression pacing algorithms can be used to prevent and/or reduce atrial arrhythmia burden (the consistent atrial pacing algorithm from Medtronic [8], and dynamic atrial overdrive pacing from St. Jude Medical [9]).

In conclusion, current guidelines for the management of AF predominantly encompass pharmacologic strategies; particularly, in AF and HF patients, the first step is to optimize HF therapy. Implantable devices are likely to have an increasing role in the near future, particularly when they are used in combination with other treatments, even though, in patients with AF and HF, specific studies are needed.

References

1. Kannel WB, Abbott RD, Savage DD et al (1982) Epidemiologic features of chronic atrial fibrillation: the Framingham study. N Engl J Med 306:1018-1022
2. Goldenberg IF, Lewis WR, Dias VC et al (1994) Intravenous diltiazem for the treatment of patients with atrial fibrillation or flutter and moderate to severe congestive cardiac failure. Am J Cardiol 74:884-889

3. Clemo HF, Wood MA, Gilligan DM et al (1998) Intravenous amiodarone for acute heart rate in critically ill patients with atrial tachyarrhythmias. Am J Cardiol 81:594-598
4. Deedwania PC, Singh BN, Ellenbogen FA et al (1998) Spontaneous conversion and maintenance of sinus rhythm by amiodarone in patients with heart failure and atrial fibrillation. Circulation 98:2574-2579
5. Andersen HR, Nielsen JC, Thomsen PEB, Thuesen L, Mortensen PT, Vesterlund T, Pedersen AK (1997) Long-term follow-up of patients from a randomized trial of atrial versus ventricular pacing. Lancet 350:1210-1216
6. Padeletti L, Porcioni C, Michelucci A et al (1999) Long-term efficacy in prevention of paroximal atrial fibrillation (abstract). Pacing Clin Electrophysiol 22:A14
7. Daubert G, Gras D, Leclerq C, Baisser FV, Mabo P (1995) Biatrial synchronous pacing: a new terapeutic approach to prevent refractory atrial tachyarrhythmia. J Am Coll Cardiol 25:754-761
8. Boriani G, Biffi M, Padeletti L et al (1999) Consistent atrial pacing (CAP) and atrial rate stabilization (ARS): new algorithm to suppress recurrent atrial fibrillation. G Ital Cardiol 29 [Suppl 5]:88-90
9. A new stimulation algorithm for suppression of atrial fibrillation: dynamic atria overdrive (DAO) (2000) DEVICE 4:1

Can Ventricular Resynchronization Reduce Atrial Fibrillation Recurrences?

M.G. Bongiorni[1], G. Giannola[2], E. Soldati[1], G. Arena[1], E. Hoffmann[2], M. Mariani[1]

In recent years a new pacing therapy has been proposed for patients affected by heart failure (HF) in order to reduce inter- [1, 2], intra- [3, 4], and atrioventricular [5] (AV) dyssynchrony. Cardiac resynchronization therapy (CRT) has the goal of correcting these hemodynamic disorders, thus improving left ventricular (LV) performance. The benefits of CRT have been evaluated in a series of clinical trials [6-10]. Although the impact of this treatment on survival is still unclear, CRT was demonstrated to improve LV and aortic pressure, to shorten mitral diastolic regurgitation, to synchronize LV and atrial systole, and to reduce LV volume and myocardial oxygen consumption; in patients treated by CRT, quality of life and peak oxygen uptake and functional capacity were improved and the number of hospitalizations was reduced.

The incidence and prevalence of atrial fibrillation (AF) are higher in patients with HF. The incidence of AF and HF increases with age [11-13], as well as HF. In HF patients the prevalence of AF ranges from 10% to 30%, and it shows a direct correlation with NYHA class: AF is estimated to be present in 10% of patients in NYHA class II and in 40%-50% of patients in NYHA class IV. In patients with LV dysfunction the presence of AF, whether symptomatic or not, is independently associated with an increased rate of all-cause mortality, it may worsen LV dysfunction [14, 15], and it is linked to a poor prognosis. HF morbidity is highly influenced by the coexistence of AF, independently of NYHA functional class. The prevalence of AF in the most important trials [16-21] on HF is shown in Fig. 1 [22].

There are many possible mechanisms whereby AF may adversely influence HF. They include:

1. Loss of atrial contraction, leading to AV dyssynchrony and to a reduction in stroke volume (up to 20%), causing an increase in mean diastolic pressure in the atria and then valvular regurgitation and consequently a reduced time interval for passive diastolic filling

[1]Cardiothoracic Department, Cisanello Hospital, University of Pisa; [2]Division of Cardiology, Polyclinic Hospital, University of Palermo, Italy

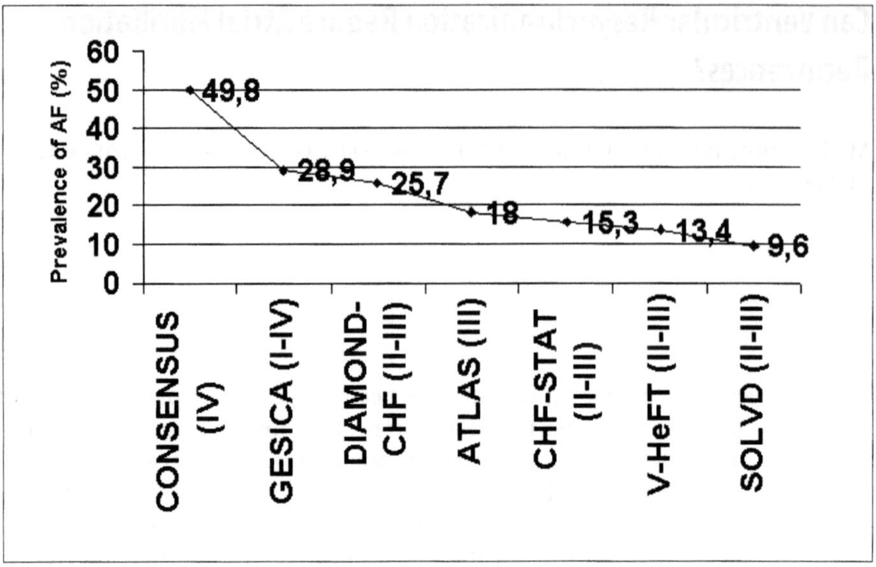

Fig. 1. Prevalence of AF in the most important trials on HF. Predominant NYHA class is shown in parentheses

2. The chronically fast heart rate, which reduces diastolic filling time, increases mean atrial diastolic pressure and induces biochemical and histological changes (myocardial ischemia, abnormalities of cardiac intracellular calcium regulation, myocyte and extracellular matrix remodeling, and reduction of serum concentration of ANP and *N*-ANP), possibly leading to the development of tachycardia-induced cardiomyopathy
3. Variation in ventricular cycle lengths (RR intervals)
4. Adverse effects of drugs commonly used in these patients to prevent recurrences of AF or to control heart rate during AF
5. Increased risk of thromboembolic events

On the other hand, the development of HF may be responsible for the occurrence of AF, as suggested by the epidemiological association between HF and AF. The increase in mean atrial pressure and the presence of mitral regurgitation may induce an increase in atrial size, thus producing the substrate for the development of AF.

Data currently available show that in HF patients affected by left intraventricular delay or ventricular desynchronization CRT is an effective therapy [23]; the benefits seem to be independent of the presence of AF or sinus rhythm [23-24]. Moreover, in patients with HF CRT could favorably influence the incidence and prevalence of AF both by the effect of atrial pacing on the recurrences of AF and by the hemodynamic effect on ventricular dysfunction.

The role of atrial pacing in preventing AF is well documented. After pacemaker implantation, more than 50% of patients with sick sinus syndrome and

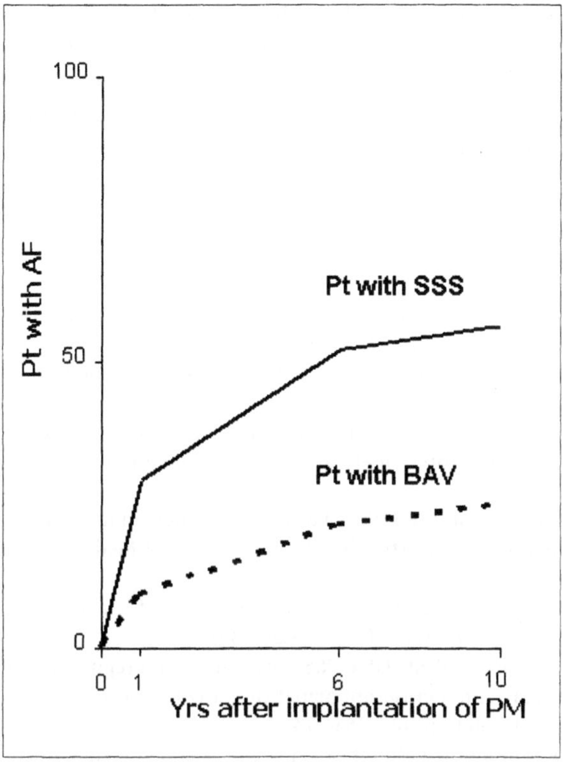

Fig. 2. Incidence of atrial fibrillation after implantation of a pacemaker (without pre-existent history of atrial fibrillation)

25% of patients with AV block develop AF within 6 years [25] (Fig. 2). Triggers for AF may be bradycardia and tachycardia, premature ventricular beats, supraventricular tachyarrhythmias (AV nodal or AV re-entrant, atrial flutter), focal activity in pulmonary veins, the influence of the autonomic nervous system activity, and others. Atrial pacing may prevent AF by several mechanisms: by stimulation in nonconventional or multiple sites (e.g., biatrial pacing, dual-site atrial pacing, stimulation of distal coronary sinus, or apex of Koch's triangle) [26-32] or by using pacing prevention algorithms (overdrive pacing, atrial ectopy suppression, rate smoothing) [33, 34].

Moreover, CRT may add the effects of LV stimulation to those of conventional pacing. CRT could prevent recurrences of AF by improving synchronized atrial and LV systole, reducing LV volume, increasing LV and aortic systolic pressure, and shortening mitral diastolic regurgitation. All these changes lead to an increase in stroke volume with a consequent decrease in mean diastolic pressure in the atria and in valvular regurgitation. The increased time for passive diastolic filling has a positive effect on atrial and ventricular remodeling and on reactive influence of the autonomic nervous system activity. All these mechanisms are very important to prevent the electrophysiological changes that happen during AF in the setting of HF, such as the changes in calcium, potassium, and sodium channels.

Data supporting the true impact of CRT on the reduction of AF recurrences are lacking, as most of the clinical trials on CRT were not designed to address this question. Some ongoing trials, such as the MASCOT, could provide more data to support this hypothesis, but new trials for the evaluation of this important aspect of HF therapy are required.

References

1. Wolferth CC, Margolies A (1935) Asynchronism in contraction of the ventricles in the so-called common type of bundle-branch block: its bearing on the determination of the side of the significant lesion and on the mechanism of split first and second heart sound. Am Heart J 10:425-452
2. Haber E, Letham A (1965) Splitting of heart sounds from ventricular asynchrony in bundle branch block, ventricular ectopic beats and artificial pacing. Br Heart J 27:691-696
3. Herman MV, Heinle RA, Klein MD, Gorlin R (1967) Localised disorders in myocardial contraction. Asynergy and its role in congestive heart failure. N Engl J Med 277:222-232
4. Gibson DG, Greenbaum RA, Pridie RB, Yacoub MH (1988) Correction of left ventricular asynchrony by coronary artery surgery. Br Heart J 59:304-308
5. Panidis IP, Ross J, Munley B, Nestico P, Mintz GS (1986) Diastolic mitral regurgitation in patients with atrioventricular conduction abnormalities: a common finding by Doppler echocardiography. J Am Coll Cardiol 7:768-774
6. Leclercq C, Kass DA (2002) Retiming the failing heart: principles and current clinical status of cardiac resynchronization. J Am Coll Cardiol 39:194-201
7. Witte K, Thackray S, Clark A, Cooklin M, Cleland JGF (2000) Clinical trials update. IMPROVEMENT-HF, COPERNICUS, MUSTIC, ASPECT-II and APRICOT. Eur J Heart Fail 2:455-461
8. Louis A, Cleland JGF, Crabbe S, Ford S, Thackray S, Houghton T et al (2001) Clinical trials update. CAPRICORN, COPERNICUS, MIRACLE, STAF, RITZ-2. RECOVER and RENAISSANCE and cachexia and cholesterol in heart failure. Highlights of the scientific sessions of the American College of Cardiology 2001. Eur J Heart Fail 3:381-387
9. Thackray S, Coletta A, Jones P, Dunn A, Clark AL, Cleland JGF (2001) Clinical trials update. Highlights of the scientific sessions of Heart Failure 2001, a meeting of the Working Group on Heart Failure of the European Society of Cardiology. CONTAK CD, CHRISTMAS, OPTIME-CHF. Eur J Heart Fail 3:491-494
10. Auricchio A, Stellbrink C, Sack S, Block M, Vogt J, Bakker P et al (2000) The pacing therapies for congestive heart failure (PATH-CHF) study. Circulation 102 [Suppl 2]:693 (abstract)
11. Benjamin EJ, Wolf PA, D'Agostino RB et al (1998) Impact of atrial fibrillation on the risk of death: the Framingham Heart Study. Circulation 98:946-952
12. Stevenson WG, Stevenson LW, Middlekauff HR et al (1996) Improving survival for patients with atrial fibrillation and advanced heart failure. J Am Coll Cardiol 28:1458-1463
13. Kannel WB, Abbott RD, Savage DD (1982) Epidemiologic features of chronic atrial fibrillation: the Framingham study. N Engl J Med 306:1018-1022

14. Middlekauff HR, Stevenson WG, Stevenson LW (1991) Prognostic significance of atrial fibrillation in advanced heart failure. A study of 390 patients. Circulation 84:40-48
15. Benjamin EJ, Levy D, Vaziri FM et al (1994) Independent risk factors for atrial fibrillation in a population-based cohort. JAMA 271:840-844
16. The CONSENSUS Trial Study Group (1987) Effect of enalapril on mortality in severe congestive heart failure. Results of the Cooperative North Scandinavian Enalapril Survival Study (CONSENSUS). N Engl J Med 316:1429-1435
17. Doval HC, Nul DR, Grancelli HO et al, for Grupo de Studio la Obrevida en la Insuficienca Cardiaca en Argentina (GESICA) (1994) Randomised trial of low dose amiodarone in severe congestive heart failure. Lancet 344:493-498
18. Pedersen OD, Bagger H, Keller N et al (2001) Efficacy of dofetilide in the treatment of atrial fibrillation-flutter in patients with reduced left ventricular function: a Danish Investigation of Arrhythmia and Mortality ON Dofetilide (DIAMOND) substudy. Circulation 104:292-296
19. Deedwania PC, Singh BN, Ellenbogen KA et al (1998) Spontaneous conversion and maintainance of sinus rhythm by amiodarone in patients with heart failure and atrial fibrillation. Observation from the Veterans Congestive Heart Failure Trial on Antiarrhythmic Therapy (CHF-STAT). Circulation 98:2574-2579
20. Carson PE, Johnson DR, Dunkman WB et al (1993) The influence of atrial fibrillation on prognosis in mild to moderate heart failure. The V-HeFT Studies. Circulation Suppl VI:VI102-110
21. Dries DL, Exner DV, Gersh BJ et al (1998) Atrial fibrillation is associated with an increased risk for mortality and heart failure progression in patients with asymptomatic and symptomatic left ventricular systolic dysfunction: a retrospective analysis of the SOLVD Trials. J Am Coll Cardiol 32:695-703
22. Ehrlich JR, Nattel S, Hohnloser SH (2002) Atrial fibrillation and congestive heart failure: specific considerations at the intersection of two common and important cardiac disease sets. J Cardiovasc Electrophysiol 13:399-405
23. Leclerq C, Kass DA (2002) Retiming heart failure: principles and current clinical status of cardiac resynchronization. J Am Coll Cardiol 39:194-201
24. Linde C, Leclercq C, Rex S et al (2002) Long-term benefits of biventricular pacing in congestive heart failure: results from the MUltisite STimulation in cardiomyopathy (MUSTIC) study. J Am Coll Cardiol 40(1):111-118
25. Etienne Y, Mansourati J, Gilard M et al (1999) Evaluation of left ventricular based pacing in patients with congestive heart failure and atrial fibrillaiton. Am J Cardiol 83(7):1138-1140
26. Saksena S, Prakash A, Hill M et al (1996) Prevention of recurrent atrial fibrillation with chronic dual-site right atrial pacing. J Am Coll Cardiol 28(3):687-694
27. Katsivas A, Manolis A, Lazaris E et al (1998) Atrial septal pacing to synchronize atrial depolarisation in patients with delayed interatrial conduction. Pacing Clin Electrophysiol 21:2220-2225
28. Spencer WH, Zhu DW, Markowitz T et al (1997) Atrial septal pacing: a method for pacing both atria simultaneously. Pacing Clin Electrophysiol 20:2739-2745
29. Delfaut P, Saksena S, Prakash A, Krol RB (1998) Long term outcome of patients with drug refractory atrial flutter and fibrillation after single- and dual-site right atrial pacing for arrhythmia prevention. J Am Coll Cardiol 32(7):1900-1908
30. Padeletti L, Porciani MC, Michelucci A et al (1999) Interatrial septum pacing: a new approach to prevent recurrent atrial fibrillation. J Interv Card Electrophysiol 3:35-43

31. Levy T, Walker S, Rochelle J, Paul V (1999) Evaluation of biatrial pacing, right atrial pacing, and no pacing in patients with drug refractory atrial fibrillation. Am J Cardiol 84:426-429
32. Becker R, Klinkott R, Bauer A et al (2000) Multisite pacing for prevention of atrial tachyarrhythmias: potential mechanisms. J Am Coll Cardiol 35:1939-1946
33. Garrigue S, Barold SS, Cazeau S, Gencel L, Jaïs P, Haissaguerre M (1998) Prevention of atrial arrhythmias during DDD pacing by atrial overdrive. Pacing Clin Electrophysiol 21:1751-1759
34. Blommaert D, Gonzalez M, Macumbitsi J et al (2000) Effective prevention of atrial fibrillation by continuous atrial overdrive pacing after coronary artery bypass surgery. J Am Coll Cardiol 35:1411-1415

Management of Atrial Fibrillation Suppression in AF-HF Comorbidity Therapy (MASCOT) Trial

M.G. Bongiorni[1], G. Giannola[2], G. Arena[1], E. Soldati[1], L. Padeletti[3], A. Puglisi[4], A. Curnis[5], S. Favale[6], A. Carboni[7], E. Hoffmann[2], M. Mariani[1]

Background

Inter- [1, 2], intra- [3, 4], and atrioventricular [5](AV) dyssynchrony are not new concepts, but only recently have attempts been made to correct these disorders in an effort to treat heart failure (HF). A series of trials [6] has addressed partial or comprehensive cardiac resynchronization in patients with severe HF and evidence of cardiac dyssynchrony. Cardiac resynchronization should improve left ventricular (LV) performance; several trials [7-10] have demonstrated improvement in many hemodynamic parameters (LV and aortic pressure, shortening of mitral diastolic regurgitation, synchronized LV and atrial systole, LV volume, reduced myocardial oxygen consumption) and clinical end-points (quality of life, peak oxygen uptake, functional capacity, reduced number of hospitalizations). The incidence of atrial fibrillation (AF) double every 10 years in adults: there are 2-3 new cases/1000 annually in the age group of 55-64 years and 35 new cases/1000 annually between the age of 85 and 94 years [11-13]. The Framingham study demonstrated that AF is an independent risk factor for mortality with a relative risk of 1.5 for men and 1.9 for women. In patients with HF, the prevalence of AF is directly related to NYHA class: AF is present in 10% of patients in NYHA class II and 40% of patients in NYHA classes III-IV. However, HF morbidity is highly influenced by the coexistence of AF, independently of functional class. Moreover, the presence of symptomatic or asymptomatic AF in patients with LV dysfunction is linked to a poor prognosis and is independently associated with a higher risk of death from all causes and from progressive pump failure [14, 15]. The prevalence of AF in most trials [16-22] on HF is shown in Fig. 1.

[1]Cardiothoracic Department, Cisanello Hospital, University of Pisa; [2]Division of Cardiology, Polyclinic Hospital, University of Palermo; [3]Ospedale Careggi, Florence; [4]Ospedale Fatebenefratelli, Rome; [5]Spedali Civili, Brescia; [6]Policlinico Consorziale, Bari; [7]Ospedale Civile, Parma, Italy

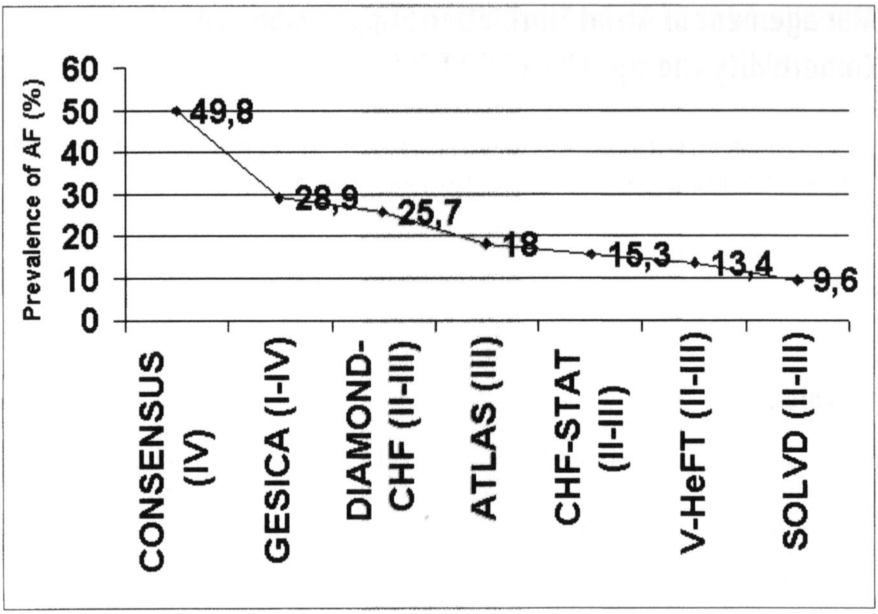

Fig. 1. Prevalence of AF in the most important trials on HF. Predominant NYHA class is shown in parentheses

The possibility of reducing morbidity in HF by treating AF is the main reason for keeping sinus rhythm rather than controlling heart rate, and forms the background of the MASCOT trial.

Recently, algorithms to prevent AF based on continuous atrial stimulation at a rate just a little higher than the spontaneous rate have been implemented in some commercially available pacemakers. St. Jude Medical Cardiac Rhythm Management has developed a cardiac resynchronization system implemented with the DAO (dynamic atrial overdrive) algorithm: the pacemaker adapts the pacing rate to the spontaneous rhythm when it is turned on, giving an overdrive atrial stimulation only after sensing two consecutive P waves.

Materials and Methods

Each patient will receive a Genesis system with a St. Jude Medical Frontier 3x2 model 5510 pacemaker, an atrial bipolar lead, a right ventricular bipolar lead, and an Aescula LV 1055 unipolar lead for LV stimulation.

End-Points

The trial will compare the effects on quality of life of cardiac resynchronization therapy with and without the DAO algorithm switched on. Secondary end-points are the observational features shown in Table 1.

Table 1. MASCOT trial end-points

Primary end-point: quality of life	
Secondary end-points:	
Incidence and onset of AF	Number of cardioversions
Functional capacity[a]	Number of hospitalizations
Echocardiographic parameters	Number of AF episodes
NYHA class and QRS duration	Risk of thromboembolic events
1-year and 2-year mortality	Rate of success of Genesis implantation
Performance of Aescula lead	Complications related to implantation

[a]6-min walking test

Organization of the Trial

At the time of implantation every patient will be randomized to cardiac resynchronization therapy (biventricular pacing) with DAO switched on or off (Fig. 2). Follow-up procedures will be at 3 months, 6 months, and than every 6 months to the end of 2 years. Each follow-up appointment will include a clinical assessment, an electrocardiogram, a Minnesota Living With Heart Failure test, two 6-min walking tests, an echocardiogram, and a pacemaker report.

The trial will enrol at least 200 patients, with no upper limit, and have a minimum follow-up of 2 years. Patients will be eligible for the study if they fulfill the following criteria: HF due to LV dysfunction with optimal and stable pharmacological therapy, NYHA class II-IV disease, QRS duration >140 ms in spontaneous rhythm or normal QRS with echocardiographic evidence of mechanical delay more than 50 ms, ejection fraction < 35%, LV end-diastolic diameter >54 mm, ability to perform a 6-min walking test, >18 years old. Exclusion criteria are: unstable angina or myocardial infarction less than 3 months ago, coronary artery bypass graft or percutaneous transluminal coronary angioplasty less than 3 months ago, chronic AF, life expectancy less than 6 months, neoplastic disease, and pregnancy.

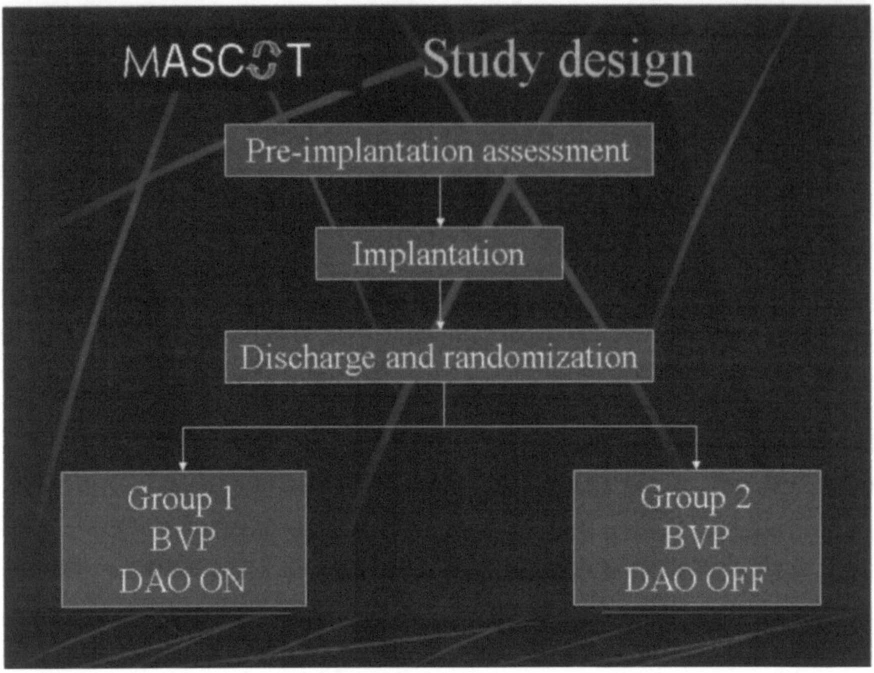

Fig. 2. The MASCOT Study design. BVP, biventricular pacing; DAO; dynamic atrial overdrive algorithm

References

1. Wolferth CC, Margolies A (1935) Asynchronism in contraction of the ventricles in the so-called common type of bundle-branch block: its bearing on the determination of the side of the significant lesion and on the mechanism of split first and second heart sound. Am Heart J 10:425-452
2. Haber E, Letham A (1965) Splitting of heart sounds from ventricular asynchrony in bundle branch block, ventricular ectopic beats and artificial pacing. Br Heart J 27:691-696
3. Herman MV, Heinle RA, Klein MD, Gorlin R (1967) Localised disorders in myocardial contraction. Asynergy and its role in congestive heart failure. N Engl J Med 277:222-232
4. Gibson DG, Greenbaum RA, Pridie RB, Yacoub MH (1988) Correction of left ventricular asynchrony by coronary artery surgery. Br Heart J 59:304-308
5. Panidis IP, Ross J, Munley B, Nestico P, Mintz GS (1986) Diastolic mitral regurgitation in patients with atrioventricular conduction abnormalities: a common finding by Doppler echocardiography. J Am Coll Cardiol 7:768-774
6. Leclercq C, Kass DA (2002) Retiming the failing heart: principles and current clinical status of cardiac resynchronization. J Am Coll Cardiol 39:194-201

7. Witte K, Thackray S, Clark A, Cooklin M, Cleland JGF (2000) Clinical trials update. IMPROVEMENT-HF, COPERNICUS, MUSTIC, ASPECT-II and APRICOT. Eur J Heart Fail 2:455-461
8. Louis A, Cleland JGF, Crabbe S et al (2001) Clinical trials update. CAPRICORN, COPERNICUS, MIRACLE, STAF, RITZ-2. RECOVER and RENAISSANCE and cachexia and cholesterol in heart failure. Highlights of the scientific sessions of the American College of Cardiology 2001. Eur J Heart Fail 3:381-387
9. Thackray S, Coletta A, Jones P, Dunn A, Clark AL, Cleland JGF (2001) Clinical trials update. Highlights of the scientific session of Heart Failure 2001, a meeting of the Working Group on Heart Failure of the European Society of Cardiology. CONTAK CD, CHRISTMAS, OPTIME-CHF. Eur J Heart Fail 3:491-494
10. Auricchio A, Stellbrink C, Sack S et al (1998) The pacing therapies for congestive heart failure (PATH-CHF) study. Circulation 102 [Suppl 2]:693 (abstract 3352)
11. Benjamin EJ, Wolf PA, D'Agostino RB et al (1998) Impact of atrial fibrillation on the risk of death: the Framingham Heart Study. Circulation 98:946-952
12. Stevenson WG, Stevenson LW, Middlekauff HR et al (1996) Improving survival for patients with atrial fibrillation and advanced heart failure. J Am Coll Cardiol 28:1458-1463
13. Kannel WB, Abbott RD, Savage DD (1982) Epidemiologic features of chronic atrial fibrillation: the Framingham study. N Engl J Med 306:1018-1022
14. Middlekauff HR, Stevenson WG, Stevenson LW (1991) Prognostic significance of atrial fibrillation in advanced heart failure. A study of 390 patients. Circulation 84: 40-48
15. Benjamin EJ, Levy D, Vaziri FM et al (1994) Independent risk factors for atrial fibrillation in a population-based cohort. JAMA 271:840-844
16. The CONSENSUS Trial Study Group (1987) Effect of enalapril on mortality in severe congestive heart failure. Results of the Cooperative North Scandinavian Enalapril Survival Study (CONSENSUS). N Engl J Med 316:1429-1435
17. Doval HC, Nul DR, Grancelli HO et al (1994) For Grupo de Studio la Obrevida en La Insuficienca Cardiaca En Argentina (GESICA). Randomised trial of low dose amiodarone in severe congestive heart failure. Lancet 344:493-498
18. Pedersen OD, Bagger H, Keller N et al (2001) Efficacy of dofetilide in the treatment of atrial fibrillation-flutter in patients with reduced left ventricular function: a Danish Investigations of Arrhythmia and Mortality ON Dofetilide (DIAMOND) substudy. Circulation 104: 292-296
19. Deedwania PC, Singh BN, Ellenbogen KA et al (1998) Spontaneous conversion and mantainance of sinus rhythm by amiodarone in patients with heart failure and atrial fibrillation. Observation from the Veterans Congestive Heart Failure Trial on Antiarrhythmic Therapy (CHF-STAT). Circulation 98:2574-2579
20. Carson PE, Johnson DR, Dunkman WB et al (1993) The influence of atrial fibrillation on prognosis in mild to moderate heart failure. The V-HeFT Studies. Circulation Suppl VI:VI102-110
21. Dries DL, Exner DV, Gersh BJ et al (1998) Atrial fibrillation is associated with an increased risk for mortality and heart failure progression in patients with asymptomatic and symptomatic left ventricular systolic dysfunction: a retrospective analysis of the SOLVD Trials. J Am Coll Cardiol 32:695-703
22. Ehrlich JR, Nattel S, Hohnloser SH (2002) Atrial fibrillation and congestive heart failure: specific considerations at the intersection of two common and important cardiac disease sets. J Cardiovasc Electrophysiol 13:399-405

Risk-Stratification in Heart Failure Patients with Varying Disease Severity

I. Can, K. Aytemir, A. Oto

Introduction

Heart failure (HF) is one of the major cardiovascular problems, affecting 15 million people worldwide [1, 2]. Despite declining mortality from heart disease, the number of patients affected by HF is still increasing [3]. There is an overall 5-year mortality of 50%, and in severe cases this percentage reaches 35%-40% in 1 year [4]. The rates for total mortality and sudden death vary by functional class. In mild HF [New York Heart Association (NYHA) functional class II], the overall annual mortality is 5%-15%, with approximately one-half to two-thirds being classified as sudden. In NYHA class III, the annual mortality increases to 20%-50% and in class IV it often exceeds 50% [5]. Considering the wide spectrum of disease severity in patients with HF, a risk stratification strategy is reasonable to identify those at high risk of cardiac events, in whom more aggressive management may be beneficial. This is especially important for ambulatory patients with moderate-to-severe congestive heart failure (CHF). In this respect, a number of variables have been thorougly investigated. A review of the most commonly used ones will be discussed in this chapter.

Clinical Evaluation

Once a diagnosis of HF has been established, symptoms may be used to classify its severity. The most widely used one is the NYHA functional classification (Table 1). In general, male gender [6], the presence of coronary artery disease as the etiology of HF [7], the presence of audible S3, low pulse and systolic arterial pressure, a high NYHA class [8], and reduced exercise capacity have each been shown to be a high risk factor for death [9]. However, among these several clinical potential predictive variables, exercise capacity, as defined by

Department of Cardiology, Faculty of Medicine Hacettepe University, Ankara, Turkey

Table 1. New York Heart Association classification of heart failure

Class I	No limitation: ordinary physical exercise does not cause undue fatigue, dyspnea or palpitations.
Class II	Slight limitation of physical activity: comfortable at rest but ordinary physical activity results in fatigue, palpitations or dyspnea.
Class III	Marked limiation of physical activity: comfortable at rest but less than ordinary activity results in symptoms.
Class IV	Unable to carry out any physical activity without discomfort: symptoms present at rest.

direct measurement of maximal oxygen consumption ($\dot{V}O_2$), has emerged as one the most consistent and powerful predictors of death [10, 11].

A peak $\dot{V}O_2$ value of 14 ml/kg or less per minute is a widely accepted high risk indicator [12]. Patients with preserved exercise capacity (peak $\dot{V}O_2 \geq 18$ ml/kg per minute) have a good prognosis and those with severe reduction of exercise tolerance (peak $\dot{V}O_2 \leq 10$ ml/kg per minute) have a poor outcome [12, 13].

For patients with intermediate exercise tolerance (peak $\dot{V}O_2$ between 10 and 18 ml/kg per minute) Corra et al. used ventilatory response ($\dot{V}E/\dot{V}CO_2$), defined as the ratio of minute ventilation ($\dot{V}E$) to carbon dioxide production ($\dot{V}CO_2$), for risk stratification [14]. The patient group consisted of NYHA class II-III patients with a mean left ventricular ejection fraction (LVEF) of 35±7%. $\dot{V}E/\dot{V}CO_2$ slope with a best cut-off value of 35 was the strongest independent predictor of outcome in the patients with intermediate exercise capacity. Total mortality was 30% in patients with a $\dot{V}E/\dot{V}CO_2$ slope of 35 or greater and 10% in those with a $\dot{V}E/\dot{V}CO_2$ slope below 35. Patients with a $\dot{V}E/\dot{V}CO_2$ slope of 35 or greater had a similar mortality to those with peak $\dot{V}O_2$ of 10 ml/kg or less per minute (30% vs 37%, p=ns).

Robbins et al. [15] assessed the prognostic value of chronotropic response to exercise in addition to ventilatory response in patients with severe heart failure and compared these with the peak $\dot{V}O_2$ values. During a follow-up period of 1.5 years, only an abnormally high $\dot{V}E/\dot{V}CO_2$ and a low chronotropic index were independently predictive of death. Although a low peak $\dot{V}O_2$ was a predictor of death in univariate analysis, it was not a predictor of death in multivariate analysis.

Although peak $\dot{V}O_2$ has been one of the gold standards by which patients with HF are risk-stratified and is considered by many to be the key component of initial evaluation for heart transplantation, better prognostic parameters, in particular ventilatory response and chronotropic index, will be used for this purpose in the near future.

Left Ventricular Ejection Fraction

Reduced LVEF remains one of the most important risk factors in respect of overall mortality and sudden cardiac death in patients with HF. When it is severely depressed (<15%-20%), the prevailing mode of cardiac death is nonsudden [16]. The meta-analysis of pooled data from the EMIAT, CAMIAT, SWORD, TRACE, and DIAMOND-MI studies in post-myocardial infarction (MI) patients confirmed that LVEF predicts 2-year all-cause, arrhythmic, and cardiac mortality [17]. A 10% increase in EF reduced the mortality at 2 years with a hazard ratio of 0.61 (95% CI: 0.48-0.78, $p<0.001$). The arrhythmic mortality figures per person-year were 3.2%, 7.7%, and 9.4% for EF of 31%-40%, 21%-30%, and <20% respectively [17]. For the prediction of cardiac death, an EF below 35% had a 40% sensitivity, 78% specificity, and 14% positive predictive accuracy [18]. In the study of the Multicenter Postinfarction Research Group there was a progressive increase in cardiac mortality during one year as the LVEF fell below 40%. An LVEF less than 40% was an independent predictor of mortality [19]. In another study, the mortality of the patients with EF below 40% was 20% over 3.5 years, and that half of these deaths sudden [20]. In the TIMI II trial 1-year mortality was found to correlate to resting LVEF as shown by radionuclide ventriculography obtained within 14 days of MI. The mortality was highest (9.9%) in patients with an LVEF below 30%. The mortality in those with an LVEF of 30% or above was 1.2%-1.3 %, and there was little difference in mortality between those with an LVEF of 30%-49% and those whose LVEF was 50% or greater [21]. For the prediction of cardiac death, an EF below 35% has a sensitivity of 48%, a specificity of 78% and a positive predictive accuracy of 14 % [22]. LVEF is usually combined with other risk factors. The risk is substantially increased when a low LVEF is combined with nonsustained ventricular tachycardia (NSVT) [23, 24]. The ATRAMI study demonstrated that a combination of low values of autonomic markers and reduced EF identified a group of post-MI patients at highest risk of sudden and nonsudden cardiac death [25].

Right Ventricular Ejection Fraction

Recently a number of studies have provided evidence that right ventricular ejection fraction (RVEF), either directly measured (by radionuclide angiography or rapid response thermodilution) or indirectly estimated (by echocardiography), is an independent prognostic factor in patients with moderate-to-severe heart failure [26, 28]. Ghio et al. [29] further investigated the prognostic value of RV systolic function and pulmonary artery pressure (PAP) in 377 patients with a mean LVEF of 21.8±6.7% and NYHA functional class II-IV disease. They performed right heart catheterization and measured RVEF with the thermodilution method. These authors found that in patients with heart failure and normal PAP, the assessment of RV function did not improve the prognostic stratification. In contrast, when PAP was high at rest despite optimized medical therapy, the prognosis of the patients was strongly related to RV function. A reduced RVEF was a harbinger of high risk of death or urgent transplantation, whereas preserved RVEF implied a prognosis that was very similar to that of patients with normal PAP .

Mitral Inflow Pattern

Transmitral flow patterns characterized by short isovolumetric relaxation times and dominant early diastolic inflow velocities have been found in the presence of severely impaired LV compliance and elevated end-diastolic filling pressures [30, 31]. This restrictive pattern of mitral inflow has been recognized as a strong predictor of mortality in advanced heart failure [32] . Furthermore, Hansen et al. [33] provided further prognostic information in HF patients that is incremental to cardiopulmonary exercise testing, the most widely used clinical selection criterion for directing patients toward heart transplantation [12]. In their patient group, a peak $\dot{V}O_2$ of 14 ml/kg or less per minute and the presence of a restrictive filling pattern (E/A>2 or 1-2, but a deceleration time of early flow ≤140 ms) were found to be associated with a poorer outcome than was their absence (2-year survival rate 52% vs 80%). Similarly, despite peak $\dot{V}O_2$ levels above 14 ml/kg per minute, the outcome was less favorable in the presence of a restrictive filling pattern (2-year survival rate 80% vs 94%). In risk model based on noninvasive predictive factors, low-, medium- and high-risk groups were identified by the presence of ≤1, 2, or 3 risk factors (peak $\dot{V}O_2$ ≤ 14 ml/kg per minute, atrial fibrillation or restrictive mitral inflow pattern, and LVEDD >65 mm), respectively. The 2-year survival rates in these risk groups were 95% in the low- 65% in the intermediate- and 39% in the high-risk groups.

Pulmonary Venous Doppler Signal

Although a restrictive filling pattern as assessed by pulsed wave Doppler imaging of the mitral flow identifies advanced heart disease associated with a poor prognosis, many patients with LV systolic dysfunction display a nonrestrictive filling pattern [34, 35]. In this respect, assessment of the difference in duration of pulmonary venous flow (PVF) and mitral inflow at atrial contraction (AR_d-A_d) provides valid information which can be used for prognostic stratification of the patients with LV dysfunction [36]. A PVF reversal wave exceeding mitral A wave duration at atrial contraction is associated with elevated LV filling pressures [37, 38]. Dini et al. [36] evaluated the additive prognostic role of AR_d-A_d in a group of patients with a mean EF of 31±7%. Based on the mitral E wave deceleration time (DT) and AR_d-A_d, they classified the patients as nonrestrictive (DT >130 ms) and AR_d-A_d <30 ms, nonrestrictive and AR_d-A_d ≥30ms, and restrictive (DT ≥130 ms). They showed that 24-month cardiac event-free interval was best (86.3%) for the group in the nonrestrictive and AR_d-A_d <30 ms group, intermediate (37.9%) in the nonrestrictive and AR_d-A_d ≥30 ms group, and worst (22.9%) in the group with restrictive flow pattern. On multivariate analysis, AR_d-A_d ≥30 ms was independently asociated with both cardiac mortality and HF events (cardiac events excluding sudden death), and it was the most powerful predictor of cardiac events (cardiac mortality and hospitalization) for worsening HF.

Biochemical Parameters

The observation that there is activation of the neurohumoral axis in HF has prompted examination of the relations between a variety of biochemical measurements and clinical outcome. Strong inverse correlations have been reported between survival and plasma levels of norepinephrine [39, 40], renin [41], arginine vasopressin [41], atrial and brain natriuretic peptide (ANP, BNP) [42, 43], endothelin-1 [44] and interleukin-6 [45]. The concentrations of these substances reflect the severity of the underlying impairment of cirulatory function.

Atrial Natriuretic Peptide

ANP is primarily released from the atria in response to volume expansion, which appears to be sensed as an increase in atrial stretch. ANP release is increased in HF and is more dependent on atrial filling volume than on filling pressure [46]. Plasma ANP levels have been used as a marker for the diagnosis of asymptomatic LV dysfunction [47], but most subsequent studies have focused on the plasma BNP concentration. Yu and Sanderson [48] found plasma BNP levels to be the most important prognostic factor predicting death in the patients admitted with an episode of acute HF. ANP levels were not predictive of prognosis. However, in another study a precursor of ANP (N-ANP) was found to be an independent predictor of event-free survival in patients with CHF [49].

Brain Natriuretic Peptide

Plasma BNP levels are not only useful in diagnosis, but also, when measured at initial presentation, provide prognostic information in patients with HF, including those receiving therapy with a β-blocker and an ACE inhibitor [50, 51], and those with asymptomatic or minimally symptomatic LV dysfunction [43, 52].

Koglin et al. [52] tested the role of plasma BNP in the risk stratification of patients with CHF as well as its prognostic value for the clinical course of the disease. The study group included patients with NHYA functional class I-IV disease (42% class II) with a mean LVEF of 36±15%. Plasma levels of BNP increased as NYHA functional class increased (class I: 21.6±2.8 pg/ml; class II: 108.6±16.3 pg/ml; class III: 197.1±27.2 pg/ml; class IV: 363.0±67.8 pg/ml). For the clinical events defined as progression of a cardiovascular disability or patient death, BNP was able to discriminate patients with from those without clinical events, with a sensitivity of 88% and a specificity of 75%. In this study they also assessed the Heart Failure Survival Score (HFSS), which is used for risk stratification of patients with advanced CHF to identify potential candidates for heart transplantation [53]. HFSS and plasma BNP levels showed a significant inverse correlation, with the highest HFSS, indicating low risk, related with low plasma BNP levels. BNP was found to be as powerful a prognostic indicator as HFSS, though it did not add prognostic information independent of HFSS. Ishii et al. [54] used the combination of cardiac troponin T (cTnT) and BNP for risk stratification of patients hospitalized for worsening chronic HF. They found that a cTnT level above 0.033 μg/l and/or a BNP concentration above 440 pg/ml on admission correlated with an incremental increase in in-hospital cardiac mortality, overall cardiac mortality, and cardiac-event rate which reliably risk-stratified the patients into low-, intermediate-, and high-risk groups.

Plasma BNP levels have prognostic value not only in CHF but also in recent-onset HF. Yu and Sanderson [48] measured plasma ANP and BNP levels in patients following an episode of acute HF who had a mean LVEF of 34.6±0.9%. In multivariate analysis, plasma BNP level was the only significant predictor of 1-year mortality.

Cardiac Troponins

Cardiac troponins, which are the markers of cellular injury, are increased in patients with advanced HF. They are mostly suggested for use in the risk stratification of the patients in NYHA functional classes III and IV, which remains a difficult problem [53, 55, 56].

Setsuta et al. [57] evaluated the levels of cTnT in patients admitted with chronic HF of NYHA classes II-IV, and found them to be elevated in patients with severe HF (classes III and IV). In the 12 months of follow-up, the cardiac event rate defined as death or rehospitalization because of worsening HF was 65.8% in the patients with a cTnT concentration of 0.05 ng/ml or more on admission and 14.8% for the patients whose admission level of cTnT was below 0.05 ng/ml. The elevated cTnT levels in the patients with advanced HF decreased after effective medical therapy, suggesting that an elevated level of cTnT reflects decompensation in patients with chronic HF and that the progression of myocardial damage may be inhibited by appropriate medical therapy. Vecchia et al. [58] measured cardiac troponin I (cTnI) in patients admitted with severe CHF and found that compared to the cTnI- group, the cTnI± group had a significantly lower LVEF (20±5% vs 26±7%, p=0.023). Ischemic etiology was equally present in the two groups. In cTnI± patients who improved after admission, cTnI became undetectable, whereas it persisted in patients with refractory HF who were hospitalized until death. A positive cTnI was the most powerful predictor of mortality at 3 months.

Cardiac troponin elevations reflect ongoing myocardial cell injury associated with the progression of chronic HF. A recent hypothesis suggests that apoptosis, or programmed cell death, in the myocardium of patients with end-stage cardiomyopathy may be the underlying mechanism for the loss of cardiomyocytes [59, 60] Interestingly, the loss of viable cardiac myocytes is considerably less in chronic HF.

The release of cardiac troponins in HF may create a new approach to patient evaluation and the risk stratification of patients with HF into groups at high or low risk of future cardiac events, and adding BNP measurements could help to improve risk stratification.

Electrophysiological Evaluation

Autonomic Markers

These markers provide information about autonomic balance. Usually, risk is increased when there are signs of reduced vagal activity to the heart.

Heart Rate Variability

Profound abnormalities in autonomic control, characterized by generalized sympathetic overactivity and parasympathetic withdrawal, are typical features of neuroendocrine activation in CHF [61]. The analysis of beat-beat variations in heart rate (heart rate variability, HRV) has been used to investigate sympathovagal balance within the cardiovascular system [62]. In CHF, a decreased HRV has been reported, indicating this derangement in cardiac autonomic control [63, 64].

The usefulness of HRV in the risk stratification of CHF patients has been evaluated in a number of studies (Table 2). The UK-HEART study examined the predictive value of HRV as measured by the standard deviation of normal-to-normal RR intervals (SDNN) in a group of patients with NYHA functional class I-III disease and an LVEF below 45% [65]. The majority of the patients had ischemic heart disease. Along with cardiothoracic ratio, left ventricular end-systolic diameter, and serum sodium, SDNN was found to be a significant predictor of all-cause mortality. The annual mortality rate for the study population in SDNN subgroups was 5.5% for an SDNN above 100 ms, 12.7% for 50-100 ms, and 51.4% for less than 50 ms. In the UK-HEART study, a reduction in SDNN was the best predictor of death due to progressive HF, however, it was not found to be a predictor of sudden cardiac death.

Sudden cardiac death accounts for 40% of the deaths in end-stage HF and one of the investigated predictors has been HRV measures. Bilchick et al. studied HRV in CHF with EF below 40% and functional class II-III disease [70]. Ischemic cardiomyopathy was the underlying etiology in more than $^3/_4$ of the patients. They found a SDNN below 65.3 ms to be the sole independent factor

Table 2. Studies investigating the predictive value of standard deviation of normal-to-normal RR intervals (SDNN) in heart failure. (From [70], with permission)

	Patients characteristics	Mortality	Sudden death
Brouwer et al. [66]	EF 0.29 ± 0.09 75% ischemic CM	No[a]	No[a]
Szabo et al. [67]	EF 0.27 75% ischemic CM	Yes (cardiac death)	Yes (cardiac death)
Ponikowski et al. [68]	EF 26 ± 11 %76 ischemic CM	Yes	Not available
Nolan et al. (UK-HEART) [65]	EF 0.41 ± 0.17 76% ischemic CM	Yes	No
Fauchier et al. [69]	EF 0.34 ± 0.12 100% idiopathic dilated CM	Yes	No
Bilchick et al. [70]	EF 26 ± 9 76% ischemic CM	Yes	Yes

CM, Cardiomyopathy; [a]Poincare plots were predictive of mortality

predictive of survival in patients with CHF in NYHA functional class II or III and EF below 40% (Fig. 1). LVEF was not a predictor of survival in multivariate analysis. Furthermore, patients with an SDNN below 65.3 ms had a significantly increased risk of sudden death (p=0.016; Fig. 2).

Thus, HRV is a significant predictive variable in CHF patients both for overall mortality and in some studies for sudden death.

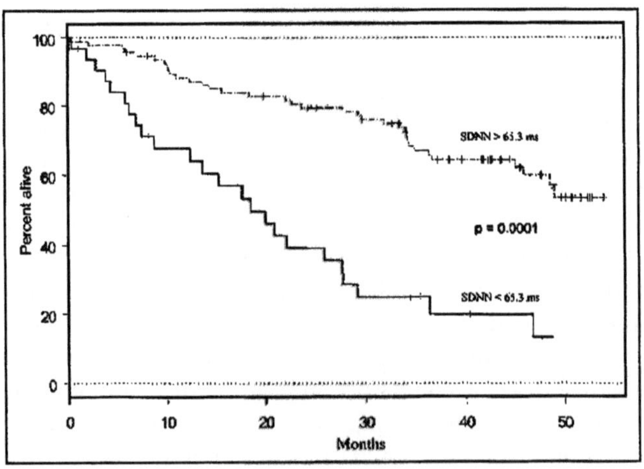

Fig. 1. Overall mortality of patients with SDNN in the lowest quartile versus the remainder. (From [71], with permission)

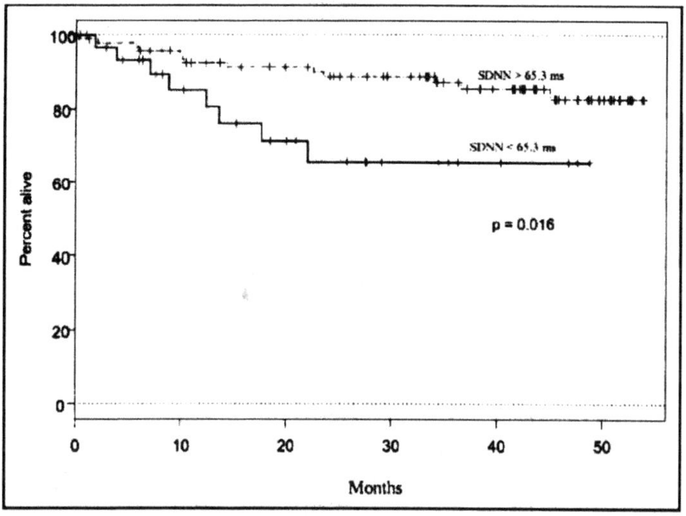

Fig. 2. Sudden death in patients with SDNN in the lowest quartile versus the remainder. (From [71], with permission)

Baroreflex Sensitivity

Sinoaortic and cardiopulmonary baroreceptors normally exert a restraining influence on resting central sympathetic activity. In patients with CHF, these normal tonic inhibitory reflexes are depressed, contributing to sympathetic excitation [71-74]. Baroreflex abnormalities in CHF patients have been reported in association with a prolonged exposure to low cardiac output and reduced blood pressure [72, 73]. Baroreflex sensitivity (BRS) which is defined as the absolute increase in RR interval produced by a 1-mmHg rise in systolic blood pressure, has been safely quantified by the phenylephrine method [75] and it has been proposed as a valid index of the capability to reflexively increase parasympathetic activity [76]. In patients with recent MI, a decreased BRS has been regarded as a powerful marker of poor prognosis [25, 77]. In the ATRAMI trial, a depressed BRS when associated with an LVEF below 35% identified a group of post-MI patients at highest risk of sudden and nonsudden cardiac death [25].

Mortara et al. [78] assessed the prognostic value of BRS in CHF patients who had a mean LVEF of 23±6% and functional class I-IV disease. BRS was found to be significantly associated with symptoms of CHF, and patients in class III or IV had a significantly more depressed BRS than those in class I or II. During 12 months follow-up, mortality was higher among the patients with a BRS below 1.3 ms/mmHg than in patients with better preserved BRS (58% vs 27%, $p<0.002$), showing the prognostic value of this autonomic marker. At multivariate analysis, BRS was an independent predictor of death after adjustment for NYHA class, LVEF, baseline RR interval, and maximum $\dot{V}O_2$, but not when hemodynamic indices (cardiac index and pulmonary capillary wedge pressure) were also considered. In CHF patients with severe mitral regurgitation, however, BRS remained a strong prognostic marker, being independent of hemodynamic function. The test was more informative in patients with ischemic rather than idiopathic cardiomyopathy (adjusted RR 2.0 vs 0.6).

Heart Rate Turbulence

Attenuation of the autonomic reflex modulation of the heart rate predicts a poor outcome after MI and in patients with chronic CHF [79, 80]. This modulation of heart rate can be examined from spontaneous HRV measurements of a 24-h ambulatory electrocardiographic Holter monitoring. Recently, a new method has been described that evaluates "heart rate turbulence" (HRT), a measure of the fluctuations in sinus-rhythm cycle length after a single ventricular premature beat (VPB). Almost all of the discriminant prognostic power of HRV was obtained by studying only the few beats that follow a premature complex. In low-risk patients, the sinus rhythm after a VPB shows a characteristic pattern of early acceleration and subsequent deceleration [81], whereas in high-risk patients no such characteristic pattern appears. Two parameters have been used for the evaluation of HRT:

- Turbulence onset (TO): The difference between the mean of the first two sinus RR intervals after a VPB and the last two sinus RR intervals before the VPB divided by the mean of the last two sinus RR intervals before the VPB:
- Turbulence onset= (RR1±RR2)-(RR-1±RR-2)/ RR-1±RR-2
- Turbulence slope (TS): the maximum positive slope of a regression line assessed over any sequence of five consecutive sinus-rhythm RR intervals within the first 20 sinus-rhythm intervals after a VPB.

Schmidt et al. [81] evaluated HRT in a group of post-MI patients with an LVEF below 30% and found that the combination of abnormal turbulence onset (≥0) and an abnormal slope (≤ 2.5 ms per RR interval) was the strongest mortality predictor. The 2-year mortality rates were 9%, 18%, and 34% in the patients with both normal TO and TS, with either factor abnormal, and with both factors abnormal, respectively. The other independent predictors of mortality were history of previous MI, LVEF, and mean heart rate. The relative hazard of the combination TO and TS was 3.2 compared to 1.7 for LVEF.

Recently, Davies et al. [82] evaluated the relation of HRT and blood pressure turbulence to BRS in a group of patients with chronic CHF with a mean LVEF of 33%. They defined blood pressure turbulence as the slope of the regression line over the five pulses corresponding to the RR intervals used for HRT, with the blood pressure data series shifted one beat to account for the delay of the baroreflex. Patients in NYHA classes I and II had a significantly higher HRT slope than patients in NYHA class III. The etiology of HF had no effect on HRT slope. They showed that, using the ratio of heart rate and blood pressure turbulence slope, turbulence-derived BRS can be estimated which showed good correlation with the α-index method of estimating BRS (BRSα). HRT correlated strongly with BRSα, but there was no correlation between blood pressure turbulence and BRSα. They showed that HRT can be used to assess BRS in patients with chronic HF.

The mechanism linking the absence of HRT to mortality is that the turbulence onset and slope assessment reflect specific aspects of cardiac autonomic status. Preserved vagal tone is known to be antiarrhythmic and probably constitutes autonomic antiarrhythmic protection [83, 84]. Thus, by measuring of the HRT, a direct manifestation of this protection can be captured when the heart is responding to a potentially proarrhythmic VPB.

HRT, the new prognostic parameter shown to have a better predictive power than other presently available factors, can be used in risk stratification.

Depolarization and Repolarization Variables

QRS Duration

A QRS duration of more than 120 ms has been shown to have 99% specificity for LV dysfunction. Recently, Iuliano et al. [85] investigated the relation of QRS duration (<120 ms or ≥ 120 ms) and mortality in 669 CHF patients. They classified patients into two groups with EF below 30% and EF between 30% and 40%. During a median follow-up of 45 months, in patients with an EF below 30% QRS prolongation was associated with a significant increase in mortality (51.6% vs 41.1%, p=0.01) and sudden death (28% vs 21.1%, p=0.02). In those with an EF of 30%-40%, QRS prolongation was associated with a significant increase in mortality (42.7% vs 23.3%, p=0.003) but not in sudden death (13.3% vs 12%, p=0.625). The independent predictors of mortality were the prolongation of QRS, LVEF below 30%, and NYHA class III or IV. Although there are studies with small numbers of patients that do not confirm this finding, a report of a large survey of 3654 patients confirms the direct association of QRS duration with 1-year mortality rate in patients with CHF [86].

Left Bundle Branch Block

Left bundle branch block (LBBB) has a deleterious effect on LV systolic and diastolic function of the persons without heart disease [87] and in patients with dilated cardiomyopathy [88]. The controversial issue has been whether mortality is increased independently with a widening of QRS. Baldasseroni et al. [89] studied the prognostic significance of LBBB in patients with CHF and found that LBBB develops in as many as 25% of patients with CHF. In multivariate analysis, after adjustments were made for age, underlying cardiac disease, CHF severity, and the effect of ACE inhibitors, LBBB was found to be associated with 1-year total mortality and sudden death (36% and 35%, respectively).

In patients with CHF, cardiac resynchronization with multisite cardiac pacing has been one of the treatment modalities that can improve LV contractility and mitral valve regurgitation [90]. Several studies have recently shown that left ventricular or biventricular cardiac pacing of patients with CHF and complete bundle branch block can improve exercise tolerance, clinical status, and health-related quality of life and can reduce the hospitalization rate [91, 92]. However, there is still a need for studies whether correction of LV asynchrony caused by intraventricular conduction defect may reduce the increased mortality.

QT Interval

Within the last decade, QT dispersion has been proposed as a descriptor of ventricular repolarization inhomogeneity and, as such, as a potential prognostic tool in the detection of future ventricular tachyarrhythmic events and death [93]. Since half of the very high mortality in patients with CHF is described as sudden death [94] and is assumed to be associated with ventricular arrhythmias, QT dispersion has been one of the most extensively studied prognostic parameters. Several earlier studies pointed toward a greater QT dispersion in CHF patients prone to ventricular tachyarrhythmias and sudden death [95-97], although this was not a consistent finding in all studies [98]. However, a recent large study examining the prognostic value of QT dispersion in 1518 patients with an LVEF below 30% did not find any difference between survivors and nonsurvivors. Moreover, QT dispersion had no prognostic value regarding all-cause mortality, cardiac mortality, or arrhythmic mortality [99].

Thus, QT dispersion, since it lacks demonstrable prognostic value, is better not taken into account in the risk stratification of patients with CHF.

T Wave Alternans

About half of the deaths in patients with CHF are sudden, resulting from ventricular arrhythmias [100]. Measurement of μV-level T wave alternans (TWA) in the surface electrocardiogram (ECG) has been introduced as a new way to assess the risk of ventricular arrhythmias [101]. TWA is a subtle change in T wave morphology that occurs in every alternate beat. TWA is thought to reflect the occurrence of localized action potential alternans, which creates dispersion of recovery, which in turn promotes the development of reentrant arrhythmias [102].

Clinical studies have convincingly shown that TWA is closely related to arrhythmia induction in the electrophysiology laboratory as well as to the occurrence of spontaneous ventricular tachyarrhythmias in patients undergoing electrophysiological study [101]. The first large clinical study of TWA was performed by Rosenbaum et al. [101], who observed 83 patients undergoing both electrophysiological study and TWA measured during atrial pacing. TWA was equivalent to electrophysiological study as a predictor of arrhythmic events. More recently, Gold et al. [103] reported on a multicenter study of TWA measured in 313 patients referred for electrophysiological study. Structural heart disease was present in 70% of subjects including 34% with CHF. Cox regression analysis revealed that TWA was the only significant independent predictor of events in this heterogenous population. Klingenheben et al. studied 107 patients with a mean EF of 28±7% and no prior sustained ventricular arrhythmia. During 18 months of follow-up review, TWA was the only independent statistical predictor of arrhythmic events (Fig. 3). Other measures of

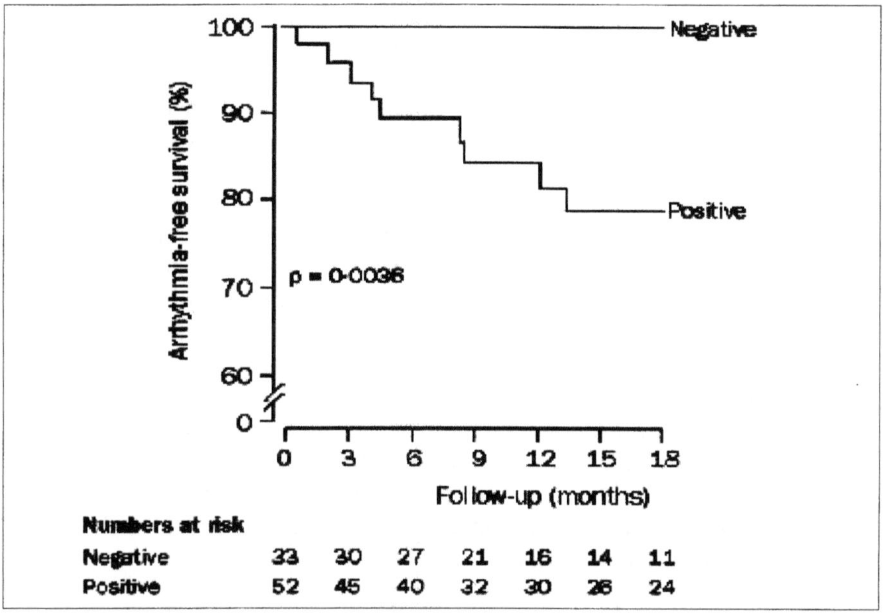

Fig. 3. Kaplan-Meier analysis of event-free survival for patients with positive or negative results in T wave alternans (TWA) measurements. The rate of arrhythmic evetns at 18 months was 21% (SE 6%) among patients with TWA and zero among those who did not show TWA. (From [114], with permission)

arrhythmic risk studied (LVEF 30%, nonsustained ventricular tachycardia, BRS ≤3.0 ms/mmHg, signal-averaged ECG, SDNN ≤70 ms, mean RR ≤ 700 ms) did not achieve statistical significance [104].

Ventricular Premature Beats and Nonsustained Ventricular Tachycardia

Ambient ventricular arrhythmia is a frequent accompaniment of LV dysfunction and increases with HF severity [105-107]. Ventricular premature beats and nonsustained vetricular tachycardia (VT) have been demonstrated to be predictors of total mortality in patients with HF associated with reduced ventricular function [105, 107-109]. However, whether the presence of complex ventricular ectopy including nonsustained VT is a specific predictor of sudden risk is controversial. Some studies have suggested that the presence of nonsustained VT is an independent risk factor that specifically predicts sudden death in HF and others have not. The Argentinean Study Group for the Prevention of Cardiac Insufficiency (GESICA) and the GEMA investigators analyzed the effect of nonsustained VT (≥ 3 consecutive ventricular premature beats at a rate >100 beats/min) detected by 24-h Holter monitoring in 516 patients with severe HF before open-label randomization to amiodarone or no antiarrhythmic therapy [107]. Nonsustained VT was detected in 33.5% of the patients. The presence of nonsustained VT was associated with a higher total mortality and sudden death rate. The combination of ventricular premature beats and nonsustained VT conferred the highest risk of total mortality. However, there was no correlation between the number of episodes of nonsustained VT noted on Holter and outcome. The prognostic significance was independent of the cause of HF (ischemic or nonischemic).

More recently, the effect of ambient ventricular arrhythmia on total mortality and sudden death rate was anlyzed in the PROMISE trial [105]. A total of 1080 patients with class III or IV HF and LVEF 35% were enrolled. There were 290 deaths of which 139 (48%) were sudden. The presence of more than 30 ventricular premature beats per hour, any nonsustained VT, and nonsustained VT of more than 10 beat duration were all potent univariate predictors of total mortality, nonsudden death, and sudden death. The frequency of nonsustained VT episodes was the most powerful predictor of mortality. However, multivariate analysis demonstrated that ventricular ectopy did not specifically predict sudden death. In summary, the presence of ventricular arrhythmias is a predictor of increased mortality in HF but does not specifically predict risk of sudden death in the individual patient.

Late Potentials

Patients with chronic HF are at a greater risk of sudden death than any other subset of patients in cardiovascular medicine [108, 109]. Although the survival of patients with nonischemic dilated cardiomyopathy is slightly better than that of patients with coronary artery disease, the incidence of sudden death is comparable.

The signal-averaged ECG (SAECG) allows the detection of late potentials, which have been associated with delayed and disorganized ventricular activation, a substrate for reentrant VT [110]. Studies in patients with prior MI have demonstrated that an abnormal SAECG has predictive value for future ventricular events [111, 112]. However, in patients with HF SAECGs have been found to be prognostic in some studies, but not in others. Galinier et al. [113] in a prospective study of 151 patients with CHF have demonstrated that the incidence of late potentials is independent of the etiology of heart failure. Although SAECG findings improved risk stratification in relation to sustained VT, they did not identify patients with CHF at high risk of sudden death. Middlekauff et al. [114] did not find SAECG to be predictive of sudden death or ventricular arrhythmias in a group of patients with ischemic and idiopathic cardiomyopathy, whereas Mancini et al. [115] found that the SAECG identified patients with nonischemic dilated cardiomyopathy at high risk of death and/or VT. Silverman et al. [116] assessed the importance of the etiology of HF on the prognostic importance of SAECG. Patients with nonischemic cardiomyopathy who had an abnormal SAECG did not have a worse prognosis than those with a normal SAECG. However, among patients with ischemic cardiomyopathy those with an abnormal SAECG tended to have poorer survival than those with a normal SAECG (73% versus 81% 1-year mortality, respectively). Thus, the etiology of HF affected the prognostic importance of an abnormal SAECG.

Electrophysiological Testing

A number of studies have evaluated the role of electrophysiological testing to select patients with ventricular arrhythmias who are at high risk of sudden cardiac death and might benefit from antiarrhythmic therapy [117-119]. One large, multicenter, prospective study (Multicenter Unsustained Tachycardia Trial (MUSTT), involved 704 patients with coronary disease with or without a remote MI, asymptomatic nonsustained VT, and LVEF ≤40% [120]. The rate of mortality was increased in patients with inducible sustained monomorphic VT (SMVT) compared to those without SMVT. The rates of cardiac arrest were 18% versus 12% at 2 years and 32% versus 24% at 5 years. Overall mortality rates at 5 years in those with and without inducible SMVT were 48% and 44%, respectively (p=0.005); death among those without inducible SMVT was less likely to be arrhythmic in origin (45% versus 54% in those with inducible SMVT). Results were similar in another study of 93 patients with nonsustained VT on Holter monitoring who did not have inducible SMVT; although the overall mortality was high, especially in those with a LVEF of 35% or less (15% and 34% at 1 and 3 years, respectively), the sudden death mortality rates were only 4% and 18%, respectively [121].

Heart Failure Survival Score

Recently, Aaronson et al. proposed a prospectively validated clinical index, the Heart Failure Survival Score (HFSS), as an instrument to improve risk stratification in patients with advanced HF [543] .The seven noninvasively determined variables included in the HFSS incorporate multiple features of CHF pathophysiology: presence of ischemic cardiomyopathy (etiology of CHF); systolic dysfunction and mean arterial pressure (hemodynamics); heart rate and serum sodium concentration (neurohumoral activation); intraventricular conduction delay (IVCD; myocardial injury/fibrosis); and peak VO_2 (functional capacity). Zugck et al. [122] prospectively evaluated the performance of HFSS in a sample of ambulatory patients with HF (LVEF 22±9% and mean NYHA class 2.3±0.7). Additionally, a 6-min walk test instead of determination of peak VO_2 was also used in order to simplify the evaluation. During a total follow-up of 28±14 months, the HFSS was able to discriminate the patients into low, medium, and high risk groups, with mortality rates of 16%, 39%, and 50%, respectively. However, the prognostic power of the HFSS was inferior to that of a two-variable model consisting only of LVEF and peak VO_2 or 6-min walk test. The HFSS also failed to reliably differentiate 1-year survival in NYHA class III patients, the potential candidates for cardiac transplantation.

Conclusions

Despite significant advances in the therapy of HF, the mortality for this disease remains high and increases with the severity of the disease. A number of clinical, hemodynamic, echocardiographic, biochemical, and electrophysiological parameters have been used to risk-stratify these patients into low, intermediate, and high risk groups. Although a number of new parameters have been introduced, LVEF, which is one of the oldest recognized prognostic variables did not lose its importance in risk stratification of the patients. A notable point that emerges from studies is the greater predictive value to be achieved by combining variables rather than evaluating then singly. These models will not only help us by guiding medical therapy but will also enable us to answer the questions asked by patients and their families about the predicted survival of such-and-such a high-risk group.

References

1. Erikson H (1995) Heart Failure: growing public health problem. J Intern Med 237:135-141
2. Ho KKL, Pinsky JL, Kannel WB et al (1993) The epidemiology of heart failure: the Framingham Study. J Am Coll Cardiol 22[Suppl]:6A-13A
3. Kelly DT (1997) Paul Dudley White International Lecture. Our future society: a global challenge. Circulation 95:2459-2464
4. Braunwald E, Zipes DP, Libby P (2001) Heart disease: a textbook of cardiovascular medicine, 6th ed. W.B. Saunders Company, Pennsylvania, pp 534-561
5. Uretsky BF, Sheahan RG (1997) Primary prevention of sudden cardiac death in heart failure: will the solution be shocking? J Am Coll Cardiol 30:1589-1597
6. Adams KF, Dunlap SH, Suteta CA et al (1996) Relation between gender, etiology and survival in patients with symptomatic heart failure. J Am Coll Cardiol 28:1781-1788
7. Bart BA, Shaw LK, McCants CB et al (1997) Clinical determinants of mortality in patients with angiographically diagnosed ischemic or nonischemic cardiomyopathy. J Am Coll Cardiol 30:1002- 1008
8. Young JB (1999) Assessment of heart failure. In: Colucci WS (ed) Cardiac function and dysfunction, 2nd ed. In: Braunwald E (series ed) Atlas of heart diseases. vol 4. Philadelphia, Current Medicine, pp 7.1-7.9
9. Chomsky DB, Lang CC, Rayos GH et al (1996) Hemodynamic exercise testing: a valuable tool in the selection of cardiac transplantation candidates. Circulation 94:3176-3183
10. Myers J, Gullestad L (1998) The role of exercise testing and gas-exchange measurement in the prognostic assessment of patients with heart failure. Curr Opin Cardiol 13:145-155
11. Myers J, Gullestad L, Vagelos R et al (1998) Clinical, hemodynamic, and cardiopulmonary exercise test determinants of survival in patients referred for evaluation of heart failure. Ann Intern Med 129:286-293
12. Mancini DM, Eisen H, Kussmaul W et al (1991) Value of peak oxygen consumption for optimal timing of cardiac transplantation in ambulatory patients with heart failure. Circulation 83:778-786

13. Kao W, Winkle EM, Johnson MR et al (1997) Role of maximal oxygen consumption in establishment of heart transplantation candidacy for heart failure patients with intermediate exercise tolerance. Am J Cardiol 79:1124-1127
14. Corra U, Mezzani A, Bosimini E et al (2002) Ventilatory response to exercise improves risk stratification in patients with chronic heart failure and intermediate functional capacity. Am Heart J 143:418-426
15. Robbins M, Francis G, Pashkow FJ et al (1999) Ventilatory and heart rate responses and exercise: better predictors of heart failure mortality than peak oxygen consumption. Circulation 100:2411-2417
16. Priori SG, Aliot E, Blomstrom-Lundqvist C et al (2001) Task Force on Sudden Cardiac Death of the European Society of Cardiology. Eur Heart J 22:1374-1450
17. Yap Y, Duong T, Bland M et al (2000) Left ventricular ejection fraction in the thrombolytic era remains a powerful predictor of long-term but not short-term all-cause, cardiac and arrhythmic mortality after myocardial infarction - a secondary meta-analysis of 2828 patients. Heart 83:55
18. Copie X, Hnatkova K, Staunton A et al (1996) Predictive power of increased heart rate versus depressed left ventricular ejection fraction and heart rate variability for risk stratification after myocardial infarction. Results of a two-year follow-up study. J Am Coll Cardiol 27:270-276
19. The Multicenter Postinfarction Research Group (1983) Risk stratification and survival after myocardial infarction. N Engl J Med 309-331-336
20. Stevenson WG, Ridker PM (1996) Should survivors of myocardial infarction with low ejection fraction be routinely referred to arrhythmia specialists ? JAMA 14:481-485
21. Zaret BL, Wackers FJ, Terrin ML et al (1995) Value of radionuclide rest and exercise left ventricular ejection fraction in assessing survival of patients after thrombolytic therapy for acute myocardial infarction: results of Thrombolysis in Myocardial Infarction (TIMI) phase II study. The TIMI Study Group. J Am Coll Cardiol 26:73-79
22. Copie X, Hnatkova K, Staunton A et al (1996) Predictive power of increased heart rate versus depressed left ventricular ejection fraction and heart rate variability for risk stratification after myocardial infarction. Results of a two year follow-up study. J Am Coll Cardiol 27:270-276
23. Mukharji J, Rude RE, Poole WK et al (1984) Risk factors for sudden death after acute myocardial infarction: Two year follow-up. Am J Cardiol 54:31-36
24. Bigger JT (1986) Prevalence, characteristics and significance of ventricular tachycardia detected by 24 hour continuous electrocardiographic recordings in the late post hospital phase of acute myocardial infarction. Am J Cardiol 58:1151-1160
25. La Rovere MT, Mortara A, Bigger JT Jr et al (1998) The prognostic value of baroreflex sensitvity and heart rate variability after myocardial infarction: ATRAMI (Autonomic Tone and Reflexes After Myocardial Infarction) Investigators. Lancet 351:478-484
26. Polak JF, Holman L, Wynne J, Colucci WS (1983) Right ventricular ejection fraction: an indicator of increased mortality in patients with congestive heart failure associated with coronary artery disease. J Am Coll Cardiol 2:217-224
27. De Groote P, Millaire A, Foucer-Hossein C et al (1998) Right ventricular ejection farction is an independent predictor of survival in patients with moderate heart failure. J Am Coll Cardiol 32:948-954
28. Gavazzi A, Berzuini C, Campana C et al (1997) Value of right ventricular ejection fraction in predicting short-term prognosis of patients with severe chronic heart failure. J Heart Lung Transplant 16:774-785
29. Ghio S, Gavazzi A, Campana C et al (2001) Independent and additive prognostic value of right ventricular systolic function and pulmonary artery pressure in patients with chronic heart failure. J Am Coll Cardiol 37:183-188

30. Lavine SJ, Arends D (1989) Importance of left ventricular filling pressure on diastolic filling in idiopathic dilated cardiomyopathy. Am J Cardiol 64:61-65
31. Channer KS, Wilde P, Culling W et al (1986) Estimation of left ventricular end-diastolic pressure by pulsed Doppler ultrasound. Lancet 3:1005-1007
32. Shen WF, Tribouilloy C, Rey JL et al (1992) Prognostic significance of Doppler-derived left ventricular filling variables in dilated cardiomyopathy. Am Heart J 124:1524-1533
33. Hansen A, Haass M, Zugck C et al (2001) Prognostic value of Doppler echocardiographic mitral inflow patterns: implications for risk stratification in patients with chronic congestive heart failure. J Am Coll Cardiol 37:1049-1055
34. Takenada K, Dabestani A, Gardin JM et al (1986) Pulsed Doppler echocardiographic study of left ventricular filling in dilated cardiomyopathy. Am J Cardiol 58:143-147
35. Masuyama T, Popp RL (1997) Doppler evaluation of left ventricular filling in congestive heart failure. Eur Heart J 18:1548-1556
36. Dini FK, Michelassi C, Micheli G. et al (2000) Prognostic value of pulmonary venous flow doppler signal in left ventricular dysfunction. J Am Coll Cardiol 36:1295-1302
37. Rossvol O, Hatle LK (1993) Pulmonary venous flow velocities recorded by transthoracic Doppler ultrasound: relation to left ventricular diastolic pressures. J Am Coll Cardiol 21:1679-1700
38. Cecconi M, Manfrin M, Zanoli R et al (1996) Doppler echocardiographic evaluation of left-ventricular end-diastolic pressure in patients with coronary artery disease. J Am Soc Echocardiogr 9:241-250
39. Cohn JN, Levine TB, Olivari MT et al (1984) Plasma norepinephrine as a guide to prognosis in patients with chronic congestive heart failure. N Engl J Med 311:819-823
40. Cohn JN, Johnson GR, Shabetai R et al (1993) Ejection fraction, peak exercise oxygen consumption, cardiothoracic ratio, ventricular arrhythmias, and plasma norepinephrine as determinants of prognosis in heart failure. The V-HeFT VA Cooperative Studies Group. Circulation 87:V15-V16
41. Packer M, Lee WH, Kessler PD et al (1987) Role of neurohumoral mechanisms in determining survival in patients with severe chronic heart failure. Circulation 75: IV80-IV92
42. Gottlieb SS, Kukin ML, Ahern D et al (1989) Prognostic importance of atrial natriuretic peptide in patients with chronic heart failure. J Am Coll Cardiol 13:1534-1539
43. Tsutamoto T, Wada A, Maeda L et al (1997) Attenuation of compensation of endogenous cardiac natriuretic peptide system in chronic heart failure: prognostic role of plasma brain natriuretic peptide concentration in patients with chronic symptomatic left ventricular dysfunction. Circulation 96:509-516
44. Hulsmann M, Stanek B, Frey B et al (1998) Value of cardiopulmonary exercise testing and big endothelin plasma levels to predict short-term prognosis in patients with chronic heart failure. J Am Coll Cardiol 32:1695-1700
45. Tsutamoto T, Hisanaga T, Wada A et al (1998) Interleukin-6 spillover in the peripheral circulation increases with the severity of heart failure, and the high plasma level of interleukin-6 is an important prognostic predictor in patients with congestive heart failure. J Am Coll Cardiol 31:391-398
46. Globits S, Frank H, Pacher B et al (1998) Atrial natriuretic peptide release is more dependent on atrial filling volume than on filling pressure in chronic congestive heart failure. Am Heart J 135:592-597
47. Lerman A, Gibbons RJ, Rodeheffer RJ et al (1993) Circulating N terminal atrial natriuretic peptide as a marker for symptomless left ventricular dysfunction. Lancet 341:1105-1109
48. Yu CM, Sanderson JE (1999) Plasma brain natriuretic peptide-independent predictor of cardiovascular mortality in acute heart failure. Eur J Heart Failure 1:59-65

49. Hülsmann M, Berger R, Sturm B et al (2002) Prediction of outcome by neurohormonal activation, the six-minute walk and the Minnesota Living with Heart Failure Questionairre in an outpatient cohort with congestive heart failure. Eur Heart J 23:886-891
50. Dao Q, Krishnaswamy P, Kazanegra R et al (2001) Utility of B-natriuretic peptide in the diagnosis of congestive heart failure in an urgent care setting. J Am Coll Cardiol 37:379-385
51. Stanek B, Frey B, Hulssman M et al (2001) Prognostic evaluation of of neurohormonal plasma levels before beta-blocker therapy in advanced left ventricular dysfunction. J Am Coll Cardiol 38:436-442
52. Koglin J, Pehlivanli S, Schwaiblmair M et al (2001) Role of brain natriuretic peptide in risk stratification of patients with congestive heart failure. J Am Coll Cardiol 38:1934-1941
53. Aaronson KD, Schwartz JS, Chen TM et al (1997) Development and prospective validation of a clinical index to predict survival in ambulatory patients referred for cardiac transplant evaluation. Circulation 95:2660-2667
54. Ishii J, Nomura M, Nakmura Y et al (2002) Risk stratification using a combination of cardiac troponin T and brain natriuretic peptide in patients hospitalized for worsening chronic heart failure. Am J Cardiol 89:691-695
55. Likoff MJ, Chandler SL, Kay MR (1987) Clinical determinants of mortality in chronic congestive heart failure secondary to idiopathic dilated or to ischemic cardiomyopathy. Am J Cardiol 59:634-638
56. Campana C, Gavazzi A, Berzuini C et al (1993) Predictors of prognosis in patients awaiting heart transplantation J Heart Lung Transplant 12:756-765
57. Setsuta K, Seino Y, Takahashi N et al (1999) Clinical significance of elevated levels of cardiac troponin T in patients with chronic heart failure. Am J Cardiol 84:608-611
58. Vecchia LL, Mezzena G, Zonalla L et al (2000) Cardiac troponin I as diagnostic and prognostic marker in severe heart failure. J Heart Lung Transplant 19:644-652
59. Narula J, Haider N, Virmani R et al (1996) Apoptosis in myocytes in end-stage heart failure. N Engl J Med 335:1182-1189
60. Olivetti G, Abbi R, Quaini F et al (1997) Apoptosis in the failing human heart. N Engl J Med 336:1131-1141
61. Floras JS (1993) Clinical aspects of sympathetic activation and parasympathetic withdrawal in heart failure. J Am Coll Cardiol 87[Suppl VI]:VI40-VI48
62. Task Force of The European Society of Cardiology and the The North American Society of Pacing and Electrophysiology (1996) Heart rate variability: standards of measurement, physiological interpretation and clinical use. Eur Heart J 17:354-381
63. Casolo G, Balli E, Taddei T et al (1989) Decreased spontaneous heart rate variability in congestive heart failure. Am J Cardiol 64:1162-1167
64. Kienzle MG, Ferguson DW, Birkett CL et al (1992) Clinical, hemodynamic and sympathetic neural correlates of heart rate variability in congestive heart failure. Am J Cardiol 69:761-767
65. Nolan J, Batin PD, Andrews R et al (1998) Prospective study of heart rate variability and mortality in chronic heart failure. Circulation 98:1510-1516
66. Brouwer J, van Veldhuisen DJ, Man in 't Veld AJ et al (1996) Prognostic value of heart rate variability during long-term follow-up in patients with mild to moderate heart failure. The Dutch Ibopamine Multicenter Trial Study Group. J Am Coll Cardiol 28:1183-1189
67. Szabo BM, van Veldhuisen DJ, van der Veer N et al (1997) Prognostic value of heart rate variability in chronic congestive heart failure secondary to idiopathic or ischemic dilated cardiomyopathy. Am J Cardiol 79:978-980

68. Ponikowski P, Aker DS, Chua TP et al (1997) Depressed heart rate variability as an independent predictor of death in chronic congestive heart failure secondary to ischemic or idiopathic dialted cardiomyopathy. Am J Cardiol 79:1645-1650
69. Fauchier L, Babuty D, Cosnay P et al (1999) Prognostic value of heart rate variability and major arrhythmic events in patients with idiopathic dilated cardiomyopathy. J Am Coll Cardiol 33:1203-1207
70. Bilchick KC, Fetics B, Djoukeng R et al (2002) Prognostic value of heart rate variability in chronic congestive heart failure (Veterans Affairs' survival trial of of antiarrhythmic therapy in congestive heart failure). Am J Cardiol 90:24-28
71. Shepherd JT (1990) Heart failure: role of cardiovascular reflexes. Cardioscience 1:7-12
72. Thames MD, Kinugawa T, Smith ML et al (1993) Abnormalities of baroreflex control in heart failure. J Am Coll Cardiol 22A:56A-60A
73. Marin-Neto JA, Pintya AO, Gallo L Jr et al (1991) Abnormal baroreflex control of heart rate in decompensated congestive heart failure and reversal after compensation. Am J Cardiol 67:604-610
74. Ellenbogen KA, Mohanty PK, Szentpetery S et al (1989) Arterial baroreflex abnormalities in heart failure: reversal after orthotropic heart transplantation. Circulation 79:51-58
75. La Rovere MT, Mortara A, Schwartz PJ (1995) Baroreflex sensitivity. J Cardiovasc Electrophysiol 6:761-774
76. Levy MN, Schwartz PJ (eds) (1994) Vagal control of the heart: experimental basis and clinical implications. Futura, Armonk, NY, pp 644
77. La Rovere MT, Specchia G, Mortara A et al (1988) Baroreflex sensitivity, clinical correlates and cardiovascular mortality among patients with a first myocardial infarction: a prospective study. Circulation 78:816-824
78. Mortara A, La Rovere MT, Pinna DG et al (1997) Arterial baroreflex modulation of heart rate in chronic heart failure. Circulation 96:3450-3458
79. Yap YG, Camm AJ (1998) The importance of the autonomic nervous system for risk stratification of post-myocardial infarction patients. Coron Artery Dis 9:353-358
80. Ponikowski P, Chua TP, Piepoli M et al (1997) Augmented peripheral chemosensitivity as a potential input to baroreflex impairment and autonomic imbalance in chronic heart failure. Circulation 96:2586-2594
81. Schmidt G, Malik M, Barthel P et al (1999) Heart-rate turbulence after ventricular premature beats as a predictor of mortality after myocardial infarction. Lancet 353:1390-1396
82. Davies LC, Francis DP, Ponikowski P et al (2001) Relation of heart rate and blood pressure turbulence following premature ventricular complexes to baroreflex sensitivity in chronic congestive heart failure. Am J Cardiol 87:737-742
83. Lown B, Verrier RL (1976) Neural activity and ventricular fibrillation. N Engl J Med 294:1165-1170
84. Corr PB, Yamada KA, Witkowski FX (1986) Mechanisms controlling cardiac autonomic function and their relation to arrhythmogenesis. In: Fozzard HA, Haber E, Jennings RB, Katz AN, Morgan HD (eds) The heart and cardiovascular system. Raven, New York pp 1343-1403
85. Iuliano S, Fischer SG, Karasik PE et al (2002) QRS duration and mortality in patients with congestive heart failure. Am Heart J 143:1085-1091
86. Gottipaty V, Krelis S, Lu F et al (1993) The resting electrocardiogram provides a sensitive and inexpensive marker of prognosis in patients with chronic congestive heart failure. J Am Coll Cardiol 33[Suppl A]:145A
87. Grines CL, Bashore TM, Boudoulas H et al (1989) Functional abnormalities in isolated left bundle-branch block. The effect of interventricular asynchrony. Circulation 79:845-853

88. Xiao HB, Lee CH, Gibson DG et al (1991) Effect of left-bundle branch block on diastolic function in dilated cardiomyopathy. Br Heart J 66:443-447
89. Baldasseroni S, Opasich C, Gorini M et al (2002) Left bundle-branch block is associated with increased 1-year sudden and total mortality rate in 5517 outpatients with congestive heart failure: a report from the Italian Network of Congestive Heart Failure. Am Heart J 143:398-405
90. Blanc JJ, Etienne Y, Gilard M et al (1997) Evaluation of different ventricular pacing sites in patients with severe heart failure: results of an acute hemodynamic study. Circulation 96:3273-3277
91. Saxon LA, Boehmer JP, Hummel J et al (1999) Biventricular pacing in patients with congestive heart failure: two prospective randomized trials. The VIGOR CHF and VENTAK CHF Investigators. Am J Cardiol 83:120D-3
92. Cazeau S, Leclercq C, Lavergne T et al (2001) Effects of multisite biventricular pacing in patients with heart failure and intraventricular conduction delay. N Engl J Med 344:873-880
93. Day CP, McComb JM, Campbell RW et al (1990) QT dispersion: an indication of arrhythmia risk in patients with long QT intervals. Br Heart J 63:342-344
94. Kannel WB, Plehn JF, Cupples LA (1998) Cardiac failure and sudden death in the Framingham Study. Am Heart J 115:869-875
95. Barr CS, Naas A, Freeman M et al (1994) QT dispersion and sudden unexpected death in chronic heart failure. Lancet 343:327-329
96. Pye M, Quinn AC, Cobbe SM (1994) QT interval dispersion: a non-invasive marker of susceptibility to arrhythmia in patients with sustained ventricular arrhythmias ? Br Heart J 71:511-514
97. Grimm W, Steder U, Menz V et al (1996) QT dispersion and arrhythmic events in idiopathic dilated cardiomyopathy. Am J Cardiol 78:458-461
98. Brendorp B, Elming H, Jun Li et al (2001) QT dispersion has no prognostic information for patients with advanced congestive heart failure and reduced left ventricular systolic function. Circulation 103:831-835
99. Fei L, Goldman JH, Prasad K et al (1996) QT dispersion and RR variations on 12-lead ECGs in patients with congestive heart failure secondary to idiopathic dilated cardiomyopathy. Eur Heart J 17:258-263
100. Ho KLL, Anderson KM, Kannel WB et al (1993) Survival after the onset of congestive heart failure in Framingham Heart Study subjects. Circulation 88:107-115
101. Rosenbaum DS, Jackson LE, Smith JM et al (1994) Electrical alternans and vulnerability to ventricular arrhythmias. N Engl J Med 330:235-241
102. Hohnloser SH, Klingenheben T, Li Y-G et al (1998) T wave alternans as a predictor of recurrent ventricular tachyarrhythmias in ICD recipients: prospective comparison with conventional risk markers. J Cardiovasc Electrophysiol 9:1258-1268
103. Gold MR, Bloomfield Dm, Anderson KP et al (2000) A comparison of T wave alternans, signal averaged electrocardiogarphy and programmed ventricular stimulation for arrhythmia risk stratification. J Am Coll Cardiol 36:2247-2253
104. Klingenheben T, Zabel M, D'Agostino RB et al (2000) Predictive value of T wave alternans for arrhythmic events in patients with congestive heart failure. Lancet 356:651-652
105. Teerlink JR, Jalaluddin M, Anderson S et al, on behalf of the PROMISE (Prospective Randomized Milrinone Survival Evaluation) Investigators (2000) Ambulatory ventricular arrhythmias among patients with heart failure do not specifically predict an increased risk of sudden death. Circulation 101:40-46
106. Wilson J, Schwartz S, St John Sutton M et al (1983) Prognosis in severe heart failure: relation to hemodynamic measurements and ventricular ectopic activity. J Am Coll Cardiol 2:403-410

107. Doval HC, Nul DR, Grancelli HO et al, for the GESICA-GEMA Investigators (1996) Nonsustained ventricular tachycardia in severe heart failure: independent marker of increased mortality due to sudden death. Circulation 94:3198-3203
108. Packer M (1985) Sudden unexpected death in patients with congestive heart failure: a second frontier. Circulation 72:681-685
109. Kannel W, Plehn J, Cupples LA (1988) Cardiac failure and sudden death in the Framingham Study. Am Heart J 115:869-875
110. Simson MB, Untereker WJ, Spielman SR et al (1983) Relation between late potentials on the body surface and directly recorded fragmanted electrograms in patients with ventricular tachycardia. Am J Cardiol 51:105-112
111. Kuchard D, Thorburn C, Sammel N (1987) Prediction of serious arrhythmic events after myocardial infarct: signal averaged electrocardiogram, Holter monitoring, and radionuclide ventriculography. J Am Coll Cardiol 9:531-538
112. Breithart G, Schwarzmaier M, Borgreffe M et al (1983) Prognostic significance of late ventricular potentials after acute myocardial infarction. Eur Heart J 4:487-495
113. Galinier M, Albenque J-P, Afchar N et al (1996) Prognostic value of late potentials in patients with congestive heart failure. Eur Heart J 17:264-271
114. Middlekauff H, Stevenson W, Woo M et al (1990) Comparison of frequency of late potentials in idiopathic dilated cardiomyopathy and ischemic cardiomyopathy with advanced congestive heart failure and their usefulness in predicting sudden death. Am J Cardiol 66:1113-1117
115. Mancini D, Wong K, Simson M (1993) Prognostic value of an abnormal signal-averaged electrocardiogram in patients with non-ischemic congestive cardiomyopathy. Circulation 87:1083-1092
116. Silverman ME, Pressel MD, Brackett JC et al (1995) Prognostic value of the signal-averaged electrocardiogram and a prolonged QRS in ischemic and nonischemic cardiomyopathy. Am J Cardiol 75:460-464
117. Poll DS, Marchlinski FE, Buxton AE et al (1986) Usefulness of programmed stimulation in idiopathic dilated cardiomyopathy. Am J Cardiol 58:992-997
118. Stamato NJ, O'Connell JB, Murdock DK et al (1986) The response of patients with complex ventricular arrhythmias secondary to dilated cardiomyopathy to programmed ventricular stimulation. Am J Cardiol 112:505-508
119. Das SK, Morady F, DiCarlo L Jr et al (1986) Prognostic usefulness of programmmed ventricular stimulation in idiopathic dilated cardiomyopathy without symptomatic ventricular arrhythmias. Am J Cardiol 58:998-1000
120. Buxton AE, Lee KL, DiCarlo L et al (2000) Electrophysiological testing to identify patients with coronary artery disease who are at risk for sudden death. Multicenter Unsustained Tachycardia Trial Investigators. N Engl J Med 342:1937-1945
121. Schmidt H, Hurst T, Coch M et al (2000) Nonsustained, asymptomatic ventricular tachycardia in patients with coronary artery disease: Prognosis and incidence of sudden death of patients who are noninducible by electrophysiologic testing. Pacing Clin Electrophysiol 23:1220-1225
122. Zugck C, Krüger C, Kell R et al (2001) Risk stratification in middle-aged patients with congestive heart failure: prospective comparison of the Heart Failure Survival Score (HFSS) and a simplified two-variable model. Eur J Heart Failure 3:577-585

Risk Stratification in Atrial Fibrillation and Congestive Heart Failure

G. BORIANI, C. CAMANINI, A. BRANZI, C. RAPEZZI

Atrial Fibrillation and Heart Failure: Epidemiologic and Clinical Connections

Atrial fibrillation (AF) and heart failure are two common cardiac diseases, affecting 1%-2% of the population [1, 2] with a prevalence that rises steeply with age. AF and heart failure are conditioned by common risk factors and frequently coexist [3]; indeed, the prevalence of left ventricular dysfunction and/or congestive heart failure among patients with AF may be as high as 40% [4], and in the Framingham Study the presence of congestive heart failure implied a 6.6-fold increased risk of developing AF in a 2-year period. On the other side, the strong association between AF and congestive heart failure is further attested by the high prevalence of AF found in major heart failure trials dealing with patients in more advanced NYHA functional classes [3].

In clinical practice the relationship between AF and heart failure, or left ventricular dysfunction, is intriguing. AF may indeed cause congestive heart failure, particularly when there is a fast uncontrolled ventricular response. This form of heart failure may be reversible after rhythm or rate control [5]. At first observation of a patient it may be quite difficult to distinguish this condition from the most common phenomenon of AF facilitated by the mechanical, electrophysiological, and neurohormonal derangements caused by heart failure in a substrate characterized by primary ventricular dilation and hypokinesia.

Hemodynamic Effects of Atrial Fibrillation

The hemodynamic consequences of AF are related to loss of atrial contribution to cardiac output, to increase in heart rate with shortening of the duration of diastole, and to irregularity of diastolic intervals. The loss of atrial contribu-

Institute of Cardiology, University of Bologna, Italy

tion to ventricular filling may be well tolerated in a healthy heart but may have adverse consequences in the presence of left ventricular dysfunction. Loss of atrial transport is particularly significant if there is impairment in left ventricular filling due to reduced diastolic compliance or to mitral stenosis. In such patients a high or a irregular heart rate with frequent short diastolic intervals will also be poorly tolerated.

In the long term a sustained uncontrolled tachycardia with heart rate higher than 120 beats/min gives rise to an impairment of left ventricular function to varying degrees which may result in significant worsening of the clinical condition unless the heart rate can be controlled or sinus rhythm restored. This clinical condition has been called "tachycardiomyopathy" or "tachycardia-induced cardiomyopathy" [5-10].

The knowledge that incessant or chronic tachyarrhythmias may lead to reversible ventricular dysfunction is the result of a series of clinical observations and, in the last 10 years, of focused interest which has led to clear experimental and clinical evidence. The first experimental model of tachycardia-induced cardiomyopathy was described by Whipple et al. in 1962 [11]. Experimental models allow study of both the effects of chronic rapid pacing on ventricular function and the recovery phase associated with discontinuance of rapid pacing, mimicking the development and treatment of tachycardia-induced cardiomyopathy in humans. The most commonly used animals are pigs and dogs who undergo atrial or ventricular pacing at chronic rates of 210 to 240 beats/min for durations of 3-6 weeks [10]. Chronic pacing tachycardia results in progressive severe biventricular systolic and diastolic dysfunction over a 3- to 4-week period. Pacing at a slower rate or for a shorter period results in a lesser degree of ventricular dysfunction.

The main hemodynamic changes observed in animal models are [9]: (1) markedly elevated ventricular filling pressures; (2) severe impairment of left ventricular (up to 55% reduction) and right ventricular systolic function; (3) severe reduction in cardiac output; (4) increase in left ventricular systolic wall stress; (5) reduction in intrinsic myocardial contractility; (6) impairment of intrinsic myocardial relaxation; (7) diminished cardiac sympathetic responsiveness; and (8) development of moderate mitral regurgitation.

In tachycardia-induced cardiomyopathy a series of cardiac structural changes occur [9]. Left ventricular dilation is more marked for end-systolic than for end-diastolic volumes and produces a spherical chamber geometry. This marked cardiac dilation is accompanied by right and left ventricular wall thinning or preservation of wall thickness without hypertrophy. A differential response between the ventricles has been demonstrated with evidence of pacing-induced right ventricular hypertrophy without associated left ventricular hypertrophy.

The development and recovery of hemodynamic impairment has a typical chronology of onset and recovery. After 24 h of rapid pacing, systemic arterial pressure and cardiac output are reduced. With longer pacing durations cardiac filling and pulmonary artery pressures increase and systemic arterial pressures decrease, with a plateau at 1 week. Cardiac output, ejection fraction, and cardiac volumes may progressively deteriorate for up to 3-5 weeks with development of end-stage heart failure [9]. The recovery from pacing-induced heart failure is the proof that the myopathic process associated with rapid heart rates is largely reversible. Within 48 h after termination of pacing, right atrial and mean arterial pressures, cardiac index, and systemic vascular resistance approach control levels [9, 12]. Left ventricular ejection fraction shows significant recovery by 24-48 h and normalizes after 1-2 weeks. Within 4 weeks, all hemodynamic variables return to control levels; yet end-systolic and end-diastolic volumes remain elevated at 12 weeks after termination of pacing, a finding indicating extensive ventricular remodeling. Diastolic dysfunction remains measurable 4 weeks after pacing [13]. Interestingly, left ventricular hypertrophy develops in the 4 weeks after discontinuation of pacing, and may be related either to inability to respond to triggers for hypertrophy during pacing itself or to compensatory remodeling [9].

Tachycardia-Induced Cardiomyopathy in Humans

In clinical practice an important problem is the evaluation of patients with "chronic" AF with high ventricular rates and ventricular dysfunction: in several cases it remains unclear at first observation whether left ventricular dysfunction is the result of chronic high rates or merely represents aggravation of a coexisting cardiomyopathy. This "chicken-egg dilemma" [8] has important practical implications because all the therapeutic possibilities currently available, including radiofrequency ablation of the AV node, are indicated to control the ventricular rate in cases of tachycardia-induced cardiomyopathy. Proof that ventricular dysfunction is secondary to high ventricular rates may be obtained in the individual case only by treating the tachycardia [14]. However, complete reversion of a clinical picture of congestive heart failure has been reported [5] for patients with left ventricular dysfunction initially believed to have idiopathic dilated cardiomyopathy.

The diagnosis of tachycardiomyopathy remains a difficult issue in clinical practice. It may be suspected on the basis of the coexistence of chronic AF and left ventricular dysfunction with improvement in cardiac performance following rate control or rhythm control. The degree of regression of ventricular dysfunction with rate control depends on several factors; it may be total, partial, or absent. An even more intriguing issue is the possibility that a tachycardiomyopathy component may exist in patients with heart failure dependent on a specific substrate but associated with AF with fast ventricular response. In these cases a vicious circle may develop, with heart failure facilitating AF with subsequent worsening of cardiac function by a rate-related mechanism. This condition facilitates arrhythmia persistence and atrial dilation.

Tachycardia-induced cardiomyopathy is now a well recognized clinical entity which stresses the complex interplay between AF and congestive heart failure. However, characterization of patients with pure reversible tachycardia-induced cardiomyopathy and their differentiation from other patients with dilated cardiomyopathy is really difficult "a priori" and constitutes the so-called "chicken-and-egg dilemma." Until more precise clinical data are available from prospective controlled evaluations, rate or rhythm control should be pursued in all patients with a clinical picture of unexplained and previously unrecognized ventricular dysfunction coupled with AF at a relatively fast ventricular response. All the pharmacological and nonpharmacological treatments currently available can be considered for this purpose.

References

1. Kannel WB, Abbott RD, Savage DD, McNamara PM (1982) Epidemiologic features of chronic atrial fibrillation. The Framingham Study. N Engl J Med 306:1018-1022
2. Krahn AD, Manfreda J, Tate RB, Mathewson FA, Cuddy TE (1995) The natural history of atrial fibrillation: incidence, risk factors, and prognosis in the Manitoba Follow-Up Study. Am J Med 98:476-484
3. Khand AU, Rankin AC, Kaye GC, Cleland JG (2000) Systematic review of the management of atrial fibrillation in patients with heart failure. Eur Heart J 21:614-632
4. Middlekauff HR, Stevenson WG, Stevenson LW (1991) Prognostic significance of atrial fibrillation in advanced heart failure. A study of 390 patients. Circulation 84:40-48
5. Grogan M, Smith HC, Gersh BJ, Wood DL (1992) Left ventricular dysfunction due to atrial fibrillation in patients initially believed to have idiopathic dilated cardiomyopathy. Am J Cardiol 69:1570-1573
6. Peters KG, Kienzle MG (1988) Severe cardiomyopathy due to chronic rapidly conduced atrial fibrillation: complete recovery after restoration of sinus rhythm. Am J Med 85:242-244
7. Packer DL, Bardy GH, Worley SJ, Smith MS, Cobb FR, Coleman RE, Gallagher JJ, German LD (1986) Tachycardia-induced cardiomyopathy: a reversible form of left ventricular dysfunction. Am J Cardiol 57:563-570
8. Gallagher JJ (1985) Tachycardia and cardiomyopathy: the chicken-egg dilemma revisited. J Am Coll Cardiol 6:1172-1173
9. Shinbane JS, Wood MA, Jensen DN, Ellanbogen KA, Fitzpatrick AP, Scheinman MM (1997) Tachycardia-induced cardimyopathy: a review of animal models and clinical studies. J Am Coll Cardiol 29:709-715
10. Iannini JP, Spinale FG (1996) The identification of contributory mechanisms for the development and progression of congestive heart failure in animal models. J Heart Lung Transplant 15:1138-1150
11. Whipple GH, Sheffield LT, Woodman EG (1962) Reversible congestive heart failure due to chronic rapid stimulation of the normal heart. Proc N Engl Cardiovasc Soc 20:39-40
12. Schumacher B, Luderitz B (1998) Rate issue in atrial fibrillation. Consequences of tachycardia and therapy for rate control. Am J Cardiol 82(8A):29N-36N
13. Tomita M, Spinale FG, Crawford FA, Zile MR (1991) Changes in left ventricular volume, mass, and function during the development and regression of supraventricular tachycardia-induced cardiomyopathy. Disparity between recovery of systolic versus diastolic function. Circulation 83:635-644
14. Ueng KC, Tsai TP, Tsai CK, Wu DJ, Lin CS, Lee SH, Chen SA (2001) Acute and long term effects of atrioventricular junction ablation and VVIR pacemaker in symptomatic patients with chronic lone atrial fibrillation and normal ventricular response. J Cardiovasc Electrophysiol 12:303-309

Physiopathology of Sudden Cardiac Death

S. Nodari, M. Metra, N. Pezzali, C. Giovannelli, G. Milesi, L. Dei Cas

Epidemiology and Etiology

Sudden cardiac death (SCD) is unexpected natural death due to cardiac causes, with abrupt loss of consciousness within 1 h of the onset of acute symptoms, with or without pre-existing heart disease. It is very hard to assess the exact incidence of SCD because of variability in the definition of the concept of "sudden" [1, 2]. We are not discussing death occurring 1 h after syncope in a healthy subject, but the definition is not completely clear in a cardiopathic patient with ventricular fibrillation as the end-stage event in a worsened clinical status.

Estimates for the United States show a mean incidence of 300 000 case of SCD per year, 0.1%-0.2% of the whole population. In Italy there are almost 50 000 events per year (about 1/1000 subjects per year) [2]. These estimates are related to the whole population, thus including both SCD as a primary cardiac event and that occurring in high-risk patients. Thus it is important to analyze the problem in depth with a view to the therapeutic options: with an incidence of SCD in the whole population of 1/1000 each year, we cannot treat 999 healthy subjects without risk for SCD to save one person from a probable event [2, 3]. Myerburgh et al. analyzed the incidence of SCD in different subgroups of patients with cardiac diseases: in the population as a whole the number of events per year is high, but the percentage is very low, so it is difficult to identify subjects at high risk [4, 5]. If we consider different subgroups, the percentage progressively increases, being 35% in patients after acute myocardial infarction (AMI) and in subjects with a history of malignant ventricular tachyarrhythmias (Fig. 1) [4]. In a Framingham study review, coronary artery disease risk factors are statistically related to SCD incidence: the percentile of patients with more risk factors shows an incidence 60 times higher than the one in the percentile with only one risk factor [7] (Fig. 2). This is much more

Cattedra di Cardiologia, Università degli Studi di Brescia, Brescia, Italy

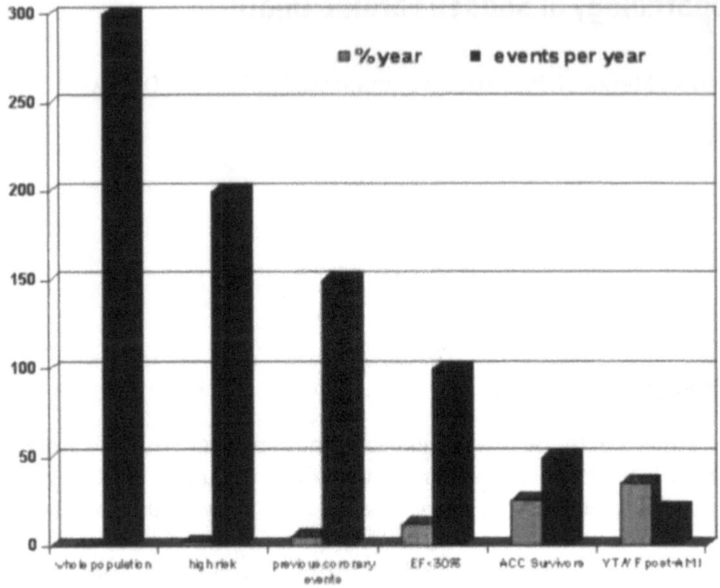

Fig. 1. Incidence of sudden cardiac death in the whole population and in different subgroups

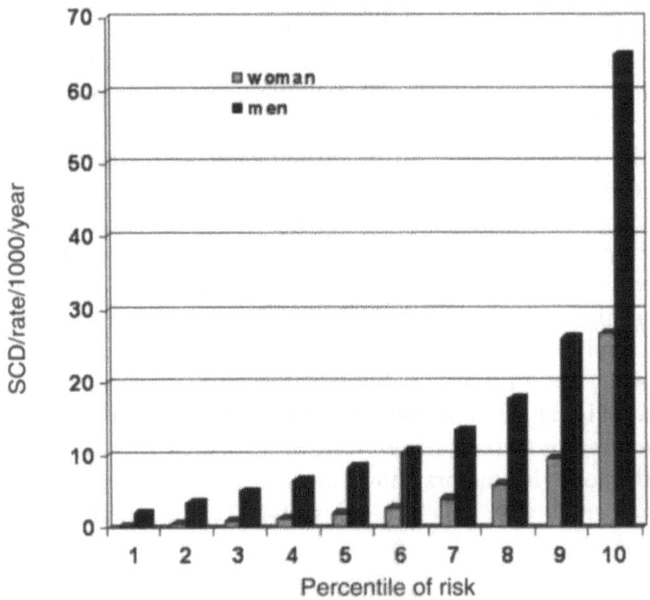

Fig. 2. Relation of sudden cardiac death incidence with multivariate risk percentile: Framingham study (26-years follow-up)

evident if we consider that coronary artery disease is the structural basis in 80% of SCDs and increases the importance of primary and secondary prevention of congestive heart disease.

Following the international guidelines for prevention of lethal and nonlethal ischemic events, the control of risk factors and pharmacological treatment are very important according to evidence-based medicine [8]. In the last 30 years pharmacological and nonpharmacological approaches have improved prognosis in post-AMI patients: β-blockers and cardiac defibrillation in intensive care units (ICU) significantly reduced the early mortality from 30%-35% to 15%-18%; thrombolysis and primary percutaneous transluminal coronary angioplasty additionally lowered mortality, which is now 6%-8%, in patients with an acute myocardial infarction [9]. Ventricular fibrillation, the most frequent early complication, is now almost totally controlled in protected areas (ICU), even though 40%-50% of patients with AMI suffer arrhythmic death before reaching hospital. However, malignant arrhythmias are still the most significant cause of late mortality, thus also underlining the importance of secondary prevention. Scandinavian trials on post-AMI patients showed that β-blocker therapy reduced total mortality by lowering the incidence of SCD. In chronic heart failure, which is associated with a high risk of arrhythmia, β-blockers such as carvedilol (US Carvedilol trial), bisoprolol (CIBIS II), and metoprolol (MERIT HF) also significantly improved the prognosis, reducing above all SCD.

New interventional strategies and pharmacological approaches have reduced early mortality but increased the incidence of late complications such as ischemic cardiomyopathy and heart failure so there is a change in the trend of post-AMI mortality, which is delayed, with a linear progression. Chronic ischemia and post-AMI heart failure are associated with ventricular hyperkinetic arrhythmias like ventricular sustained tachycardia, ventricular flutter, and torsades de pointes, often degenerating into ventricular fibrillation and cardiac arrest. It is well understood that the majority of SCDs in adults - about 80% - are caused by a known or unknown coronary artery disease, and that the mortality in patients with an AMI is about 50% in the so-called door-to-needle time. In 25% of cases SCD is the first event of acute ischemia, while more often it is a late complication of AMI or post-infarction cardiopathy, explaining 75% of deaths in patients with a previous myocardial infarction. Fibrosis and hypoperfusion in perinecrotic areas induced elecrophysiological changes, promoting reentrant arrhythmias and increasing automaticity [6, 10].

Among cardiac causes, coronary artery disease is the most frequent (80%-90%) in western societies: myocardial infarction, angina, chronic myocardial ischemia, and post-AMI cardiomyopathy are often complicated by fatal arrhythmic events. Among noncoronary cardiac causes (5%-10%), cardiomyopathies and congenital cardiopathies may be mentioned. Primary electrical disturbances such as long QT syndrome (LQTS), Brugada's syndrome, right ventricular arrhythmogenic dysplasia, and preexcitation syndrome are causes of SCD as well.

In patients with heart failure, too, sudden death is the final event in 50% of cases. Mortality is positively related to clinical severity (12% in NYHA class II, 24% in class III, and 36% in class IV), while SCD is the most frequent cause of mortality in NYHA class II (64%) and III (59%) patients [11-13].

Other causes of death are the absence of ventricular activation, primary and secondary conduction system alterations, and subsequent asystole (10%). Electromechanical uncoupling or acute heart failure may also be involved, whereby electrical activation is normal but ventricular systole is inefficient, as in pulmonary embolism, aortic dissection, cardiac tamponade, and extensive AMI.

Physiopathology

Arrhythmogenic mechanisms can be divided in two groups: abnormal impulse initiation and abnormal impulse conduction. The first group includes automaticity, both normal and abnormal; triggered activity, early afterdepolarizations, and delayed afterdepolarizations. The second group includes conduction block leading to ectopic pacemaker escape, unidirectional block, and reentry and reflection. Automaticity is the property of myocytes to undergo spontaneous diastolic depolarization and initiate an electrical impulse in the absence of external electrical stimulation. Spontaneous depolarization is the result of the development of a net inward ionic current during phase 4 of the action potential. "Normal automaticity" refers to situations in which spontaneous depolarization is the result of ionic currents, which are involved in impulse initiation during physiological conditions. Ionic currents, which are not normally involved in the initiation of spontaneous impulses, may become pacemaker currents as a result of experimental interventions or diseases, resulting in abnormal automaticity, which causes arrhythmias. Triggered activity describes impulse initiation in cardiac fibers that is dependent on afterdepolarizations. These are oscillations in membrane potential that follow the upstroke of an action potential. Early afterdepolarizations are a sudden change in the time course of repolarization of an action potential so that the membrane potential does not follow the trend of normal repolarization, but suddenly shifts in a depolarization direction. Recently interest has been growing in the effects of gene mutation on repolarizing membrane currents in relation to congenital LQTS, which are associated with polymorphic ventricular tachycardia. These tachycardias are possibly initiated by early afterdepolarizations and triggered activity, although reentry may also be involved. Gene mutations may be responsible for altered sodium (SCN5A) and potassium (HERG and KVLQT1) currents. The SCN5A mutation causes defective sodium channel inactivation, while HERG and KVLQT1 mutations result in decreased potassium currents. Both result in a net decrease in outward current that prolongs action potential duration and causes early afterdepolarizations.

Unidirectional conduction block initiates and maintains reentry. There is a core of inexcitable tissue around which the wave front propagates, and the maintenance of excitable tissue ahead of the propagating wave front is facilitated by slowing of conduction, shortening of the refractory period, or both.

Ventricular fibrillation is the most frequent cause of SCD and can be triggered by a single focus or by reentrant arrhythmias. Arrhythmogenic mechanisms depend on the underlying pathologies (scar tissue infarction, acute ischemia, ventricular hypertrophy, ventricular enlargement, etc.). Transient modulating factors, such as acute myocardial ischemia, adrenergic stimulation, and hypokalemia, play an important role as well, particularly in patients with severe left ventricular dysfunction.

In addition to plaque rupture, intracoronary thrombosis, piastrinemic emboli, coronary spasm-induced flow reduction, and postischemic reperfusion damage, changes in membrane ionic currents and adrenergic hyperstimulation are also very important arrhythmogenic mechanisms [10, 11, 14].

Adrenergic hyperactivation increases automatism and reentrant arrhythmias. Acute myocardial ischemia alters biochemical and biophysical myocyte features, thus changing transmembrane ionic currents and electrophysiological status. These can increase automatism- and reentrant-triggered arrhythmias; thus, prolonged acute ischemia may be associated with sustained ventricular tachycardia and ventricular fibrillation.

The most important electrophysiological effect during ischemia is a reduction of membrane potential and changes in ionic currents. Acute ischemia induces a shift from fast-Na^+ dependent into slow-Ca^{2+} dependent response fibers, with changes in local conductance promoting reentrant hyperkinetic arrhytmias. Sympathetic stimulation reduces the threshold of ventricular fibrillation onset. During AMI it increases the phase 4 action potential slope and triggers Ca^{2+} dependent fibers. AMI associated with infarction scar tissue enhances ventricular vulnerability. Sympathetic hyperactivity, like renin-angiotensin system (RAS) system activation, is characteristic in myocardial dysfunction. Chronic sympathetic hyperactivity enhances ventricular hyperkinetic arrhythmias, both through α- and β-receptor stimulation and by increased cellular remodeling and electrolytic changes. Sympathetic hyperactivity induces L-type Ca^{2++}-channel stimulation, with an increase in early and late afterdepolarizations and in triggered activity; K^+-channel stimulation, with faster repolarization and refractory time shortening; and Na^+-K^+-ATPase stimulation, with membrane hyperpolarization, which induces inhomogeneous conductance and repolarization, generating reentrant mechanisms. Ischemia/reperfusion-linked arrhythmogenic mechanisms, electrolytic disturbances, drug use (digitalis, diuretics, antiarrhythmic drugs) and sympathetic hyperactivity increase susceptibility towards arrhythmias.

Antiarrhythmogenic Effects of n3-Polyunsaturated Fatty Acids

β-Blockers prevent SCD by reducing myocardial oxygen consumption and counteracting ventricular remodeling and neuroendocrine activation.

β-Blocker and amiodarone therapy is fundamental in the guidelines for SCD prevention [15]. ACE-inhibitors and antialdosterone drugs are also important in preventing ventricular remodeling, interstitial myocardial fibrosis, and arrhythmias [16].

A new pharmacological option in the prevention of SCD is represented by n3-polyunsaturated fatty acids (n3-PUFA). These drugs act by opposing cellular remodeling, counteracting membrane structural changes and cellular electric instability. They also influence sympathovagal balance and have anti-ischemic characteristics [17-21] (Fig. 3). However, they cannot be considered antiarrhythmic drugs, as we do not yet know of any proarrhythmic effect like those of drugs acting on cellular action potential.

A possible explanation of the antiarrhythmogenic effects of n3-PUFA is sympathovagal balance modulation. These drugs increase heart rate variability in high-arrhythmic-risk patients (post-AMI patients with left ventricular dysfunction, patients with chronic renal failure undergoing dialysis, and patients with diabetes mellitus), and in healthy subjects this is associated with a higher n3-PUFA membrane concentration [22-25].

Many studies have shown a decrease in heart rate variability after an AMI, an expression of increased sympathetic influence on cardiac activity, associated with increased arrhythmic risk and mortality [26]. The antiarrhythmogenic

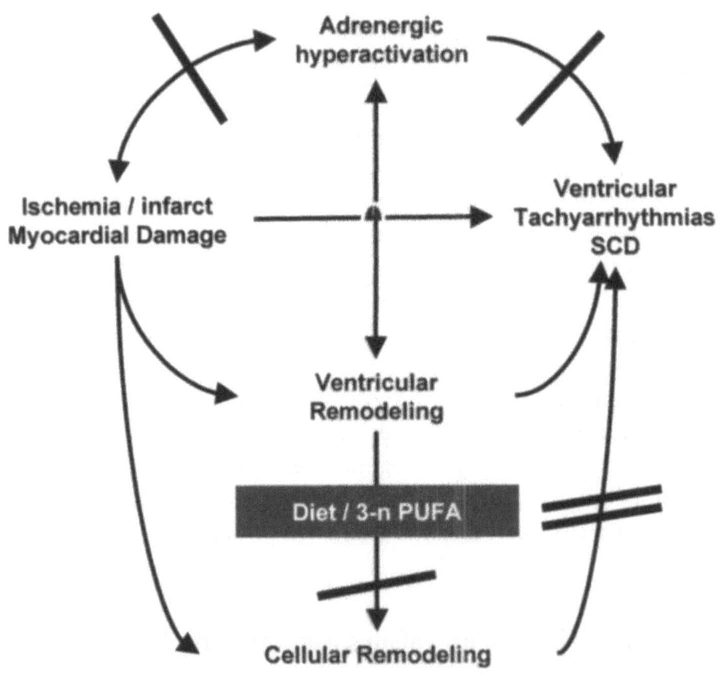

Fig. 3. Effects of n3-PUFA on arrhythmogenic mechanisms

effect of n3-PUFA has been demonstrated in isolated myocytes and animal experiments studies as well. It is caused by a changed concentration of phospholipids in cell membranes. A higher concentration of n3-PUFA (eicosapentenoic acid and docosohexaenoic acid) versus n6-PUFA (arachidonic acid) causes TXA3 and LTB5 production during ischemia. These eicosanoids have a less vasoconstrictive and inflammatory effect. There is a consequent reduction of infarct size and reduced superoxide radical production, which reduces electrical instability in peri-infarction areas [20, 21].

N3-PUFA also modulate membrane ionic channel conductance, by modulating the double-layer lipid fluid features. With regard to Na^+ ion channels, n3-PUFA increase the opening threshold so that the action potential can be triggered only by a higher than 40%-50% stimulation [27, 28]. Besides cell membrane hyperpolarization, n3-PUFA also induce the cardiac cycle refractory period to lengthen. With regard to CA^{2+} ion channels, n3-PUFA inhibit L-type voltage-dependent currents, thus reducing the high cytosol CA^{2+} concentration responsible for partial membrane depolarization, arrhythmogenic postpotentials, and arrhythmias [29]. In ischemic or dysfunctional myocardium there is a cytosol NA^+ overload, because of a sarcoplasmic reticulum Ca^{++}-ATPase (SERCA) dysfunction and lower ryanodine receptor sensibility towards cytosol CA^{2+} storage. The consequence is a reduction in CA^{2+} uptake in sarcoplasmic reticulum and a nonmodulated outflow of this ion from the reticulum itself. Increased NA^+ inflow in exchange for Ca^{2+} ions enhances arrhythmogenic triggers. Experimental studies on isolated ventricular myocytes showed an n3-PUFA inhibitory effect on L-type Ca^{2+} channel currents and on SERCA activity and microsome Ca^{2+}/Mg^{2+}-ATPase stimulation, with a reduction in cytosol Ca^{2+} concentration and fluctuations, partly explaining the antiarrhythmogenic effects of n3-PUFA. The possibility that these drugs may reduce the risk of SCD is based on evidence from a prospective cohort study, a case-control study, and prospective dietary intervention trials; however, additional studies are needed to confirm and further define the health benefits of n3-PUFA supplements for both primary and secondary prevention [30].

References

1. Stoupel E, Jottrand M (2001) Sudden cardiac death. Rev Med Brux 22: 488-498
2. Myerburg RJ, Castellanos A (2001) Cardiac arrest and sudden cardiac death. In: Braunwald E, Zipes DP, Libby P (ed) Heart disease: a textbook of cardiovascular medicine, 6th edn. Elsevier Science, New York
3. Myerburg RJ (2001) Sudden cardiac death: exploring the limits of our knowledge. J Cardiovasc Electrophisiol 12:369-381
4. Myerburg RJ, Interian A Jr, Mitrani RM, Kessler KM, Castellanos A (1997) Frequency of sudden cardiac death and profiles of risk. Am J Cardiol 80(5B):10F-19F
5. Myerburg RJ, Kessler KM, Castellanos A (1993) Sudden cardiac death: epidemiology, transient risk and intervention assessment. Ann Intern Med 119:1187-1197

6. Goldstein MR (2001) Sudden death due to cardiac arrhythmias. N Engl J Med 345:1473-1482
7. Kannel WB, Schatzkin A (1985) Sudden death: lessons from subsets in population studies. J Am Coll Cardiol 5(6 Suppl):141B-149B
8. Smith SC Jr, Blair SN, Bonow RO et al (2001) AHA/ACC Scientific Statement. AHA/ACC guidelines for preventing heart attack and death in patients with atherosclerotic cardiovascular disease: 2001 update: a statement for health care professionals from the American Heart Association and the American College of Cardiology. Circulation 104:1577-1579
9. Solomon SD, Antman E (1993) Prehospital thrombolytic therapy for myocardial infarction. N Engl J Med 329:383-389
10. Disertori M, Dallafior D, Marini M (2001) Arrhythmia risk stratification based on etiological and anatomo-structural factors. Ital Heart J 2(12 Suppl):1265-1269
11. Sweeney MO (2001) Sudden death in heart failure associated with reduced left ventricular function: substrates, mechanisms and evidence-based management. Part I. Pacing Clin Electrophysiol 24:871-888
12. Bigger JT Jr, Fleiss JL, Kleiger R, Miller JP, Rolnitzky LM (1984) The relationships among ventricular arrhyhtmias, left ventricular dysfunction and mortality in the 2 years after myocardial infarction. Circulation 69:250-258
13. Kjekshus J (1990) Arrhythmia and mortality in congestive heart failure. Am J Cardiol 65:42-I
14. Zipes DP, Wellens HJ (1998) Sudden cardiac death. Circulation 98:2334-2351
15. Anonymous (1997) Effect of prophylactic amiodarone on mortality after acute myocardial infarction and in congestive heart failure: meta-analysis of individual data from 6500 patients in randomized trials. Amiodarone Trials Meta-Analysis Investigators. Lancet 350:1417-1424
16. Domanski MJ, Exner DV, Borkowf CB, Geller NL, Rosenberg Y, Pfeffer MA (1999) Effect of angiotensin converting enzyme inhibition on sudden cardiac death in patients following acute myocardial infarction. A meta-analysis of randomized clinical trials. J Am Coll Cardiol 33:598-604
17. Kim D, Duff RA (1990) Regulation of K+ channels in cardiac myocytes by free fatty acids. Circ Res 67:1040-1046
18. Pound EM, Kang JX, Leaf A (2001) Partitioning of polyunsatured fatty acids, which prevent cardiac arrhythmias, into phospholipid cell membranes. J Lipid Res 42:346-351
19. Leaf A (2001) Electrophysiologic basis for the antiarrhythmic and anticonvulsant effects of omega 3 polyunsaturated fatty acids. World Rev Nutr Diet 88:72-78
20. De Caterina R, Madonna R (2002) Antiarrhythmic effects of omega-3 fatty acids. A review. Ital Heart J 3(3 Suppl):297-308
21. Lundmark K, Abelnoor M, Urdal P et al (1998) Use of fish oils appears to reduce infarct size as estimated from peak creatinekinase and loctate dehydrogenase activities. Cardiology 89:94-102
22. Christensen JH, Dyerberg J, Schmidt EB (1999) n-3 fatty acids and the risk of sudden cardiac death assessed by 24-hour heart rate variability. Lipids 34[Suppl]:S197
23. Christensen JH, Kroup E, Aaroe J, Toft E, Moller J, Rasmussen K, Dyerberg J, Schmidt EB (1997) Fish consumption, n-3 fatty acids in cell membranes, and heart rate variability in survivors of myocardial infarction with left ventricular dysfunction. Am J Cardiol 79:1670-1673
24. Christensen HJ, Skou HA, Fog L, Hansen V, Vesterlund T, Dyerberg J, Toft E, Schmidt EB (2001) Marine n-3 fatty acids, wine intake, and heart rate variability in patients

referred for coronary angiography. Circulation 103:651-657
25. Christensen JH, Skou HA, Madsen T, Torring I, Schmidt EB (2001) Heart rate variability and n-3 polyunsaturated fatty acids in patients with diabetes mellitus. J Intern Med 249:545-552
26. Barron HV, Viskin S (1998) Autonomic markers and prediction of cardiac death after myocardial infarction. Lancet 351:461-462
27. Xiao YF, Wright SN, Wang JK, Morgan JP, Leaf A (2000) Coexpression with beta(1) subunit modifies the kinetics and fatty acid block of hH1(alpha) Na+ channels. Am J Physiol Heart Circ Physiol 279:H35-46
28. Bendahhou S, Cummins TR, Agnew WS (1997) Mechanism of modulation of the voltage-gated skeletal and cardiac muscle sodium channels by fatty acids. Am J Physiol 272(2Pt 1):C592-600
29. Pepe S, Bogdanov K, Hallaq H, Spurgeon H, Leaf A, Lakatta E (1994) Omega 3 polyunsaturated fatty acids modulate dihydropiridine effects on L-type Ca2+ channels, cytosolic Ca2+ and contraction in adult rat cardiac myocytes. Proc Natl Acad Sci USA 91(19): 8832-8836
30. Kris-Etherton PM, Harris WS, Appel LJ (2002) Fish consumption, fish oil, omega-3 fatty acids, and cardiovascular disease. Circulation 106: 2747-2757

Drugs and Implantable Cardioverter Defibrillators in Patients with Atrial Fibrillation and Heart Failure

P. Dini, F. Laurenzi

Atrial fibrillation (AF) and heart failure (HF) are two pathological conditions that frequently coexist.

The prevalence of AF in patients with HF is 10%-30%, with an increasing incidence in patients with more severe left ventricular dysfunction [1-3]. It has been noted that HF predisposes patients to developing AF. In the Framingham Study the diagnosis of HF implied a 6.6-fold increased risk of developing AF in a 2-year period [4]. Conversely, the prevalence of left ventricular dysfunction or HF among patients with AF may be up to 40% [5].

In clinical practice the relationship between AF and HF may be reciprocal and intriguing. AF may cause congestive HF in patients without structural heart disease, particularly when there is a fast ventricular response (> 120 bpm) that is uncontrolled by drugs and persistent. On the other hand, previously asymptomatic patients with left ventricular dysfunction may develop congestive HF after the onset of persistent AF.

The two most common strategies in the management of AF are rate control plus anticoagulation and rhythm control with antiarrhythmic drugs. Both approaches are far from ideal in terms of safety, efficacy, and compliance [6], especially in patients with HF, so new therapeutic options (implantable pacemakers and defibrillators) are gaining an increasing role in selected groups of patients.

The first implantable atrial defibrillator, the Metrix Atrioverter (InControl) was developed to detect and promptly cardiovert persistent AF and was particularly indicated in symptomatic patients with structurally normal hearts [7]. It has been reported that the device was able to convert, either automatically or as activated by the patient, most episodes of AF, leading to a decrease in the frequency of long-lasting episodes [8-9]. The reported efficacy of the device was 90% of the episodes, with no instances of ventricular proarrhythmia.

Department of Cardiology, S. Camillo Hospital, Rome, Italy

Patients felt moderate discomfort from the shocks, but overall good satisfaction with the device was reported.

Nowadays the Atrioverter is no longer manufactured, but the initial concept progressed in patients with a class I indication to an implantable cardioverter-defibrillator (ICD) for ventricular tachyarrhythmias. In ICD candidates, most of whom are affected by organic heart disease with left ventricular dysfunction, AF represents a significant challenge. Approximately 25% had paroxysmal AF before implantation, and more than 50% will develop a first episode thereafter, with an annual rate of 2.6% [10-11]. It has been reported that AF may lead to inappropriate ventricular shocks, may precipitate HF or thromboembolic episodes, and is associated with increased mortality when ventricular function is depressed [1, 12]. Moreover, atrial tachyarrhythmias increase the cost of care.

Antiarrhythmic drugs represent the first-line therapy for the management of these patients with AF, but the insufficient long-term efficacy and the risk of ventricular proarrhythmia set a limit on pharmacological treatment. For this reason, previous experiences with the atrial implantable device were applied to patients in whom a dual-chamber defibrillator for life-threatening ventricular tachyarrhythmias was indicated, but who were also affected by episodes of symptomatic persistent AF .

A device (Jewel AF 7250; Medtronic Inc., Minneapolis, Minn., USA) was manufactured that combined the functions of a conventional dual-chamber ICD with algorithms for the detection, prevention, and treatment of atrial tachyarrhythmias [13]. The FDA approved the ICD for treatment of either drug-refractory AF or ventricular tachyarrhythmias.

The dual-chamber ICD uses pacing and shock therapies for prevention and/or termination of cardiac arrhythmias both in the atrium and in the ventricle. The device is able to discriminate atrial tachycardia (AT) from AF on the basis of two programmable detection zones, which may overlap. In the overlap zone the rhythm is classified as AT if it is regular and as AF if it is irregular. Two prevention algorithms (atrial rate stabilization and overdrive switchback delay) and four types of termination therapies (atrial burst ±, atrial ramp, atrial 50-Hz burst pacing, and atrial shock) are available. There is a programmable delay between AT/AF detection and the onset of therapy. Any of the possible therapies can be programmed to be skipped. The atrial burst plus two premature stimuli at the end of the burst and the autodecremental atrial ramp can be delivered at programmable percentage of the AT cycle length. The atrial 50 Hz is programmable both for AT and AF. The atrial shocks are delivered over a programmable pathway at programmable energies of 0.4-27 J, independently of ventricular shock programming. All atrial shocks are synchronized to the QRS and are withheld if the RR interval preceding the QRS is less than a programmable value, in order to avoid shock delivery during ventricular repolarization.

Worldwide clinical experience with this system has demonstrated good discrimination between atrial and ventricular sustained arrhythmias, resulting in cardioversion of 76% of rhythms identified as AF [14, 15]. The study demonstrated that antitachycardia pacing terminated 48% of AT/AF episodes. The efficacy was significantly greater for episodes classified as AT (59%) than for those classified as AF (30%). ATP therapy efficacy was a function of median PP interval and of a delay from the detection of AT/AF to the onset of pacing of less than 5 min.

The combined use of atrial pacing and shock therapies resulted in a reduction of atrial tachyarrhythmia burden from a mean of 58.5 h to 7.8 h per month [16].

There is debate about the role of an ICD in patients who only have AF. The subject has been evaluated in a prospective, nonrandomized trial that included patients with symptomatic episodes of paroxysmal (35%) or persistent (65%) AF and/or AT, refractory to or intolerant of one or more antiarrhythmic drugs, but without a history of sustained ventricular tachycardia of fibrillation [17]. One hundred forty-four patients were implanted with the Jewel AF device and followed for a mean of 12.6 months. Use of antiarrhythmic drugs was 63% at baseline and was stable over time. The overall antitachycardia pacing efficacy for episodes detected as AT was 48.7%, versus 22.7% for AF episodes. Cardioversion efficacy of the AT/AF was 86.7%. Early recurrence of AF within 1 min of a successful cardioversion was 20%. One year after the implant, 94% of the patients were in sinus rhythm, and 91% still had atrial therapies enabled. An indicator of the good patient acceptance of the device was that about half of the patients used the patient-initiated modality to deliver shock. It is of interest to note that after the implantation 11 patients (7.6%) had a first spontaneous episode of VT/VF that was appropriately detected and treated by the ICD. Most of these patients had coronary disease with an ejection fraction below 30%. All-cause survival was 98.6% at 12 months. Deaths were considered to be non-device related. Mortality and morbidity rates reflected similar results to those of other ICD trials and of AF patients in the Framingham Study.

Although the study [16] demonstrated the safety and the efficacy of an atrioventicular ICD used in combination with drugs to detect and treat AF in patients with no history of ventricular tachyarrhythmias, there is still some concern about extrapolating these results to a larger population of AF patients because it is well known that AF may originate from a variety of pathophysiological mechanisms with different natural histories and responses to treatment.

Future trials should aim to select, in patients with drug-refractory, symptomatic persistent or paroxysmal AF, the best nonpharmacological option, such as: ablate and pace, focal ablation including pulmonary vein isolation, and ICD. Nowadays the dual-chamber ICD appears a valid option in patients with a clinical indication for a conventional ventricular defibrillator and with previous documented episodes of symptomatic persistent AF. Antiarrhythmic drugs and anticoagulants remain the mainstay of AF management even in these patients and should be given in conjunction with the device in order to reduce the tachyarrhythmia burden and the thromboembolic risk. The worldwide

Jewell AF-only study suggests that if an atrial cardioverter-defibrillator is to be implanted in a patient with organic heart disease and left ventricular dysfunction, it is imperative that the device should be a dual-chamber ICD. Further studies should try to identify subjects at risk of highly symptomatic AF who are likely to benefit from an atrial defibrillator, such as patients with hypertrophic cardiomyopathy, in whom rapid conduction of AF may induce ventricular fibrillation [18]. Future trials should also aim to determine the cost-effectiveness of this strategy.

References

1. Dries DL, Exner DV, Gersh BJ, Domanski MJ, Waclawiw MA, Stevenson LW (1998) Atrial fibrillation is associated with an increased risk for mortality and heart failure progression in patients with asymptomatic and symptomatic left ventricular systolic dysfunction: a retrospective analysis of the SOLVD trials. Studies of left ventricular dysfunction. J Am Coll Cardiol 32:695–703
2. Feinberg WM, Blackshear JL, Laupacis A, Kronmal R, Hart RG (1995) Prevalence, age distribution, and gender of patients with atrial fibrillation. Analysis and implications. Arch Intern Med 155:469–473
3. Ryder KM, Benjamin EJ (1999) Epidemiology and significance of atrial fibrillation. Am J Cardiol 84:131R–138R
4. Kannel WB, Abbott RD, Savage DD, McNamara PM (1982) Epidemiologic features of chronic atrial fibrillation: the Framingham study. N Engl J Med 306:1018–1022
5. Middlekauff HR, Stevenson WG, Stevenson LW (1991) Prognostic significance of atrial fibrillation in advanced heart failure. A study of 390 patients. Circulation 84:40-48
6. Jung F, Di Marco JP (1998) Treatment strategies for atrial fibrillation. Am J Med 104:272-286
7. Wellens HJ, Lau CP, Luderitz B et al (1998) Atrioverter: an implantable device for treatment of atrial fibrillation. Circulation 98:1651-1656
8. Daoud EG, Timmermanns C, Fellows C et al (2000) Initial clinical experience with ambulatory use of an implantable atrial defibrillator for conversion of atrial fibrillation. Metrix investigators. Circulation 102:1407-1413
9. Timmermanns C, Levy S, Ayers G et al (2000) Spontaneous episodes of atrial fibrillation after implantation of the Metrix Atrioverter: observations on treated and non-treated episodes. Metrix investigators. J Am Coll Cardiol 35:1428-1433
10. Schmitt C, Montero M, Melichercik J (1998) Significance of supraventricular tachyarrhhythmias in patients with implanted pacing cardioverter defibrillators. Pacing Clin Electrophysiol 17:295-302
11. Best PJ, Hayes DL, Stanton MS (1999) The potential usage of dual chamber pacing in patients with implantable cardioverter defibrillators. Pacing Clin Electrophysiol 22:79-85
12. Grimm W, Flores B, Marchlinski FE (1995) Electrocardiographically documented unnecessary, spontaneous shocks in 241 patients with implantable cardioverter defibrillators. J Cardiovasc Electrophysiol 6:832-851
13. Swerdlow C, Schoels W, Dijkman B et al (2000) Detection of atrial fibrillation and flutter by a dual-chamber implantable cardioverter-defibrillator. Circulation 101:878-885

14. Schoels W, Swerdlow DC, Jung W et al (2001) Worldwide clinical experince with a new dual-chamber implantable cardioverter defibrillator. J Cardiovasc Electrophysiol 12:521-528
15. Adler SW II, Wolpert C, Warman EN et al (2001) Efficacy of pacing therapies for treating atrial tachyarrhythmias in patients with ventricular arrhythmias receiving a dual-chamber implantable cardioverter defibrillator. Circulation 104:887-892
16. Friedman PA, Dijkman B, Warman EN, et (2001) Atrial therapies reduce atrial arrhythmia burden in defibrillator patients.Circulation 104:1023-1028
17. Gold MR, Sulke N, Schwartzman DS et al (2001) Clinical experience with a dual-chamber implantable cardioverter defibrillator to treat atrial tachyarrhythmias. J Cardiovasc Electrophysiol 12:1247-1253
18. Lopez Gil M, Arribas F, Cosio FG (2000) Ventricular fibrillation induced by rapid atrial rates in patients with hypertrophic cardiomyopathy. Europace 2:327-332

New ICD Perspectives in the Congestive Heart Failure Patient

H.-J. Trappe

Introduction

Sudden cardiac death is one of the major causes of mortality in western countries, with an incidence of 500 000 sudden deaths per year in the United States and 400 000 sudden cardiac deaths per year in Europe [1, 2]. It has been shown that the risk of sudden cardiac death increases with the severity of left ventricular (LV) dysfunction [3-5]. Although treatment for congestive heart failure (CHF) has improved markedly during the last 20 years, the prognosis is still poor in patients with severe heart failure, with an annual mortality of 50% [6]. Different studies indicate that the implantable cardioverter-defibrillator (ICD) prevents sudden cardiac death in patients with life-threatening ventricular tachyarrhythmias and impaired LV [7-9]. However, the extent of the clinical benefits of long-term survival is unclear, and it is unknown whether patients with different degrees of heart failure will benefit from ICD implantation or not. To date, it is still debatable to implant ICDs in patients with a higher degree of heart failure, and there are no available data analyzing the role of ICD therapy in patients with mild, moderate, or severe heart failure over a period of more than 10 years. In addition to this, it has been shown in recent years that technical innovations have allowed sharp reductions in pulse generator volume and mass without sacrificing longevity or clinical effectiveness. ICDs with dual-chamber pacing, sensors for rate-adaptive pacing, and biventricular pacing possibilities have been introduced in clinical cardiology, allowing atrioventricular and biventricular synchrony with an improved cardiac output. Several studies have pointed out the beneficial effect of cardiac resynchronization therapy in these patients.

Study Patients

Four hundred and ten patients (368 male, 42 female), mean age 57±11 years

Department of Cardiology and Angiology, University of Bochum, Germany (range 10-78 years), were consecutively included in this study. Coronary artery disease was present in 279 patients (68%), congestive cardiomyopathy in 76 (19%), left and/or right ventricular dysplasia in 22 (5%), and the remaining 33 patients (8%) had another underlying disease (congenital heart disease, valvular heart disease, idiopathic ventricular tachycardia/fibrillation). Symptomatic drug-refractory sustained (duration ≥ 30 s) ventricular tachycardia and/or ventricular fibrillation were present in 393 patients (96%), whereas 17 patients (4%) underwent prophylactic ICD implantation according to the MADIT or the CAT study protocol [10, 11]. Antiarrhythmic drug therapy had failed to suppress life-threatening ventricular tachyarrhythmias in all patients, with a mean of 3.3±2.7 antiarrhythmic drug trials per patient (range 1-14 drugs per patient) before ICD implantation. The degree of heart failure was assessed according to New York Heart Association (NYHA) functional class and by angiographically proven LV ejection fraction. Fifty patients (12%) were in NYHA class I-II, 151 patients (37%) in NYHA class II, 117 patients (29%) in NYHA class II-III, and the remaining 92 patients (22%) in NYHA class III. No patient underwent ICD implantation in NYHA class IV. The mean LV ejection fraction was 42±15% (range 15%-73%). The clinical characteristics of the patients are listed in Table 1.

Table 1. Clinical characteristics of 410 patients

	NYHA class			
	I-II	I	II-III	III
No. of patients	50	151	117	92
Mean ± SD Age (years)	48±15	49±10	57±10	59±11
Range	10-71	15-78	23-78	31-77
Males	43 (86%)	139 (92%)	108 (92%)	78 (85%)
Mean ± SD Follow-up (months)	26±28	24±23	25±23	26±21
Range	<1-95	<1-98	<1-114	<1-89
Underlying disease				
Coronary artery disease	16 (33%)	114 (75%)	86 (74%)	63 (68%)
Congestive cardiomyopathy	9 (17%)	25 (17%)	21 (18%)	21 (23%)
Left and/or right ventricular dysplasia	10 (20%)	5 (3%)	3 (3%)	4 (4%)
Other	15 (30%)	7 (5%)	7 (6%)	4 (4%)
Ejection Fraction				
Mean ejection fraction	47±17%	37±11%	29±12%	30±12%
Arrhythmia History				
No arrhythmia*	5 (10%)	8 (5%)	2 (2%)	2 (2%)
VT	14 (30%)	53 (35%)	39 (33%)	25 (27%)
VF	22 (43%)	44 (29%)	35 (30%)	28 (30%)
VT±VF	9 (15%)	46 (30%)	41 (35%)	37 (40%)

VT, ventricular tachycardia; VF, ventricular fibrillation

Device Implantation

After written informed consent, all patients were maintained under general anesthesia through out implantation of the ICD system. During the first 5 years (1984-1989), an epicardial defibrillation lead system was used and was implanted via a median sternotomy or left anterior thoracotomy [11]. Using this approach, the leads (two defibrillation patch electrodes, two myocardial screw-in pacing/sensing leads) were attached to the left and right ventricle. Since 1990, nonthoracotomy defibrillation lead systems have been used at our institution. The transvenous defibrillation lead electrode system (Endotak lead, CPI, St. Paul, Minn., USA; TVL lead system, St. Jude Medical., Sunnyvale, Calif., USA) is advanced via the subclavian or the cephalic vein into the right atrium and then to the right ventricle. The distal tip of the lead is lodged in the right ventricular apex. After evaluation of the defibrillation threshold (DFT) the leads are tunnelled to the abdominal pocket subcutaneously and attached to the pulse generator, which is placed submuscularly. The implantation procedure has been reported in detail recently [12-14].

Results

Perioperative Mortality

From January 1984 to May 1990, epicardial ICD implantation was performed in 209 patients (51%), and the remaining 201 patients (49%), from May 1990 onward, underwent nonthoracotomy lead implantation. Perioperative deaths (within 30 days after ICD implantation) occurred in 12 patients (3%). One patient (8%) was in NYHA class I-II, 4 patients (33%) were in NYHA class II, 5 patients (42%) in NYHA class II-III, and the remaining 2 patients (17%) were in NYHA class III. Six patients (50%) had an ejection fraction below 30% and six patients (50%) an ejection fraction of 30% or higher (p=ns). Perioperative deaths occurred significantly more frequently in patients with epicardial implantation (11 of 209 patients, 5%) than in those with nonthoracotomy ICDs (1 of 201 patients, <1%)($p<0.05$). The cause of perioperative death was CHF in 9 patients while 3 patients died from ventricular arrhythmias: 1 from recurrent ventricular fibrillation not treatable by the ICD or additional antiarrhythmic drugs, and 2 from electromechanical dissociation.

Long-Term Mortality

During a mean follow-up of 28±24 months (range <1 to 114 months), 90 patients (23%) died: 14 patients (4%) died suddenly (within 1 h after the beginning of symptoms), 9 patients (2%) died from sudden arrhythmic death, and 5 patients (1%) died suddenly but probably not from arrhythmic causes. Fifty-five patients (14%) died from cardiac causes (CHF, myocardial reinfarction) and 21 patients (5%) from noncardiac causes. We have been able to demonstrate that the incidence of sudden death was low in all groups. There was an excellent survival rate independent of the degree of LV dysfunction (Table 2). However, there was a higher cardiac death rate and a higher total mortality in patients in NYHA functional class II-III and class III than in patients in NYHA functional class I-II or class II. In addition, the survival rates with regard to cardiac or total mortality were clearly influenced by NYHA functional class. In addition, survival was significantly better in patients with

Table 2. Survival after ICD implantation in relation to the degree of heart failure

	NYHA class			
Survival	**I-II (%)**	**II (%)**	**II-III (%)**	**III (%)**
Sudden Death				
1-year	100	100	98	99
2-years	100	96	94	92
3-years	95	96	94	92
4-years	95	96	90	92
5-years	95	96	84	92
6-years	95	96	84	92
7-years	95	96	84	92
8-years	95	96	84	92
9-years	*	*	84	*
10-years	*	*	84	*
Cardiac Death				
1-year	98	97	94	95
2-years	98	96	91	86
3-years	98	89	86	79
4-years	98	89	81	70
5-years	98	84	81	57
6-years	98	84	72	57
7-years	98	84	60	28
8-years	98	42	48	28
9-years	*	*	48	*
10-years	*	*	24	*
Total Mortality				
1-year	93	95	84	89
2-years	89	90	77	72
3-years	85	81	70	67
4-years	85	81	64	57
5-years	85	71	59	46
6-years	85	71	53	40
7-years	85	71	44	20
8-years	85	36	18	20
9-years	*	*	18	*
10-years	*	*	18	*

*No patients with this follow-up

an ejection fraction (EF) of 30 or more compared to patients with an EF below 30%: we were able to demonstrate significant differences in total mortality ($p<0.001$), cardiac mortality ($p<0.001$), and incidence of sudden death ($p<0.05$).

Incidence of ICD Shocks

Over the follow-up period, 338 patients (82%) received ICD shocks, with a mean incidence of 21±43 shocks per patient (range 0-621 shocks per patient).We were able to demonstrate that patients in NYHA class II (125 of 151 patients, 83%), NYHA class II-III (98 of 117 patients, 84%), and NYHA class III (83 of 92 patients, 90%) received significantly more frequent ICD discharges than patients in NYHA class I-II (32 of 50 patients, 64%)($p<0.05$). However, we did not find significant differences in the incidence of ICD discharges between patients with coronary disease, dilated cardiomyopathy, or another disease. Similar results were observed in the mean number of shocks per patient: there was a significantly higher mean number of ICD shocks in patients with NYHA class II (18±32 shocks, range 0-233 shocks), NYHA class II-III (19±25 shocks, range 0-139 shocks) and NYHA class III disease (27±36 shocks, range 0-228 shocks) than in patients with NYHA class I-II disease (12±19 shocks, range 0-80 shocks)($p<0.05$). In addition, no significant differences were visible between patients with coronary disease, dilated cardiomyopathy, or another disease.

Survival After the First Shock

To study whether patients would survive ICD implantation and would therefore benefit from ICD therapy, the follow-up was evaluated *after* the first shock. The mean interval between the first shock and the end of our follow-up was 25±22 months (range <1 to 112 months). It was demonstrated that after the first shock the mean survival time was 27±24 months (range <1 to 106 months) in patients in NYHA class I-II , 25±19 months (range <1 to 91 months) in patients in NYHA class II, 25±25 months (range <1 to 112 months) in NYHA class II-III, and 25±21 months (range <1 to 83 months) in NYHA class III. There were no significant differences in mean survival times from first shock to the end of the follow-up between patients with mild (NYHA class I-II), moderate (NYHA class II-III), or severe left ventricular dysfunction (NYHA class III).

Additional Treatment

After ICD implantation, 153 patients (37%) received digitalis, 230 patients (56%) were treated with diuretics, and 11 patients (3%) received β-blocking agents during follow-up. Class I antiarrhythmic drugs (propafenone, mexiletine, flecainide) were given to 28 patients (7%), amiodarone therapy was performed in 47 patients (11%), and 173 patients (42%) were treated with sotalol; 217 patients (53%) received ACE inhibitors. There were significant differences in the incidence of digitalis and diuretic therapy between patients with mild, moderate, and severe heart failure ($p<0.05$). Patients in NYHA class III received ACE inhibitors more frequently than patients in NYHA class I-II, II, or II-III; however, these differences were not statistically significant. In addition, no significant differences were observed in antiarrhythmic drug therapy (class I, amiodarone, sotalol) between the different patient groups.

Discussion

There is little doubt about the efficacy of cardioverter-defibrillator therapy in terminating life-threatening ventricular tachyarrhythmias; however, the benefits of ICD therapy in patients with ventricular tachycardia and/or ventricular fibrillation and impaired LV function are still unclear [15, 16]. At the present time, only a few reports are available comparing the outcome after ICD therapy in relation to the functional class of heart failure or in relation to the degree of LV dysfunction during a relatively short follow-up period [17, 18]. In the present study we report on the outcome after ICD implantation with regard to functional class of heart failure and LV ejection fraction during a long-term follow-up of more than 10 years. There are two important aspects of ICD therapy in patients with impaired LV function: (1) to evaluate the potential benefit of ICD therapy for survival and (2) to see whether the ICD will serve as a "bridge" to heart transplantation in patients with end-stage ventricles who are awaiting a donor heart [19].

Risk of Sudden Death in Heart Failure

Previously published data on survival of patients with ventricular tachyarrhythmias treated with antiarrhythmic drugs or antitachycardia surgery suggest that LV function is an independent predictor of recurrence events and survival [20-22]. In patients with life-threatening ventricular tachyarrhythmias and severely impaired LV dysfunction 3-year arrhythmia recurrence rates have been reported to be approximately 50% [4]. In the V-Heft II trial the incidence of sudden death was reported to be as high as 30% during a follow-up of 66 months [23]. In comparison, patients with ICDs have an excellent outcome with very low sudden death rates [24, 25]. However, it is still unclear whether the ICD will prolong life, and it is unclear whether patients with moderate or severe heart failure will benefit from ICD therapy or not [26]. The discussion of such an approach has to address not only the benefit of ICD therapy on sudden death rate and survival but, of course, the risk and complication rate of ICD treatment, particularly in patients with poor LV function.

Survival After ICD Implantation in Patients with Impaired LV Function

That sudden death is one of the major problems in patients with LV dysfunction has been discussed in detail [18, 19, 22]. Cardioverter-defibrillator therapy is able to prevent sudden death both in patients with normal and in those with abnormal LV function [18]. In the present study we demonstrated 3-year, 5-year, and 7-year survival of 92%-96% in respect of arrhythmic mortality in NYHA class I, II and III, and 3-year survival of 94% and 5-year and 7-year survival of 84% in patients in NYHA class II-III. These results are in accordance with a 5-year survival of 96%-99% in respect to arrhythmic mortality in patients with a LV ejection fraction of 30% or lower [24, 27]. In contrast to the excellent results in the prevention of sudden death, the prognosis of ICD patients is clearly influenced by the underlying disease and the degree of LV dysfunction [7, 28]. Initial reports showed a survival rate (cardiac death) of 67%-87% at 2 years of follow-up [7]. Recent reports with a longer follow-up indicate a poorer prognosis in patients with an ICD and impaired LV function: Axtell et al. [27] reported a 5-year survival rate of 60% in respect of cardiac mortality while Mehta et al. [18] found 4-year survival rates of 85% in respect of cardiac mortality in patients with moderate LV dysfunction and 59% in patients with severe LV impairment. These data accord with the findings of the present study: our 4-year survival in respect of cardiac death was 81%-89% in patients with moderate (NYHA classes II, II-III) and 70% in patients with severe LV dysfunction (NYHA class III). Therefore, in addition to ICD implantation and to avoid cardiac death after ICD implantation, as the major cause of death, appropriate and aggresive treatment of heart failure is necessary [29, 30].

Incidence and Occurrence of Shocks

The incidence of appropriate ICD shocks over a 2- to 5-year follow-up period has been reported to be in the range of 33%-70% [31, 32]. In addition, the incidence of discharges was 45% in patients with an ejection fraction below 30% compared to 32% in those with an ejection fraction above 30% [31]. These observations were not confirmed by the study of Mehta et al. [18], in which ICD shocks occurred in 66% of patients with an ejection fraction above 30% and in 62% of patients with an ejection fraction of 30% or lower (p=ns). Schlepper et al. [24] found that 27 patients (31%) with an ejection fraction below 30% experienced at least one appropriate shock, compared to 48 patients (51%) with an ejection fraction of 30% or lower ($p<0.05$). In the present study, the incidence of shocks and the time from ICD implantation to first shock were studied in relation to the degree of LV dysfunction. We found that the incidence and the mean number of shocks were higher in patients with moderate or severe LV dysfunction, particularly in patients in NYHA class III, than in patients in NYHA class I-II. Similar observations were reported by Vester et al. [33]. An interesting observation is the time of the first shock after

ICD implantation: we were able to show that the period from device implantation to the first shock was shorter in patients with severe LV dysfunction (mean 16-19 months) than in patients with lesser degrees of heart failure (22 months). Similar observations have been made by Myerburg et al. [31] and Vester et al. [33].

ICDs with Biventricular Pacing Possibilities

It has been shown in several studies that the outcome of patients with ICDs is clearly related to LV dysfunction, with the worst prognosis in patients with severe CHF. The prognosis and quality of life of patients with CHF remain poor despite the use of ACE inhibitors or β-blocking agents, supporting the use of nonpharmacological therapies. It has been proposed by several authors that electrical stimulation may be useful in conjunction with pharmacological therapy to improve cardiac output and functional class. Although early studies reported benefits of right ventricular pacing on hemodynamic findings, subsequent studies did not reproduce these improvements with similar CHF patients. Consequently, the case of a patient in end-stage heart failure who improved dramatically after initiation of biventricular pacing introduced the concept of multisite pacing for patients with severe heart failure. Recently, it has been reported that patients with CHF with sufficiently wide surface QRS benefit from atrial-synchronous ventricular pacing; these authors state that LV stimulation is required for maximum acute benefit. There is no question that biventricular pacing is a very promising approach to the treatment of patients with severe heart failure [34]. However, at the present time only a few study results are available and the role of biventricular pacing in patients with ICDs is unclear [35]. Despite very promising first results in improving cardiac output and LV function, some technical problems are present: although we showed that implantation of biventricular ICD devices was possible without any problems, the implantation time was relatively long compared to a single-chamber ICD implantation [27]. For this reason, one of the most important steps to improve the implantation procedure is to develop guiding catheters for intubation of the coronary sinus with an acceptable "back-up" to introduce the Easytrack electrode more easily. In addition, at the present time the "ideal" site for LV pacing is undeteremined: Blanc et al. [36] studied different pacing sites in 23 patients with severe CHF and demonstrated that LV pacing alone and biventricular pacing resulted in similar hemodynamic improvements, whereas the hemodynamic effect of right ventricular pacing alone was low. Cazeau et al. [37] studied multiple pacing sites in eight patients and concluded that biventricular pacing was associated with rapid and sustained hemodynamic improvement. However, to the best of our knowledge no confirmed data are available as to the "ideal" site for left lateral free wall pacing, and no data are present to show the best part of the "coronary sinus tree" for definitive LV pacing. The outcome of patients with biventricular pacing modalities confirmed clinical results of improved LV function in patients with severe CHF [34-36].

However, these data are mainly observed during short term follow-up and, of course, are not representative of all patients with poor LV function [37]. Therefore, further studies with larger patient populations and longer follow-up periods are necessary to confirm or reject the preliminary excellent results of biventricular pacing in patients with severe CHF. In addition, further observations are necessary to study the mechanisms of biventricular pacing and to evaluate the role of "biventricular resynchronisation".

ICD Therapy in Patients with Poor LV Function Without Ventricular Arrhythmias

It is well known that patients with myocardial infarction and reduced LV function are at risk of CHF and sudden cardiac death [38]. Within the last few years, several studies have analyzed the role of ICD therapy to prevent sudden cardiac death in patients with ventricular tachyarrhythmias [39-41]. In the MADIT and the MUSTT study it has been pointed out that patients with coronary artery disease and reduced LV function are at high risk of sudden death; in addition, the prognostic value of invasive electrophysiological testing for the identification of patients who are at risk of ventricular tachyarrhythmias is uncertain. Recently, the MADIT II study was published and showed clearly that patients with a previous myocardial infarction and advanced LV dysfunction benefited from ICD therapy, although these patients had no spontaneous ventricular arrhythmias [42]. As compared with conventional medical therapy, defibrillator therapy was associated with a 31% reduction in the risk of death. In contrast with the earlier MADIT trial, in which the survival rate improved within the first few months after the implantation of the device, in the MADIT II study the survival benefit began approximately 9 months after the device was implanted.

Clinical Implications

In the United States, an estimated three to four million patients have coronary artery disease and advanced LV dysfunction. Approximately 400 000 new cases occur annually [43]. Since the incidence of sudden death in patients with poor LV function is high, even in patients receiving ACE inhibitors, the automatic cardioverter-defibrillator is a useful tool in the management of these patients. It has been shown in our study, and by others, that both patients with moderate and those with severe LV dysfunction benefit from ICD therapy and survive for long time after the first shock. On the other hand, it must be borne in mind that survival after ICD implant is clearly influenced by the degree of LV function. Additional aggressive treatment of heart failure is necessary to prevent cardiac death, and heart transplantation should be discussed as early as possible in selected patients.

Resynchronization therapy is an acceptable approach to improve LV function in selected patients. However, there are still other patients with coronary disease and poor LV function who are not suitable candidates for biventricular pacing. To improve survival in patients with a previously myocardial infarction and advanced LV dysfunction, prophylactic ICD implantation is recommended.

References

1. Cappucci A, Boriani G (1993) Drugs, surgery, cardioverter defibrillator: a decision based on the clinical problem. Pacing Clin Electrophysiol 16:519-526
2. Gillum RF (1989) Sudden coronary death in the United States. Circulation 79:756-765
3. Franciosa JA, Wilen M, Ziesche S et al (1983) Survival in men with severe chronic left ventricular failure due to either coronary heart disease or idiopathic dilated cardiomyopathy. Am J Cardiol 51:831-836
4. Swerdlow CD, Winkle RA, Mason JW (1983) Determinants of survival in patients with ventricular tachyarrhythmias. N Engl J Med 308:1436-1442
5. Bigger JT Jr, Fliess JL, Kleiger R et al (1984) The relationship among ventricular arrhythmias, left ventricular dysfunction and the mortality in the 2 years after myocardial infarction. Circulation 69:250-258
6. Massie BM, Conway M (1987) Survival of patients with congestive heart failure: past, present, and future prospects. Circulation 75:11-19
7. Fogoros RN, Elson JJ, Bonnet CA et al (1990) Efficacy of the automatic implantable cardioverter-defibrillator in prolonging survival in patients with severe underlying heart disease. J Am Coll Cardiol 16:381-386
8. Tchou PJ, Kadri N, Anderson J et al (1988) Automatic implantable cardioverter defibrillators and survival in patients with ventricular dysfunction and malignant ventricular arrhythmias. Ann Intern Med 109:529-534
9. Axtell K, Tchou PJ, Akhtar M (1991) Survival in patients with depressed left ventricular function treated with implantable defibrillator. Pacing Clin Electrophysiol 14:291-296
10. Moss AJ (1992) Prospective antiarrhythmic studies assessing prophylactic pharmacological and device therapy in high risk coronary patients. Pacing Clin Electrophysiol 15:694-696
11. The Cardiomyopathy Trial Investigators (1993). Cardiomyopathy trial. Pacing Clin Electrophysiol 16:576-581
12. Trappe HJ, Pfitzner P, Fieguth HG, Wenzlaff P, Kielblock B, Klein H (1997) Nonpharmacological therapy of ventricular tachyarrhythmias: observations in 554 patients. Pacing Clin Electrophysiol 17:2172-2177
13. Trappe HJ, Klein H (1994) Clinical results with implantable cardioverter-defibrillator therapy. In: Singer I (ed) Implantable cardioverter defibrillator. Futura, Mount Kisco, NY, pp 487-505
14. Trappe HJ, Klein H, Kielblock B (1994) Role of antitachycardia pacing in patients with third generation cardioverter defibrillators. Pacing Clin Electrophysiol 17:506-513
15. The Cardiac Arrhythmia Suppression Trial Investigators (1989) Preliminary report: effect of encainide and flecainide on mortality in randomized trial of arrhythmia suppression and myocardial infarction. N Engl J Med 321:406-412
16. Furman S (1989) AICD benefit (editorial). Pacing Clin Electrophysiol 12:399-400
17. Akhtar M, Jazayeri M, Sra J et al (1993) Implantable cardioverter defibrillator for prevention of sudden cardiac death in patients with ventricular tachycardia and ventricular fibrillation. Pacing Clin Electrophysiol 16:511-518

18. Mehta D, Saksena S, Krol RB, John T, Saxena A, Raju R, Kaushik R, Karanam R (1993) Device use patterns and clinical outcome of implantable cardioverter defibrillator patients with moderate and severe impairment of left ventricular function. Pacing Clin Electrophysiol 16:179-185
19. Trappe HJ, Wenzlaff P (1995) Cardioverter defibrillator therapy as a bridge to heart transplantation. Pacing Clin Electrophysiol 18:622-631
20. Wilber DJ, Garan H, Finkelstein D et al (1988) Out-of-hospital cardiac arrest: use of electrophysiologic testing in the prediction of long-term outcome. N Engl J Med 318:19-24
21. Lawrie GM, Pacifico A, Kaushik R et al (1991) Factors predictive of results of direct ablative operations for drug-refractory ventricular tachycardia: analysis of 80 patients. J Thorac Cardiovasc Surg 73:1239-1247
22. Stevenson WG, Stevenson LW, Middlekauf HR et al (1993) Sudden death prevention in patients with advanced ventricular dysfunction. Circulation 88:2953-2961
23. Cohn J, Johnson G, Ziesche S et al (1991) A comparison of enalapril with hydralazine-isosorbide dinitrate in treatment of chronic congestive heart failure: V-Heft II. N Engl J Med 325:303-310
24. Schlepper M, Neuzner J, Pitschner HF (1995) Implantable cardioverter defibrillator: effect on survival. Pacing Clin Electrophysiol 18:569-578
25. Nisam S, Kaye A, Mower MM, Hull M (1995) AICD automatic cardioverter defibrillator clinical update: 14 years experience in over 34,000 patients. Pacing Clin Electrophysiol 18:142-147
26. Böcker D, Block M, Isbruch F, Wietholt D, Hammel D, Borggrefe M, Breithardt G (1993) Do patients with implantable defibrillators live longer? J Am Coll Cardiol 21:1638-1644
27. Axtell K, Tchou PJ, Akhtar M (1991) Survival in patients with depressed left ventricular function treated with implantable defibrillator. Pacing Clin Electrophysiol 14:291-296
28. Trappe HJ, Fieguth HG, Klein H, Wenzlaff P, Weber-Conrad O, Schöhl W, Kielblock B, Lichtlen PR (1993) Role of the underlying etiology in patients with an implantable cardioverter defibrillator. Med Klinik 88:362-370
29. Swerdberg K, Idanpaan-Heikkila U, Remes J et al (1987) Effects of enalapril on mortality in severe congestive heart failure. Results of the Cooperative North Scandinavian Enalapril Survival Study (CONSENSUS). N Engl J Med 316:1429-1435
30. Ball SG, Hall AS, Mackintosh AT et al (1993) Effect of ramipril and morbidity of survivors of acute myocardial infarction with clinical evidence of heart failure. Lancet 342:821-828
31. Myerburg RJ, Luceri RM, Thurer R et al (1989) Time to first shock and clinical outcome in patients receiving an automatic implantable cardioverter-defibrillator. J Am Coll Cardiol 14:508-514
32. Kim SG, Fisher JD, Choue CW et al (1992) Influence of left ventricular function on outcome of patients treated with implantable defibrillators. Circulation 85:1304-1310
33. Vester EG, Kuhls S, Altenvoerde G et al (1994) Ten-years follow-up after automatic cardioverter/defibrillator-implantation: determining factors of survival and shock incidence (abstract) Eur J Cardiol 15:187
34. Stellbrink C, Auricchio A, Diem B, Breithardt OA, Kloss M, Schöndube FA, Klein H, Messmer B, Hanrath P (1999) Potential benefit of biventricular pacing in patients with congestive heart failure and ventricular tachyarrhythmia. Am J Cardiol 83:143D-150D

35. Auricchio A, Stellbrink C, Sack S, Block M, Vogt J, Bakker P, Mortensen P, Klein H, for the PATH-CHF Study Group (1999) The Pacing Therapies for Congestive Heart Failure (PATH-CHF) study: rationale, design, and endpoints of a prospective randomized multicenter study. Am J Cardiol 83:130D-135D
36. Blanc JJ, Etienne Y, Gilard M, Mansourati J, Munier S, Boschat J, Benditt DG, Lurie KG (1997) Evaluation of different ventricular pacing sites in patients with severe heart failure. Results of an acute hemodynamic study. Circulation 96:3273-3277
37. Cazeau S, Ritter P, Lazarus A, Gras D, Backdach H, Mundler O, Mugica J (1996) Multisite pacing for end-stage heart failure: early experience. Pacing Clin Electrophysiol 19:1748-1757
38. Myerburg RJ (2001) Sudden cardiac death: exploring the limits of our knowledge. J Cardiovasc Electrophysiol 12:369-381
39. Moss AJ, Hall WJ, Cannom DS et al (1996) Improved survival with an implanted defibrillator in patients with coronary disease at high risk for ventricular arrhythmia. N Engl J Med 335:1933-1940
40. Trappe HJ (2001) ICD-Therapie. In: Hombach V (ed) Interventionelle Kardiologie, Angiologie und Koronarvaskularchirurgie. Schattauer, Stuttgart, pp 550-563
41. Buxton AE, Lee KL, Fisher JD, Josephson ME, Prystowsky EN, Hefley G (1999) A randomized study of the prevention of sudden death in patients with coronary artery disease. N Engl J Med 341:1882-1890
42. Moss AJ, Zareba W, Hall WJ et al (2002) Prophylactic implantation of a defibrillator in patients with myocardial infarction and reduced ejection fraction. N Engl J Med 346:877-883
43. Cohn JN, Bristow MR, Chien KR et al (1997) Report of the National Heart, Lung, and Blood Institute Special Emphasis Panel on Heart Failure Research. Circulation 95:766-770

Type of Therapy and Quality of Life in Atrial Fibrillation

B. LÜDERITZ

Introduction

Atrial fibrillation (AF) is a frequent and costly health care problem. In patients with AF, the restoration and maintenance of sinus rhythm is the primary therapeutic goal. The most frequent strategy for maintaining sinus rhythm after its restoration is the use of antiarrhythmic drugs. The efficacy of therapy in AF has been predominantly measured using objective criteria such as mortality and morbidity. In recent years, the importance of quality of life as an outcome measure has been recognized. However, few studies in the literature have examined quality of life in patients with AF using properly validated tools. In addition, the specific impact of antiarrhythmic treatment on quality of life in patients with AF has not been assessed. These issues are now being addressed in several ongoing studies. This article attempts to define quality of life, makes recommendations on how quality of life might be assessed, and reviews our current knowledge regarding quality of life in patients with AF.

AF is the most frequently experienced cardiac arrhythmia, affecting an estimated 2.2 million people in the United States and approximately 6 million in Europe. Approximately 1.2 million patients suffer from paroxysmal AF, and about 0.6 million from persistent AF. A transition from paroxysmal AF to persistent AF of 30% of patients is anticipated [1]. The prevalence of AF increases with age [2], ranging from less than 1% at 50-59 years to nearly 9% at 80-89 years [3]. In addition to palpitations, patients with AF are at an increased risk of stroke and can develop reduced exercise tolerance and left ventricular dysfunction [4]. All of these problems may be reversed with restoration and maintenance of sinus rhythm. Thus, treatment of AF is warranted in the hope of eliminating symptoms, preventing complications, and possibly reducing the excess mortality associated with this arrhythmia [5]. The primary intervention for maintaining sinus rhythm after restoration is the use of antiarrhythmic

Department of Cardiology, Faculty of Medicine, University of Bonn, Germany

drugs. However, many of the existing drugs have only limited efficacy and are associated with considerable unexpected adverse effects. Current treatment is therefore suboptimal [6].

Therapeutic Goals

As already mentioned, in patients with AF the restoration and maintenance of sinus rhythm is the primary therapeutic goal. Once sinus rhythm is maintained, physiological rate control is restored and left ventricular ejection fraction, cardiac output, and exercise capacity are increased. If sinus rhythm is reestablished, quality of life as defined by the New York Heart Association is usually increased (Fig. 1). This improved cardiovascular performance thus enhances the patient's ability to perform the functions of normal daily life. Effective treatment of AF is based on these objective criteria, but subjective criteria such as quality of life are important. To address the quality-of-life issues, rigorous, yet practical approaches are needed to allow a comprehensive understanding of quality of life in patients with AF [7]. Different instruments can be used to measure various parameters reflecting quality of life. The most important items to be considered for endpoints and outcome events for the assessment of therapy for AF as agreed by the European Society of Cardiology Atrial Fibrillation Endpoints Working Group in June 2000 are depicted in Table 1 [8-12].

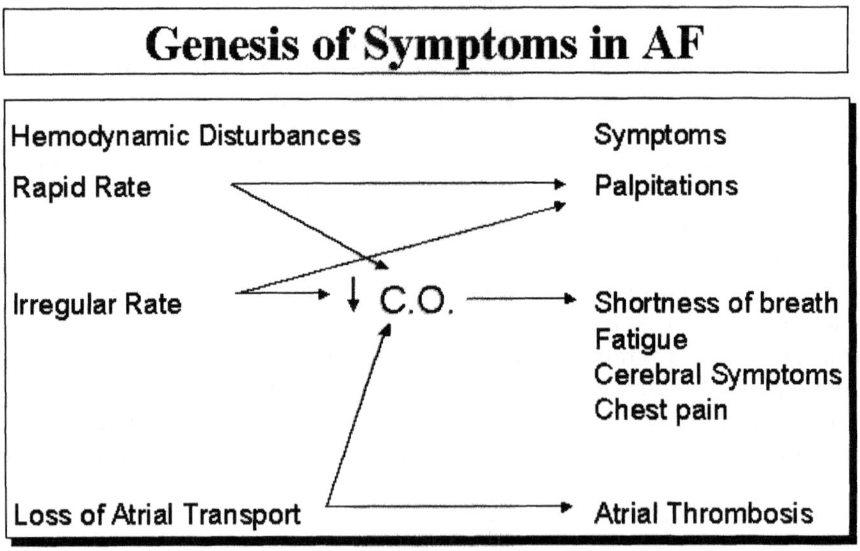

Fig. 1. Genesis of symptoms in AF: relationship of symptoms to hemodynamic change. CO, cardiac output

Table 1. Meaningful endpoints for quality of life evaluation in AF patients

Frequency of episodes Duration of episodes Hospitalizations Frequency of symptoms Type of AF: "paroxysmal, persistent, permanent" vs "initial, recurrent, established" AF and NYHA classification General life satisfaction (general health and well being) Cardiac symptom frequency/cardiac symptom severity (symptom burden) SF-36 category Mental health/social functioning (emotional/social functioning) Physical role, vitality (physical functioning) Somatization	Gender men/women (SF-36) Outcome scores (follow-up) Silent AF vs symptomatic AF Age <50 years vs age >50 years Comparison to other settings (post myocardial infarction, implantable cardioverter/defibrillator, congestive heart failure) Therapeutic interventions: radiofrequency catheter and atrioventricular node ablation Medical therapy vs ablation AV junction ablation Cardiac output-change (rest, exercise) after cardioversion Effects of Maze operation New technology for therapy (new leads, new algorithms, ATP, stabilization features)

Quality of Life in Patients with Silent Atrial Fibrillation

In a very recent trial, quality of life in patients with silent AF was studied. Patients with AF had substantially impaired quality of life compared with healthy subjects [13]. Although the conventional "objective" measures of illness severity were similar in patients with silent AF (group 1) and symptomatic AF patients (group 2), the latter reported significantly lower scores on all SF-36 scales ($p < 0.005$). Symptomatic AF patients had a significantly increased illness intrusiveness compared with asymptomatic patients ($p < 0.001$). Total functional capacity and global life satisfaction were significantly lower in symptomatic patients than in asymptomatic patients ($p < 0.005$).

Although most SF-36 scale scores did not differ much between normal subjects and asymptomatic AF patients, and total functional capacity was similar in both groups, the perception of general health was significantly poorer in the latter ($p < 0.003$). Global life satisfaction was significantly decreased in asymptomatic patients compared with normal subjects ($p < 0.003$) [13].

Rhythm Control or Rate Control and Anticoagulation

The clinical categorization concerning quality of life of patients who present with AF is a major determinant of the most appropriate strategy for rhythm management. For patients with recurrent AF that has not become permanent, the two available strategies are rhythm control and anticoagulation or rate control and anticoagulation. There is no clear evidence that either of these strategies is superior to the other [14]. Our knowledge of the efficacy and safety of various therapeutic strategies is insufficient, especially with respect to the direct comparison of re establishment of sinus rhythm by drugs versus rate control [14].

Ventricular Rate Control by AV Junction Ablation

Hemodynamic effects of complete atrioventricular (AV) junction ablation with subsequent regular ventricular pacing are exclusively consequences of rate control and regularization of ventricular contraction rather than consequences of atrial contractile function and AV synchrony. Several studies have been published that underline the beneficial effects of complete AV junction ablation in patients with AF, fast ventricular response, and depressed left ventricular function (Table 2) [9, 15-21].

Table 2. Impact of complete AV junction ablation and pacemaker implantation on left ventricular hemodynamics, exercise capacity, and quality of life

Author	No. of patients	Hemo-dynamics	Exercise capacity	Quality of life
Heinz et al [15]	10 (10/0)	±	0	-
Twidale et al [16]	14 (7/7)	±	±	-
Rodriguez et al [17]	30 (3/27)	±	-	-
Brignole et al [18]	23 (23/0)	±	±	±
Edner et al [19]	29 (17/12)	±	±	-
Fitzpatrick et al [20]	90 (54/36)	±	±	±
Natale et al [21]	29 (17/12)	±	±	±
Schumacher and Lüderitz [9]	45 (27/18)	±	±	±

±, significant improvement; 0, no significant improvement; -, no data available

Radiofrequency Catheter Ablation

The frequency of hospital admission and emergency room visits and number of antiarrhythmic drugs used decreased significantly after radiofrequency catheter ablation and pacemaker implantation. Activity capacity improved significantly after ablation in patients with depressed left ventricular function. All improvements after ablation were maintained over 6 months follow-up. However, compared to patients without AF, those with AF had less improvement in general quality of life, frequency of significant symptoms, and symptoms during attacks [22].

In summary, it has been shown that not only pharmaceutical, but, even more, electrical treatment can enhance quality of life in patients with AF [23].

References

1. Feinberg WM, Blackshear JL, Laupacis A, Kronmal R, Hart RG (1995) Prevalence, age distribution, and gender of patients with atrial fibrillation: analysis and implications. Arch Intern Med 155:469-473
2. Benjamin EJ, Levy D, Vaziri SM, D'Agostino RB, Belanger AJ, Wolf PA (1994) Independent risk factors for atrial fibrillation in a population-based cohort: the Framingham Heart Study. JAMA 271:840-844
3. Kannel WB, Wolf PA, Benjamin EJ, Levy D (1998) Prevalence, incidence, prognosis, and predisposing conditions for atrial fibrillation: population-based estimates. Am J Cardiol 82:2N-9N
4. Krahn AD, Manfreda J, Tate RB, Mathewson FA, Cuddy TE (1995) The natural history of atrial fibrillation: incidence, risk factors, and prognosis in the Manitoba Follow-Up Study. Am J Med 98:476-484
5. Benjamin EJ, Wolf PA, D'Agostino RB, Silbershatz H, Kannel WB, Levy D (1998) Impact of atrial fibrillation on the risk of death: the Framingham Heart Study. Circulation 98:946-952
6. Lüderitz B, Jung W (2000) Quality of life in patients with atrial fibrillation. Arch Intern Med 160:1749-1757
7. Jung W, Lüderitz B (1998) Quality of life in patients with atrial fibrillation. J Cardiovasc Electrophysiol 9[Suppl 8]:S177-S186
8. Crijns HJGM, Van Gelder IC, Tieleman RG, Gosselink ATM, Van den Berg MP (1997) Why is atrial fibrillation bad for you? In: Murgatroyd FD, Camm AJ (eds) Nonpharmacological management of atrial fibrillation. Futura, Armonk, pp 3-13
9. Schumacher B, Lüderitz B (1998) Rate issues in atrial fibrillation: consequences of tachycardia and therapy for rate control. Am J Cardiol 82:29N-36N
10. Lönnerholm S, Blomström P, Nilsson L, Oxelbark S, Jideus L, Blomström-Lundqvist C (2000) Effects of the Maze operation on health-related quality of life in patients with atrial fibrillation. Circulation 101:2607-2611
11. Wellens JJW, Lau CP, Lüderitz B, Akhtar M, Waldo A, Camm AJ, Timmermans C, Tse HF, Jung W, Jordaens L, Ayers G, for the METRIX Investigators (1998) Atrioverter: an implantable device for the treatment of atrial fibrillation. Circulation 98:1651-1656
12. Lüderitz B, Jung W (2000) Quality of life in atrial fibrillation. J Interv Card Electrophysiol 4:201-209
13. Savelieva I, Paquette M, Dorian P, Lüderitz B, Camm AJ (2001) Quality of life in patients with silent atrial fibrillation. Heart 85:216-217
14. Wyse DG (2000) The AFFIRM trial: main trial and substudies - what can we expect? J Interv Card Electrophysiol 4:171-176
15. Heinz G, Siostrzonek P, Kreiner G, Gossinger H (1992) Improvement in left ventricular systolic function after successful radiofrequency His bundle ablation for drug refractory, chronic atrial fibrillation and recurrent atrial flutter. Am J Cardiol 69:489-492
16. Twidale N, Sutton K, Bartlett L, Booley A, Winstanley S, Heddle W, Hassam R, Koutsounis H (1993) Effects on cardiac performance of atrioventricular node catheter ablation using radiofrequency current for drug-refractory atrial arrhythmias. Pacing Clin Electrophysiol 16:1275-1284
17. Rodriguez LM, Smeets JL, Xie B, de Chillou C, Cherix E, Pieters F, Metzger J, den Dulk K, Wellens HJJ (1993) Improvement in left ventricular function by ablation of atrioventricular nodal conduction in selected patients with lone atrial fibrillation. Am J Cardiol 72:1137-1141

18. Brignole M, Gionfranchi L, Menozzi C, Bottoni N, Bollini R, Lolli G, Oddone D, Giaggioli G (1994) Influence of atrioventricular junction radiofrequency ablation patients with chronic atrial fibrillation and flutter on quality of life and cardiac performance. Am J Cardiol 74:242-246
19. Edner M, Caidahl K, Bergfeldt L, Darpö B, Edvardsson N. Rosenqvist M (1995) Prospective study of left ventricular function after radiofrequency ablation of atrioventricular junction in patients with atrial fibrillation. Br Heart J 74:261-267
20. Fitzpatrick AP, Kourouyan HD, Siu A, Lee RJ, Lesh MD, Epstein LM, Griffin JC, Scheinman NM (1996) Quality of life and outcomes after radiofrequency His-bundle catheter ablation and permanent pacemaker implantation: impact of treatment in paroxysmal and established atrial fibrillation. Am Heart J 131:499-507
21. Natale A, Zimerman L, Tomassoni G, Kearney M, Kent V, Brandon MJ, Newby K (1996) Impact on ventricular function and quality of life of transcatheter ablation of the atrioventricular junction in chronic atrial fibrillation with a normal ventricular response. Am J Cardiol 78:1431-1433
22. Steinbeck G (1996) Drug therapy of atrial fibrillation: control of heart rate versus establishing sinus rhythm (in German). Z Kardiol 85[Suppl 6]:69-74
23. Bathina MN, Mickelsen S, Brooks C, Jaramillo J, Hepton T, Kusumoto FM (1998) Radiofrequency catheter ablation versus medical therapy for initial treatment of supraventricular tachycardia and its impact on quality of life and healthcare costs. Am J Cardiol 82:589-593

IN- AND OUTHOSPITAL MANAGEMENT OF HEART FAILURE PATIENTS

Non-Invasive Evaluation and Early Treatment of Heart Failure Patients

M. Scherillo[1], F. Scotto di Uccio[2], F. Vigorito[2], D. Miceli[2], M.G. Tesorio[3], V. Monda[2], R. Calabrò[3]

The epidemiological context

The Hospital as Observation Point

The effects of the growing spreading of heart failure (HF) in Italy can be described on the basis of data from the Italian National Health Care System (www.sanita.it) relating to the number of patients discharged from Italian hospitals with the main diagnosis of HF (DRG 127) in the last 5 years (Fig. 1). From 86 235 patients discharged in 1995, the number reached 170 972 discharged with DRG 127 in 1999. In 5 years, the number of patients with HF discharged from Italian hospitals has nearly doubled, with an estimated global cost of about € 500 million per year.

Fig. 1. Data from the Italian Health System. Patients discharged from Italian hospitals (1995-99) with heart failure as principal diagnosis (DRG 127)

[1]Cardiologia Interventistica e UTIC, A.O. Rummo, Benevento; [2]Dipartimento di Cardiologia, Azienda Ospedaliera Monaldi, Naples; [3]Cattedra di Cardiologia, Seconda Università di Napoli, Naples, Italy

We also have important information from the Temistocle study (FADOI-ANMCO heart failure epidemiological study in Italian people) regarding the epidemiological-clinical profile of patients admitted to hospital for HF [1]. This was a short (12 days) observational study that took a "snapshot" of the hospitalization proceedings of 2127 patients discharged with a diagnosis of HF from 167 cardiology and 250 general medicine units distributed throughout the country. The mean age of the recruited patients was high: 76 years for those who were admitted to a general medical department and 70 years for the cardiology-assisted patients, with an average of 11 days' hospitalization. About 50% were women. Both sexes had a long history of disease, with at least one hospitalization in the previous year in about 40% of the cases. These patients also had an elevated incidence of associated diseases: chronic obstructive pulmonary disease (COPD) in 40% and diabetes in 30%.

The Temistocle study showed that patients admitted to hospital with CHF have a reduced duration and quality of life:

- 5% died during the hospital stay.
- 15% died within 6 months of hospital discharge.
- 45% were re-admitted to hospital at least once within 6 months of hospital discharge; there was no significant difference between patients admitted to cardiology department compared to those admitted to general medical departments.

This elevated mortality and morbidity of patients admitted for HF was observed despite appropriate use of pharmacological treatment as recommended by clinical guidelines:

- An ACE inhibitor was used in 72% of the patients.
- A β-blocker was prescribed on discharge for 18% of patients discharged from a cardiology department.

The Community as Observation Point

In reality the above data underestimate the real epidemiological dimensions of HF and need to be integrated with data coming from community studies. This allows a correct estimation of the percentage of the population affected by HF, from asymptomatic left ventricular dysfunction to clinically evident HF, and selection of the appropriate medical intervention strategy.

The existence of a hidden part of the HF problem has already been pointed out [2]. It may be represented by the "iceberg" or "pyramid phenomenon" (Fig. 2). Only the upper part of the pyramid is visible (patients with signs and symptoms of reduced left ventricular function) and thus recognized and managed by cardiologists, internists, and family doctors; the base of the pyramid, made up of the asymptomatic left ventricular dysfunction remains hidden or fails to be recognized.

The identification of patients with asymptomatic left ventricular dysfunction with a high risk of developing clinically manifested HF (in other words, the "platform" which feeds the top of the iceberg) can contribute to the imple-

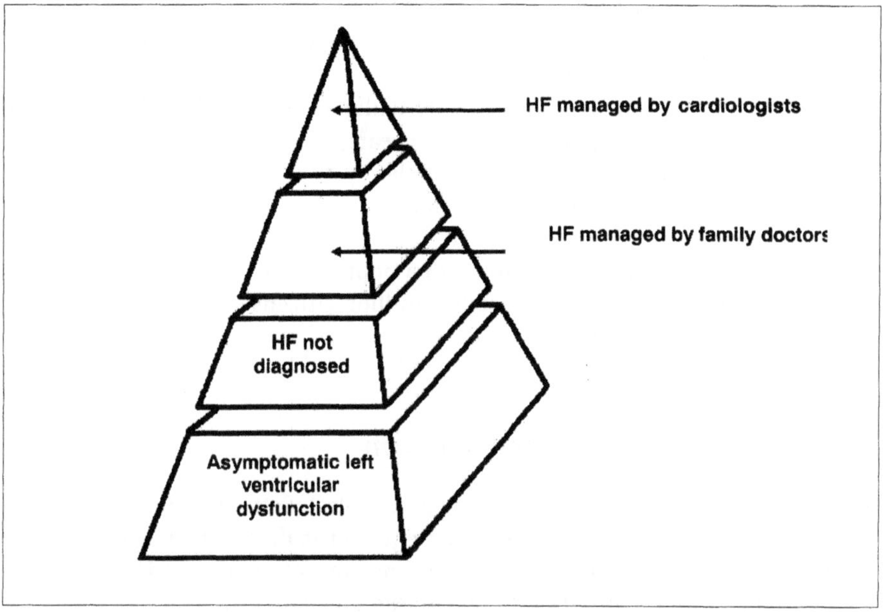

Fig. 2. The heart failure "pyramid"

mentation of strategies such as those of preventing HF development and/or improving its prognosis [3, 4]. The risk of sudden death in these patients is high and seems to be higher than that of symptomatic patients [5]. The available data are based on studies of American communities, such as the Framinghan and the Olmsted [6, 7], and European communities like Rotterdam and Glasgow [8, 9].

The prevalence of asymptomatic HF in the adult population has been estimated from echocardiographic studies at approximately 3% [10]. In people between 25 and 65 years, the prevalence of asymptomatic left ventricular dysfunction is 2%, going up to 4%-6% in those older than 65 years. Regarding HF with clinical signs of left ventricular systolic dysfunction, some studies indicate a prevalence of 0.4% which can go up to 3.6% of the adult population. Prevalence tends to increase with age, being up to 2%-5% in those older than 65 years [10].

The Total Burden of HF

It would be right to estimate the total dimensions of the HF pyramid to plan appropriate strategies for health interventions. This approach shows the complex task of the health structures, which may not be limited just to the care of hospitalized patients suffering from HF, but also to the identification – and correct treatment – of patients at high risk of developing HF.

This total burden which the healthcare service has to take care of might be estimated at approximately 5% of the general population [11]. This total percentage from is put together from:

- 1% HF with clinical signs of left ventricular systolic dysfunction (1.5% of the population aged between 25 and 75 years)
- 1% HF with asymptomatic left ventricular dysfunction
- 1% HF with preserved systolic function
- 2% HF suspected but not confirmed

This would indicate that in Italy, with a population of 57884000 inhabitants (data from ISTAT 2000), approximately 3 million citizens suffer from HF, either asymptomatic or manifest.

Risk Factors for Left Ventricular Dysfunction

The known risk factors for HF are shown in Table 1. Setting aside the powerful unchangeable risk factors such as older age and male sex, it is opportune to keep the others in mind in order to reduce or prevent the risk of HF by choosing the right screening program for asymptomatic patients.

It should be remembered that half of the patients admitted for myocardial infarction have already developed signs and symptoms of HF during their hospital stay [12], and up to 50% of these show severe left ventricular dysfunction. Approximately 75% of the latter will develop HF [13]. Furthermore, there are also signs that, in an unselected population with a previous myocardial infarction, the annual risk of developing HF could be around 2.5% [14]. Hypertension represents an absolute risk for the development of HF, and in presence of other factors even moderate rises in the pressure values can lead to multiple risk elements [15]. In the same way, smoking, especially in men, dyslipidemia, diabetes, and microalbuminuria are predictive elements of independent risk [5, 16, 17]. Other factors have also been observed: low or reduced vital capacity, increased cardiac frequency at rest, and obesity have all been associated with an increased risk of HF development [15].

Taking all this together, we can now consider a global cardiovascular risk for HF. Our attention should precisely be shifted away from the patients with asymptomatic left ventricular dysfunction at risk of HF and toward choosing

Table 1. Risks factors for left ventricular dysfunction

Age
Male gender
Coronary heart disease with or without myocardial infarction
Hypertension
Left ventricular hypertrophy
Left ventricular dilatation
Diabetes

an educational program for the population to encourage the adoption of a "safe heart" lifestyle and promote among family doctors, cardiologists, and internists the adoption of appropriate diagnostic and therapeutic strategies for these kinds of patients.

Appropriate treatment of hypertension reduces the risk [18], as does therapy with statin, as deduced from the results of the 4S study [19]. Associated diseases such as diabetes identify a population of patients in whom treatment must be undertaken before the development of symptomatic ventricular dysfunction [17].

Pitfalls in the Diagnosis of HF and Left Ventricular Dysfunction

The necessity of widely recognized criteria, not only for the diagnosis and the evaluation of HF in clinical practice, but also for epidemiological purposes, led the Task Force on Heart Failure of the European Society of Cardiology to the compilation of guidelines for the diagnosis of HF [20]. According to the Task Force, the diagnosis can be made in the presence of objective symptoms and signs (at rest or during effort) with objective demonstrations of left ventricular dysfunction at rest and, only in cases where the diagnosis is still doubtful, from the response to a specific therapeutic treatment. By these criteria, a patient with suspected symptoms and/or signs of HF, for objective demonstration of left ventricular dysfunction, must undergo an electrocardiographic exam, a laboratory test, lung and thyroid functionality tests, and an echocardiographic exam, in that order. In reality, although the clinical symptoms and signs can be extremely useful for the correct diagnosis of HF, they can manifest in many other diseases, so that they are not very specific for HF, or they can be fairly precise but not very sensitive, since they can manifest themselves in the most severe phase of the disease. Thus, the clinical criteria can lead to an overestimation of the problem with more than 66% false-positive results [21].

In the clinical context of HF, the electrocardiogram (ECG) has an elevated predictive negative value, up to 98% [22]: a patient with abnormal ECG (signs of previous necrosis, left ventricular hypertrophy, complete block of the left part, atrial fibrillation) can have a 33% probability of having a left ventricular systolic dysfunction. Among the instrumental tests, echocardiography is the most commonly used method for identifying patients with an asymptomatic left ventricular dysfunction, because of its sensitivity, specificity, simplicity of execution, reproducibility, and relative cheapness. Furthermore, it has been said that correct use of echocardiography improves diagnostic and therapeutic accuracy, favorably influencing on the prognosis of HF [23]. Quiñones et al. [24] have demonstrated in 1172 patients enrolled in the SOLVD study, that there is an association between left ventricular hypertrophy, echocardiographically defined, and cardiovascular events in patients with chronic left ventricular dysfunction, independently of the presence of HF symptoms. Evidence of hypertrophy, calculated as left ventricular mass and associated with contractile dysfunction, would therefore, it is argued, identify a population of persons at risk of developing clinically evident HF.

However, as is well-known, calculation of left ventricular mass can be difficult in some patients because of the poor quality of the images. Furthermore, echocardiographic technique in general, as far as determination of ventricular volume and wall thickness is concerned, is strongly operator-dependent [25]. In addition, although calling on echocardiography is possible and indeed easy in a specifically cardiological context, it is less easily accessible in a different context. Data from the Euro-HF study [26] indicate underuse of echocardiography for the diagnosis of HF in general medicine, with lower use in consequence of the main recommended pharmacological treatments. In most cases this is due to organizational difficulties; however, in experimental models of management "open access services" with the possibility of performing an echocardiographic exam at the direct request of the family doctor [27], in nearly 75% of cases the diagnosis of HF was not confirmed [28]. Thus, proposing systematic and easier use of echocardiography for all patients where there is a suspicion of HF would cause a fruitless increase in the already tough workload of the specialized diagnostic apparatus.

The New Biohumoral Markers of Left Ventricular Dysfunction

As regards the diagnosis of HF, new determinable indicators can now be recognized at the humoral level, in particular natriuretic factors as ANP and BNP produced at a cardiac level, already known since the second half of the 1980's [29] and better known in the following years, thanks in part to the work of Japanese researchers [30]. The ANP, or atrial natriuretic peptide, is normally produced in the atria, and in smaller amounts in the ventricles. The BNP, or brain natriuretic peptide, is produced in large amounts in the ventricles. Both act on kidney function, increasing the glomeular filtration rate and inhibiting the secretion of renin and aldosterone [31]. The correlation between hypertrophy and left ventricular dysfunction and the plasma concentration of ANP and BNP has recently been well documented [32]. Japanese researchers have demonstrated that there is an increase in plasma BNP concentration in patients with hypertension and left ventricular hypertrophy and in patients with evident HF [32]. The same study showed that enalapril is able to reduce the plasma levels of ANP and BNP together with favorable effects on the regression of left ventricular hypertrophy and the reduction of ventricular mass in patients with hypertension. In the last few years, many studies have suggested possible applications of these markers in the field of HF, either diagnostic evaluation [33-39], prognostic stratification [40-43], or in the monitoring of therapy [44-47]. Particularly interesting is the possible use of these markers in emergency departments [48], where it is necessary to rapidly identify the nature of a dyspnea, where the clinical criteria can mislead, and where imaging technologies (echocardiography, myocardial scintigraphy) are more expensive and complex to use.

In 250 patients admitted to the emergency department with dyspneic symptoms, the concentration of BNP measured was higher in the 97 patients affected by HF than in the patients with dyspnea caused by other reasons: 1076+/-138 pg/ml vs 38+/-4 pg/ml ($p<0.001$). The same authors reported a study conducted in 72 patients admitted for HF in NYHA class III/IV characterized by daily measurement of BNP [42]. The BNP values were correlated with the mortality endpoint and rehospitalization at 30 days: of 72 patients with HF, 13 died and 9 were readmitted. In the latter group of 22 patients, the BNP values progressively increased during the hospital stay, and this was different to the patients who did not reach the endpoint, who showed a progressive drop in BNP values during their hospital stay.

A pivotal study was conducted to determine whether the variation in BNP concentration correlated with the acute variation of pulmonary capillary pressure in the patients with HF [49]; these results have given even greater importance to the diagnostic power of the determination of natriuretic factors in the management of patients with HF. In this study 20 patients were examined, after hospital admission for NYHA functional class III and IV HF, in whom the effect of therapy was evaluated by measuring the pulmonary capillary pressure (Swan-Ganz method) and at the same time measuring values of BNP every 2-4 h for a period of 24-48 h. The results showed a significant correlation between a drop in pulmonary capillary pressure and BNP values. As early as 1996 and 1998, respectively, Arakawa et al. [50] and Richards et al. [51] affirmed the predictive role of BNP in prognostic stratification after myocardial infarction, suggesting the possibility of individualizing patient typology through the neurohormonal profile, and most of all, pinpointing the best moment to start β-blocker therapy.

In 1999 came the publication of the first study to demonstrate the capacity on the basis of the neurohormonal factors to predict the response of the treatment with carvedilol [52]. In 415 patients with ischemic left ventricular dysfunction, BNP and norepinephrine were measured. Carvedilol reduced the death rate among the patients with the highest pretreatment level of BNP and the lowest norepinephrine activation.

Furthermore, a recent study estimated the course of the BNP values in 30 patients with idiopathic dilatative cardiomyopathy receiving carvedilol [53]. The BNP concentration showed a strong correlation with the end-diastolic diameter of the left ventricle, the ejection fraction, and the left ventricular mass index, indicating a good possibility for hormone-guided therapy. The effectiveness of BPN as prognostic indicator for HF was confirmed by the data from a Japanese study [40]. A significant correlation among successive events (another hospitalization for a new episode) and BNP values higher than 132 pg/ml has been found at the follow-up of 84 patients older than 65 years admitted for a HF instability. The authors suggest using a BNP determination as a prognostic value and, most of all, to plan better the further following-up in all discharged patients with a HF diagnosis.

But the field which makes the application of these parameters even more fascinating, and which opens new potentialities, is the diagnostic/prognostic capacity of the natriuretic factors. The final aim is to have a user-friendly test available for the early diagnosis of left ventricular dysfunction which allows:

- Evaluation of the compensation state and the prognosis of the patient with HF
- Diagnosis of the disease in a pre-clinical phase

Another aim is to be able to use an easily determinable numerical datum for verification of the current compensation state and prognosis of each patient (as with glycosylated hemoglobin in the diabetic patient) or to reveal a tendency to develop manifest disease in a preclinical stage, like the Paptest in the prediction of uterine cancer.

Particularly interesting is the possible use of these indicators for screening of the general population, where a HF diagnosis based only on clinical criteria could be uncertain, with the aim of identifying a group of patients to send for an early diagnosis by echocardiography. Cowie et al. determined the concentrations of ANP, NT-ANP (N-terminal ANP), and BNP by the radioimmunological method in an outpatient clinic where 122 patients were being checked for a suspected HF diagnosis [54]. The sensitivity, specificity, and positive predictive value for the patients in whom the clinical suspicion was confirmed were respectively 97%, 72%, and 95% for ANP, 97%, 66%, and 94% for NT-ANP, and 97%,84%, and 70% for BNP. In particular, determining ANP and NT-ANP concentrations did not lead to a significant increase of the predictive value in respect to the cases in which the BNP was separately evaluated, thus conferring on BNP the potentiality of being the most sensitive and specific marker. Determination of BNP concentration seems also to be a relatively simple method and undoubtedly cost-effective for the screening of patients with suspected left ventricular dysfunction and to start at a successive diagnostic level.

The value of BNP concentration in patients with suspected left ventricular dysfunction has also been compared with the value of the ejection fraction obtained with nuclear medicine imaging techniques [55]: Bettencourt and al. confirmed a significant correlation between ejection fractions higher than 55% and low values of BNP against values progressively higher for ejection fraction lower than 40%. Also, modest but encouraging experiences have already been reported in subgroups of patients with HF with preserved systolic function [55].

Very recently, there has also been an indication for the use of a precursor of BNP, the N-terminal pro-BNP (NT-BNP), which, besides possessing equivalent diagnostic accuracy, would be more stable and, most of all, measurable by enzyme linked immunosorbent assay, thus avoiding the radioimmuno assay necessary to extract the BNP from the plasma [56]. On the basis of this information we could also consider a "redesigned" diagnostic algorithm of HF, with the insertion, in the phase preceding an echocardiographic exam, of determination of BNP or NT-BNP. Family doctors could request BNP or NT-BNP determination to confirm the clinical diagnosis of HF and the necessity of further diagnostic study, and cardiologists could use it as a prognostic indicator or an orientation aid for appropriate therapy.

The effectiveness of this strategy of intervention for HF in the community is being evaluated by the Sicilian NT-BNP study. This is an ANMCO study of the Region of Sicily in collaboration with the ANMCO Study Center and the Mario Negri Institute, which aims to verify the predictive value of NT-BNP in the diagnosis of HF in general medicine. The project foresees the involvement of nearly 150 doctors and 5 referral centers which will examine by a visit, an ECG and an echocardiographic exam, the new cases of suspected HF referred to them by the doctors to confirm or exclude the diagnosis, and compare the findings with the NT-BNP values.

Therapeutic Strategies for Asymptomatic Left Ventricular Dysfunction

ACE Inhibitors

The effectiveness of ACE inhibitors in reducing mortality, hospitalization, and the development of symptomatic HF in patients with asymptomatic or nearly asymptomatic left ventricular dysfunction has been demonstrated by the SAVE [57], AIRE [58], and TRACE [12] studies (Table 2). The results of these three studies are homogeneous and consistent not only in respect of the total mortality primary endpoint [odds ratio (OR) 0.74; 95% confidence interval (CI) 0.66-0.83] but also for the important clinical first HF-related hospitalization endpoint (OR 0.73; 95% HF 0.63-0.85).

In the only trial conducted on HF prevention, the SOLVD trial [59], 4228 patients with asymptomatic left ventricular dysfunction were randomized to receive placebo or enalapril; enalapril did not significantly influence mortality relative risk 8%; p=0.30), but significantly reduced endpoints of symptomatic HF (29%) and hospitalization (20%). Furthermore, evidence was collected that the patients with asymptomatic left ventricular dysfunction in the placebo arm developed chronic HF in an average period of 8.3 months.

Table 2. Effects of ACE inhibitors on mortality and hospitalizations in patients with asymptomatic left ventricular dysfunction

		Risk reduction	
Trial	**Drug**	**Mortality (%)**	**Hospitalization (%)**
SAVE [57]	Captopril 50 mg × 3/die	30	35
AIRE [58]	Ramipril 50mg × 2/die	21	25
TRACE [12]	Trandolapril 4 mg/die	27	22

β-Blockers

The effectiveness of β-Blockers in the treatment of patients with asymptomatic left ventricular dysfunction has been demonstrated by the results of the CAPRICORN (Carvedilol postinfarction survival control in LV dysfunction) study [60]. This study enrolled 1959 patients with a recent acute myocardial infarction (3-21 days previously) and a left ventricular ejection fraction below or equal to 40% or a wall motion score index below or equal to 1.3 treated with an ACE inhibitor for at least 48 h, and randomized to receive carvedilol or placebo (Fig. 3). The purpose was to evaluate the effectiveness of carvedilol on the clinical outcome in patients with a left ventricular dysfunction in the post-thrombosis period after an acute myocardial infarction, on top of a standard therapy which foresaw the use of the ACE inhibitor, prescribed in 98% of the patients treated with the β-blocker. The primary endpoint was death and/or hospitalization for cardiovascular reasons. The results are shown in Table 3. Total mortality was lower in the carvedilol group than in the placebo group: 12% and 15% respectively (OR 0.77; 95% CI 0.60 –0.98, $p<0.03$). There were no relevant significant differences regarding the total mortality endpoint and hospitalization. These data suggest that patients with left ventricular dysfunction due to a myocardial infarction can be treated with an ACE inhibitor and carvedilol.

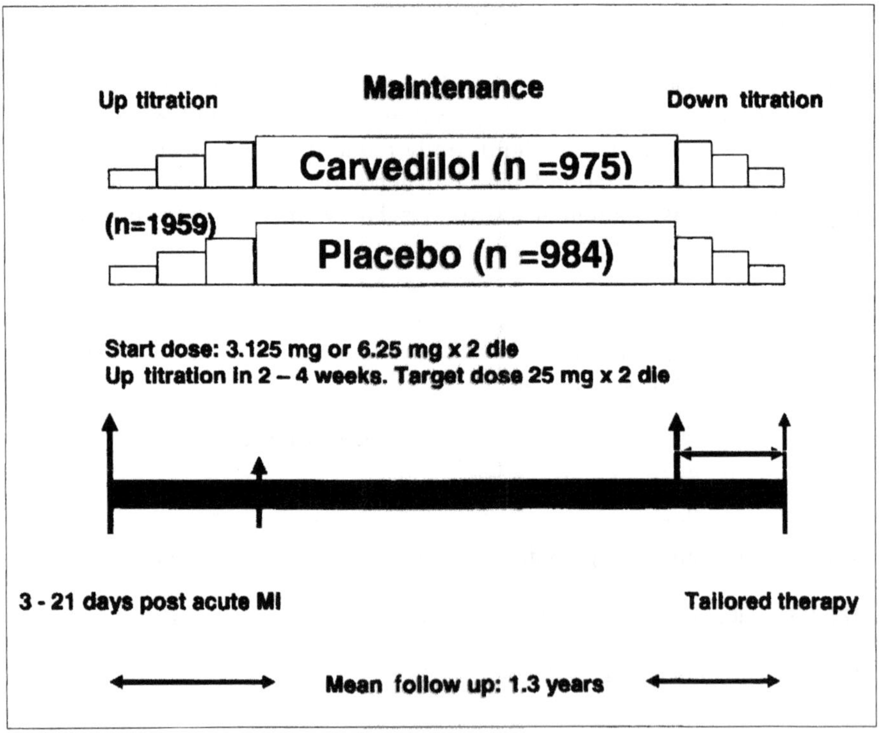

Fig. 3. CAPRICORN study design

Table 3. Results of the CAPRICORN study

	Carvedilol 25 mg X 2/die	Placebo	Odds ratio (95% CI)	*p*
All-cause mortality	12%	15%	0.77 (0.60-0.98)	0.031
All-cause mortality or hospitalization	35%	37%	0.92 (0.80-1.07)	0.296

Angiotensin Receptor Blockers

The efficacy of this category of drugs in patients with asymptomatic left ventricular dysfunction is being analyzed by the Valinat (Valsartan in acute myocardial infarction) study. This is an international multicenter trial that has enrolled 14500 patients with left ventricular dysfunction (ejection fraction less than equal to 35% or wall motion score index below or equal to 1.2) and/or clinical or radiological signs of HF. The purpose of the trial is to evaluate the efficacy and safety of long-term treatment with valsartan, captopril, or a combination of both in patients at high risk after a myocardial infarction. The design of the study is shown in Fig. 4.

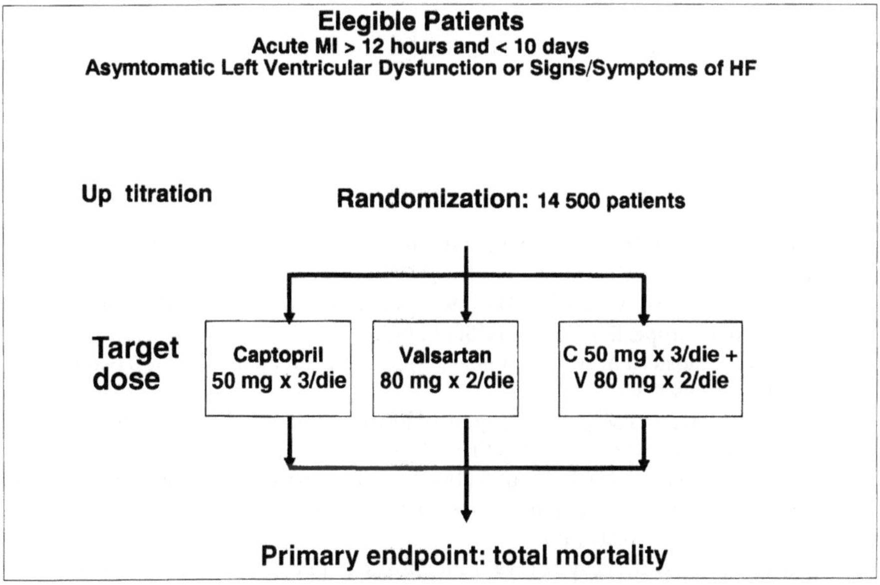

Fig. 4. The Valiant study design. Eligibility criteria include acute myocardial infarction between 12 h and 10 days ago, asymptomatic left ventricular dysfunction, and/or signs or symptoms of HF

Future Perspectives

HF represents the ultimate stage of the cardiovascular diseases; life expectation is reduced as in some other terminal diseases like cancer, but, unlike in the latter, we also know that in HF the incidence of sudden death is high, in spite of the therapeutic armamentarium that we possess. The aim in future years is to bring about a reduction in the number of HF cases. To do this, it is necessary to prevent cardiac disease from developing in the first place, to diagnose it earlier in the community, and to correct both left ventricular dysfunction in the asymptomatic phase and the predisposing risk factors. Patients at risk of HF could be entered into screening programs using NT-BNP and BNP testing, followed in the second instance by an echocardiographic exam, a method which safeguards the cost/effectiveness ratio and which will diagnose left ventricular dysfunction and allow treatment in such a way as to delay manifestation of the disease.

From the point of view of prevention, it is necessary to redefine HF on the basis of elements obtained from the pathophysiologic pattern rather than from the signs and symptoms. In this way, the aim of treatment should be to improve left ventricular function to achieve an increase in the survival of HF patients.

Future research, therefore, will be directed not only at the correction and prevention of hypertrophy and left ventricular dysfunction, but also at developing the instruments to verify the appropriateness of any treatment in terms of preventing HF and improving patients' the quality of life.

Acknowledgements: The authors thank Mr. Antonio Piccinini of the Department of Cardiology, AO Monaldi, for technical assistance in the preparation of the manuscript and the tables.

References

1. Scherillo M (2001) Oral presentation. XXXI National Congress of Italian Association Hospital Cardiologists (ANMCO), 16-19 May, Florence, Italy
2. Hoes AW, Mosterd A, Grohbee DE (1998) An epidemic of heart failure? Recent evidence from Europe. Eur Heart J 19[Suppl L]:L2-9
3. Cowie MR, Mosterd A, Wood DA et al (1997) The epidemiology of heart failure. Eur Heart J 18: 208-225
4. Yamani M, Massie BM (1993) Congestive heart failure: insights from epidemiology, implications for treatment. Mayo Clinic Proc 68:1214-1218
5. McKelvie RS, Benedict CR, Yusuf S (1999) Evidence based cardiology. Prevention of congestive heart failure and management of asymptomatic left ventricular dysfunction. Br Med J 318:1400-1402
6. Lauer MS, Evans JC, Levy D (1992) Prognostic implications of subclinical left ventricular dilatation and systolic dysfunction in men free of overt cardiovascular disease (the Framingham heart study). Am J Cardiol 70:1180-1184

7. McMurray JJ, Petric MC, Murdock DR, Davie AP (1998) Clinical epidemiology of heart failure: public and private health burden. Eur Heart J 19[Suppl P]:P 9-16
8. Mosterd A, De Bruijine MC, Hoes AW, Deckers JW, Hofman A, Grobbee DE (1997) Usefulness of echocardiography in detecting left ventricular dysfunction in population based studies (the Rotterdam study). Am J Cardiol 79:103-104
9. McDonagh T, Morrison CE, Lawrence A et al (1997) Symptomatic and asymptomatic left-ventricular systolic dysfunction in an urban population. Lancet 350:829-833
10. Cleland JGF (1997) Screening for left ventricular dysfunction and heart failure: should it be done and if so how? Dis Manag Health Outcomes 1:169-84
11. Cleland JGF, Khand A, Clark A (2001) The heart failure epidemic: exactly how big is it? Eur Heart J 22:623-626
12. Kober L, Torp-Pedersen C, Carlsen JE et al (1995) A clinical trial of the angiotensin-converting-enzyme inhibitor trandolapril in patients with left ventricular dysfunction after myocardial infarction. The Trandolapril Cardiac Evaluation (TRACE) Study Group. N Engl J Med 333:1670-1676
13. De Vita C et al (1994) GISSI-3 Effects of lisinopril and transdermal glyceryl binitrate singly and together on 6-week mortality and ventricular function after acute myocardial infarction. Lancet 343:1115-1122
14. Kannel WB et al (1979) Prognosis after initial myocardial infarction: the Framinghan study. Am J Cardiol 44:53-59
15. McKelvie RS, Benedict CR, Yusuf S (1998) Prevention of congestive heart failure and treatment of asymptomatic left ventricular dysfunction. In: Yusuf S, Cairns JA, Camm AJ, Fallen EI, Gersh BJ (eds) Evidence based cardiology. Br Med Publishing Group, London, pp 703-721
16. Shindler JM, Kostis JB, Yusuf S et al (1996) Diabetes mellitus, a predictor of morbidity and mortality in the studies of left ventricular dysfunction (SOLVD) trials ad registry. Am J Cardiol 77:1017-1020
17. Gerstein HC, FeMann J, Zinman B et al (1997) Albuminuria is highly prevalent and predicts cardiovascular events in high risk diabetic and non-diabetic patients. Circulation 96[Suppl 8]:1225
18. Psaty BM, Smith NL, Siscovick DS et al (1997) Health outcomes associated with antihypertensive therapies used as first-line agents. A systematic review and meta-analysis. JAMA 277:739-745
19. Kjekshus J, Pedersen TR, Olsson AG, Faegeman O, Pyorala K, on behalf of the 4S Study Group (1997) The effects of simvastatin on the incidence of heart failure in patients with coronary heart disease. J Cardiac Failure 3:249-254
20. Task Force on Heart Failure of the European Society of Cardiology (1995) Guidelines for the diagnosis of heart failure. Eur Heart J 16: 741
21. Stevenson LW, Perloff JK (1989) The limited reliability of physical signs for estimating hemodynamics in heart failure. JAMA 261:884-888
22. Davie AP, Francis CM, Love MP et al (1996) Value of the electrocardiogram in identifying heart failure due to left ventricular systolic dysfunction. Br Med J 312: 222
23. Senni M, Rodeheffer RJ, Triboulloy CM et al (1999) Use of echocardiography in the management of congestive heart failure in the community. J Am Coll Cardiol 33:171-173
24. Quiñones MA, Greenberg BH, Koplen HA et al (2000) Echocardiographic predictors of clinical outcome in patients with left ventricular dysfunction enrolled in the SOLVD registry and trials: significance of left ventricular hypertrophy. J Am Coll Cardiol 35-5:1237-1244

25. Mukherjee SK, Jaffe CC (1995) Left ventricular mass estimation by echocardiography: is it clinically useful? Echocardiography 12:185-193
26. Hobbs FDR, Jones MI, Allan TF, Tobias R (2000) European survey of primary care physician perceptions on heart failure diagnosis and management (Euro-HF). Euro Heart J 21:1877-1887
27. Francis CM, Caruana L, Kearney P et al (1995) Open access echocardiography in management of heart failure in the community Br Med J 310:634-636
28. Fox KF, Cowie MR, Wood DA, Coats AJS, Poole-Wilson PA, Sutton C (2000) A rapid access heart failure clinic provides a prompt diagnosis and appropriate management of new heart failure presenting in the community. Eur J Heart Fail 4:423-429
29. Phillips PA, Sasadeus J, Hodsman GP et al (1989) Plasma atrial natriuretic peptide in patients with acute myocardial infarction: effects of streptochinase. Br Heart J 61:139-143
30. Mukoyama M, Nakao K, Hosoda K et al (1991) Brain natriuretic peptide as a novel cardiac hormone in humans. J Clin Invest 87:1402-1414
31. Levin ER, Gardner DG, Samson WK (1998) Natriuretic peptides in mechanisms of disease. N Engl J Med 339:321-328
32. Khono M, Yokokawa K, Yasunari K et al (1997) Changes in plasma natriuretic peptide concentrations during 1 year treatment with angiotensin-converting enzyme inhibitor in elderly hypertensive patients with left ventricular hypertrophy. Int J Clin Pharmacol Ther 35: 38-42
33. Arad M, Elazar E, Shotan A et al (1996) Brain and atrial natriuretic peptides in patients with ischemic disease with and without heart failure. Cardiology 87:12-17
34. Masson S, Gorini M, Salio M, Lucci D, Latini R, Maggioni AP on behalf of the IN-CHF Investigators (2000) Clinical correlates of elevated plasma natriuretic peptides and Big-endothelin-1 in a population of ambulatory patients with heart failure. A substudy of the Italian Network on Congestive Heart Failure(IN-CHF) registry. Ital Heart J 4:282-288
35. Valli N, Georges A, Corcuff J, Barat J, Bordenave L (2001) Assessment of brain natriuretic peptide in patients with suspected heart failure: comparison with radionuclide ventriculography data. Clin Chim Acta 306:19-26
36. Mallamaci F, Zoccali C, Tripepi G et al (2001) Diagnostic potential of cardiac natriuretic peptides in dialysis patients. Kidney Int 59:1599-1566
37. Yamamoto K, Burnett JC Jr, Bermudez EA, Jougasaki M, Bailey KR, Redfield MM (2000) Clinical criteria and biochemical markers for the detection of systolic dysfunction. J Card Fail 6:194-200
38. McDonagh TA (2000) Asymptomatic left ventricular dysfunction in the community. Curr Cardiol Rep 2:470-474
39. Suzuki T, Yamaoki K, Nakajima O et al (2000) Screening for cardiac dysfunction in asymptomatic patients by measuring B-type natriuretic peptide levels. Jpn Heart J 41:205-214
40. Tamura K, Takahashi N, Nakatani Y, Onishi S, Iwasaka T (2001) Prognostic impact of plasma brain natriuretic peptide for cardiac events in elderly patients with congestive heart failure. Gerontology 47:46-51
41. Maisel AS, Koon J, Krishnaswamy P et al (2001) Utility of B-natriuretic peptide as a rapid, point-of-care test for screening patients undergoing echocardiography to determine left ventricular dysfunction. Am Heart J 141:367-374
42. Cheng V, Kazanagra R, Garcia A et al (2001) A rapid bedside test for B-type peptide predicts treatment outcomes in patients admitted for decompensated heart failure. Pilot study. J Am Coll Cardiol 37:386-391

43. Bettencourt P, Ferreira A, Dias P et al (2000) Predictors of prognosis in patients with stable mild to moderate heart failure. J Card Fail 6:306-313
44. Tsutamoto T, Wada A, Maeda K et al (2001) Effect of spironolactone on plasma brain natriuretic peptide and left ventricular remodeling in patients with congestive heart failure. J Am Coll Cardiol 37:1228-1233
45. Okumura H, Iuchi K, Yoshida T et al (2000) Brain natriuretic peptide is a predictor of anthracycline-induced cardiotoxicity. Acta Haematol 104:158-163
46. Tsutamoto T, Wada A, Maeda K et al (1997) Digitalis increases brain natriuretic peptide in patients with severe congestive heart failure. Am Heart J 134:910-916
47. Troughton RW, Frampton CM, Yandle TG, Espiner EA, Nicholls MG, Richards AM (2000) Treatment of heart failure guided by plasma aminoterminal brain natriuretic peptide (N-BNP) concentrations. Lancet 355:1126-1130
48. Dao Q, Krishnaswamy P, Kazanegra R et al (2001) Utility of B-type natriuretic peptide in the diagnosis of congestive heart failure in an urgent-care setting. J Am Coll Cardiol 37:379-385
49. Kazanegra R, Cheng V, Garcia A et al (2001) A rapid test for B-type natriuretic peptide correlates with falling wedge pressures in patients treated for decompensated heart failure: a pilot study. J Card Fail 7:21-29
50. Arakawa N, Nakamura M, Aoki H, Hiramori K (1996) Plasma brain natriuretic peptide concentrations predict survival after acute myocardial infarction. J Am Coll Cardiol 27:1656-1661
51. Richards AM, Nicholls MG, Yandle TG et al (1998) Plasma N-terminal pro-brain natriuretic peptide and adrenomedullin: new neurhormonal predictors of left ventricular function and prognosis after myocardial infarction. Circulation 97:1921-1929
52. Richards AM, Doughty R, Nicholls MG et al (1999) Neurohormonal prediction of benefit from carvedilol in ischemic left ventricular dysfunction. Circulation 99:786-792
53. Kawai K, Hata K, Takahoka H, Kawai H, Yokoyama M (2001) Plasma brain natriuretic peptide as a novel therapeutic indicator in idiopathic dilated cardiomyopathy during β-blocker therapy: a potential of hormone-guided treatment. Am Heart J 141:925-932
54. Cowie MR, Struthers AD, Wood DA et al (1997) Value of natriuretic peptides in assessment of patients with possible new heart failure in primary care. Lancet 350:1349-1353
55. Bettencourt P, Ferreira A, Dias P, Castro A, Martins L, Cerqueira-Gomes M (2000) Evaluation of brain natrurietic peptide in the diagnosis of heart failure. Cardiology 93:19-25
56. McDonald K, Ledwidge M, Cahill J et al (2001) Elimination of early rehospitalization in a randomized, controlled trial of multidisciplinary care in high-risk, elderly heart failure population: the potential contributions of specialist care, clinical stability and optimal angiotensin-converting enzyme inhibitor dose at discharge. Eur J Heart Fail 3:209-215
57. Pfeffer MA, Braunwald E, Moyè LA et al (1992) Effect of captopril on mortality and morbidity in patients with left ventricular dysfunction after myocardial infarction. Results of the survival and ventricular enlargement trial. The SAVE Investigators. N Engl J Med 327:669-677
58. The Acute Infarction Ramipril Efficacy (AIRE) Study Investigators (1993) Effect of ramipril on mortality and morbidity of survivors of acute myocardial infarction with clinical evidence of heart failure. Lancet 342:821-828

59. The SOLVD Investigators (1992) Effect of enalapril on mortality and development of heart failure in asymptomatic patients with reduced left ventricular ejection fractions. N Engl J Med 327:685-691
60. The CAPRICORN Investigators (2001) Effect of carvedilol on outcome after myocardial infarction in patients with left-ventricular dysfunction: the CAPRICORN randomised trial. Lancet 357:1385-1390

ACE-Inhibitors, β-Blockers, Spironolactone: Do We Need Many More Drugs to Treat Chronic Heart Failure?

G. Sinagra[1], G. Sabbadini[2], A. Perkan[1], S. Rakar[1], F. Longaro[1], L. Salvatore[1], G. Lardieri[1], A. Di Lenarda[1]

Current Heart Failure Therapies: Pathophysiological Basis and Clinical Evidence

Over the last two decades, considerable insights into the pathophysiology of chronic congestive heart failure (HF) have been gained to suggest that the overstimulation of biologically active pathways - primarily the renin-angiotensin-aldosterone and sympathoadrenergic systems - may play a key role in determining the progression of the syndrome [1]. Supporting this concept, a large body of evidence has been accumulated to show that drugs possessing the ability to counteract these up-regulated neuroendocrine mechanisms may represent an effective therapeutic strategy to improve the course of the disease [2-7].

In the setting of left ventricular dilation/systolic dysfunction cardiomyopathies, angiotensin-converting enzyme (ACE) inhibitors [2] and, more recently, β-blockers [3] have been extensively proven to reduce the rates of morbidity and mortality in a broad spectrum of HF populations, from those who are symptom-free to those who have symptoms at rest. Although no mortality trial has evaluated the effects of diuretics, it is irrefutable that such drugs represent the most effective means to relieve the pulmonary and systemic congestion and, thus, they remain a cornerstone in the treatment of HF patients with overt fluid retention [4]. Moreover, in those who have symptoms despite receiving neurohormonal antagonists and diuretics, the addition of digoxin has been shown to decrease the need of hospitalization for worsening HF, while its withdrawal adversely influences the quality of life [5].

Hospitalization and death rates can be further reduced by adding low dose of spironolactone, although these benefits have been documented only in the subset of subjects with advanced HF [6]. In NYHA class II-IV HF, significant

[1]S.C. di Cardiologia; [2]Cattedra di Geriatria, Ospedale Maggiore, Trieste, Italy

improvements in morbidity and mortality can be also attained with the use of angiotensin II type 1 receptor blockers, although they have not been proven to be superior to ACE inhibitors [7].

Future Heart Failure Therapies: Research Directions

As a result, the established treatment of symptomatic HF currently includes an ACE inhibitor (or, if not tolerated, an angiotensin II receptor blocker), a β-blocker (since a class effect has not been clearly proven, only carvedilol, long-acting metoprolol, and bisoprolol can be recommended at present), a loop diuretic such as furosemide (alone or in combination with another agent in the class in patients with marked fluid retention), digoxin, and spironolactone (in patients with advanced-stage disease) [8]. However, in the face of these successful pharmacological therapies, the progression of HF syndrome continues relentlessly and the long-term prognosis of the patients remains poor [9]. Thus, there is a general perception that new treatments are needed to further improve the course of the disease.

Why the HF syndrome advances and the patients progressively worsen despite optimal medical therapy has yet to be fully understood, but a partial explanation is that current treatments do not completely suppress the activity of biological systems that are overstimulated in HF. On this basis, great efforts are being currently directed to the search for additional neurohumoral therapies, candidate drugs including arginine-vasopressin, endothelin, and cytokine antagonists as well as antioxidant agents [10]. However, some evidence exists to suggest that too much neurohumoral antagonism might be deleterious rather than beneficial for HF patients. In this regard, the results of the VAL-HeFT trial [11] are paradigmatic. Despite a significant reduction in the composite endpoint hospitalizations/deaths with valsartan as compared to placebo, a subgroup analysis revealed that this benefit was greater in patients not treated with an ACE inhibitor because of intolerance than in those receiving an ACE inhibitor; there was even an unfavorable trend observed when valsartan was given to patients taking both an ACE inhibitor and a β-blocker.

Thus, there is now an increasing awareness that it is time to go beyond mere attempts to completely inhibit the effects of hyperactivated neurohumoral systems in HF, for two main reasons. Firstly, many biologically active pathways potentially have both favorable and unfavorable actions. For example, although it delivers a number of deleterious effects in HF, sympathetic activation may be helpful to support circulatory function when cardiac output is severely lowered. In patients with advanced HF, a too marked pharmacological antagonism (such as that exerted by moxonidine, a potent centrally acting inhibitor of sympathetic outflow) may be detrimental [12], while a blunted adrenergic withdrawal (such as that achievable combining a β-blocker with a phosphodiesterase inhibitor, the latter offsetting the myocardial depressant effects of the former) may be beneficial [13]. Secondly, some biologically active factors are overexpressed in HF to counterbalance the harmful effects of other hyperactivated neurohumoral pathways. This is the case of natriuretic peptides, which may exert favorable actions in patients with HF [14].

Thus, the pharmacological interventions should aim to carefully modulate rather than indiscriminately suppress the neurohumoral activity in HF. Looking forward, however, we must recognize that modulation of all the biologically active systems thought to play a role in the progression of the syndrome is probably unattainable. Accordingly, it is likely that the leading direction in the basic and clinical research for future HF therapies will be the development of strategies targeted at modifying the genetic mechanisms responsible for the syndrome, rather than at interfering with all the hyperactivated neurohumoral pathways which may contribute to its progression.

Can We Achieve Greater Benefits from Currently Available Drugs for Heart Failure?

As we have seen, four to six drugs can currently be considered part of the established treatment of overt HF. However, a significant proportion of patients may require in addition cardiovascular drugs (including antiplatelet drugs or anticoagulants, antiarrythmic drugs, and nitrates or other vasodilators) or pharmacological interventions to control coronary risk factors (e.g., lipid-lowering or antidiabetic agents). Furthermore, most of these patients tend to be elderly, a condition usually associated with major medical comorbidities that often require further additional therapies [15]. The need for fine adjustments or major changes in therapy to prevent or counteract episodes of acute exacerbation of the disease contributes to making the pharmacological management of HF patients more and more complex.

How long will it be possible to pursue the strategy of introducing additional therapies in patients already on such complicated pharmacological regimens? How far will the patients be able to tolerate such increasingly complex prescriptions? In fact, improvements in the management of HF can be achieved not only by adding new efficacious drugs, but also by ensuring better use of existing pharmacological options. In this regard, great efforts must be directed toward broader and more appropriate employment of potentially life-saving treatments. Drugs proven to be effective in clinical trials have not been given to all the suitable patients encountered in clinical practice, and many clinicians prescribe ACE inhibitors less frequently and at lower doses than do cardiologists, or remain reluctant to use β-blockers because of the fear of harmful side effects [16]. There is a need to close the gap between the clinical evidence and clinical practice.

The implementation of effective HF therapies can be facilitated by the development of more comprehensive management strategies. Both clinic- and home-based intervention programs may improve the ability of patients to comply with prescribed pharmacological regimens and to promptly recognize the symptoms of clinical decompensation, thus reducing the risk of hospitalization and the burden of related expenditure [17]. Along with a carefully planned follow-up program, a pivotal component of such strategies is to provide information, education, and counseling to the patients and their relatives or support persons.

More appropriate use of existing HF therapies also includes the adoption of the best pharmacological strategy for each patient, avoiding interventions which cannot lead to any benefit. A careful clinical and neurohumoral evaluation of the patient may be a useful guide by which to tailor optimal treatment and achieve the most favorable outcome for that individual patient [18]. When treating patients with end-stage HF, it should be kept in mind that drugs with the ability to slow the progression of the disease have no role, while those providing symptomatic benefits may come to meet the patients desire to feel better at the price of a greater risk of death [19]. Accurate patient profiling is required to tailor such individualized therapies.

Finally, a number of relevant questions concerning the use of currently available HF drugs have yet to be faced or fully elucidated. How much ACE inhibitor do we give to HF patients? Are different β-blocking agents equally effective in HF? Are angiotensin II or aldosterone antagonist therapies safe and effective when given to patients receiving not only an ACE inhibitor but also a β-blocker? Is the use of spironolactone beneficial in patients with mild to moderate symptoms? Is there still a place for digoxin now that β-blockade has entered as mainstay component of the standard therapy for most HF patients? What about the role of angiotensin II and aldosterone antagonists in NYHA class I patients, and that of β-blockers in those in whom asymptomatic left ventricular dysfunction does not follow myocardial infarction? Extensive clinical investigation of these issues might lead to expanding indications for currently available drugs in HF.

References

1. Packer M (1992) The neurohormonal hypothesis: a theory to explain the mechanism of disease progression in heart failure. J Am Coll Cardiol 20:248-254
2. Garg R, Yusuf S, for the Collaborative Group on ACE Inhibitor Trials (1995) Overview of randomized trials of angiotensin-converting enzyme inhibitors on mortality and morbidity in patients with heart failure. JAMA 273:1450-1456
3. Packer M (2001) Current role of beta-adrenergic blockers in the management of chronic heart failure. Am J Med 110(7A):81S-94S
4. Hampton JR (1994) Results of clinical trials with diuretics in heart failure. Br Heart J 72 [Suppl]:S68-S72
5. Soler-Soler J, Permanyer-Miralda G (1998) Should we still prescribe digoxin in mild-to-moderate heart failure? Is quality of life the issue rather than quantity? Eur Heart J 19 [Suppl P]:P26-P31
6. Pitt B, Zannad F, Remme WJ et al, for the Randomized Aldactone Evaluation Study Investigators (RALES) (1999) The effect of spironolactone on morbidity and morta-

lity in patients with severe heart failure. N Engl J Med 341:709-717
7. Jong P, Demers C, McKelvie RS et al (2002) Angiotensin receptor blockers in heart failure: meta-analysis of randomized controlled trials. J Am Coll Cardiol 39:463-470
8. Kostam MA, Mann DL (2002) Contemporary medical options for treating patients with heart failure. Circulation 105:2244-2246
9. Stewart S, MacIntrye K, Hole DJ et al (2001) More "malignant" than cancer? Five-year survival following a first admission for heart failure. Eur J Heart Fail 3:315-332
10. Givertz MM, Colucci WS (1998) New targets for heart failure therapy: endothelin, inflammatory cytokines, and oxidative stress. Lancet 352 [Suppl I]:34-38
11. Cohn JN, Tognoni G, for the Valsartan Heart Failure Trial (Val-HeFT) Investigators (2001) A randomized trial of the angiotensin-receptor blocker valsartan in chronic heart failure. N Engl J Med 345:1667-1675
12. Coats AJ (1999) Heart failure 99: the MOXCON story. Int J Cardiol 71:109-111
13. Shakar SF, Abraham WT, Gilbert EM et al (1998) Combined oral positive inotropic and beta-blocker therapy for treatment of refractory class IV heart failure. J Am Coll Cardiol 31:1336-1340
14. Colucci WS, Elkayam U, Horton DP (2000) Intravenous nesiritide, a natriuretic peptide, in the treatment of decompensated congestive heart failure. N Engl J Med 343:246-253
15. McLalsen A, Konig G, Thimme W (1998) Preventable causative factors leading to hospital admission with decompensated heart failure. Heart 80:437-441
16. Cleland JGF, Swedberg K, Poole-Wilson PA (1998) Successes and failures of current treatment of heart failure. Lancet 352 [Suppl 1]:19-28
17. Stevenson LW (1998) Inotropic therapy for heart failure. N Engl J Med 339:1848-1850
18. Troughton RW, Framptom CM, Yandle TG et al (2000) Treatment of heart failure guided by plasma aminoterminal brain natriuretic peptide (n-BNP) concentrations. Lancet 355:1126-1130
19. Horowitz JD (2000) Home-based intervention: the next step in treatment of chronic heart failure? Eur Heart J 21:1807-1809

The Problem of Recreational Sport in Patients with Mild to Moderate Heart Failure

F. Furlanello[1], F. Terrasi[2], A. Bertoldi[3], R. Cappato[1]

Background

Today some information exists on the beneficial effect of exercise training in patients with mild to moderate heart failure (HF). Consequently, the common belief that rest is the mainstay of treatment in these patients should no longer be accepted [1]. In particular, an improvement in HF patients' quality of life was observed in a prospective study, with a significant correlation between physiological and psychological improvements [2]. It has also been reported in patients with congestive heart failure (CHF) that exercise training is associated with reduction of peripheral resistance and small but significant improvements in stroke volume and reduction in cardiomegaly [3]. Exercise training results in an increase in peak heart rate and partial reversal of chronotropic incompetence in patients with CHF [4].

The Exercise Rehabilitation Trial (EXERT) in patients with HF showed significant increases in 6-min walking distance at 3 and 12 months but little further improvement over time. In addition, adherence to the exercise program was good during supervised training but reduced during home-based training [5]. All studies showed no clinical events or adverse effects on cardiac function that were related to training activity [1–7].

The aim of this presentation is to discuss the practicability of some specific sports activities in patients with nonsevere HF.

HF and Sports Activities

Contrary to previous belief, in some heart disease regular aerobic physical activity, at work or during leisure hours, has been found helpful and can have a

[1] Department of Clinical Arrhythmias and Electrophysiology, Policlinico San Donato, Milan; [2] Villa Bianca Hospital, Trento; [3] Department of Cardiology, S. Chiara Hospital, Trento, Italy

positive effect on the patient's quality of life of [8]. Mechanisms by which physical activity may protect patients from coronary events have been proposed [9, 10]. Improvement of physical performance of the patient with impaired left ventricular function has also been suggested [11].

On the other hand, in subjects with underlying heart disease or primary or secondary arrhythmic disorders [12–14], particularly those who are unaccustomed to such activity or do not take regular exercise [8, 15–18], vigorous sports activity can trigger life-threatening cardiac events such as syncope and cardiac arrest, which if resuscitation fails can lead to sudden death.

Thus, the "exercise paradox" [13] is a threat hanging over sports activity both for competitive athletes and for unsupervised persons, and has given rise to particular recommendations, expert consensus documents, and specific guidelines including suggestions for older athletes with possible cardiovascular disease [8, 14, 19–24].

Notwithstanding the widespread agreement that the overall benefits of physical exertion usually outweigh the risks [1, 15–18, 25, 26], recommendations for sports clearance eligibility in individual patients with HF must be cautious to avoid catastrophic cardiac events related to sports activity. In the clinical setting there are many limitations in the decision-making process about sports activity in a patient with HF:

- At present no exhaustive information is available out of the studies on supervised exercise training in patients with HF.
- Structural heart disease with impaired ventricular function, such as is present in HF, is incompatible with high-intensity sports. Consequently, any type of competitive sports is totally banned for these patients in accordance with current Italian and international guidelines [8, 19–22].
- Arrhythmias are very common in competitive athletes that are usually benign but in some cases can be life-threatening and can lead to arrhythmic syncope, cardiac arrest, and sudden death in the field. There is evidence to suggest that athletic activity can have a trigger effect in the induction of pathological supraventricular and ventricular tachy- and bradyarrhythmias in athletes with "silent" underlying arrhythmogenic pathologies [27–30], generally without HF. We report here some data resulting from our large experience (since 1974) in a population of arrhythmic athletes without apparent heart disease.

Study Experience with Young Arrhythmic Athletes

In our 28-year series of young competitive athletes (age <35 years and identified as having significant arrhythmias, previously considered eligible for athletic activity in agreement with Italian legislation) (Table 1), with a study protocol including invasive and noninvasive diagnostic studies, we had 53 cases of cardiac arrest, fatal in 21 (sudden death), with resuscitation in 32 [14, 27, 30]. The underlying types of heart disease were:

Table 1. Young competitive athletes with arrhythmias studied from 1974 to 2002

	No. of athletes	Male	Female	Average age	Follow-up	Sudden death	Cardiac arrest
Total athletes	2363	2024	339	21.5	3-168	21 (0.8%)	32 (1.4%)
Elite athletes	207	172	35	24.2	3-151	5 (2.4%)	6 (2.9%)

- 1 Commotio cordis
- 1 Long QT syndrome
- 1 Primary electrical heart disease
- 2 Hypertrophic cardiomyopathy
- 3 Lev–Lenègre disease
- 1 Mitral valve prolapse (2 sudden deaths)
- 3 Dilated cardiomyopathy (3 sudden deaths)
- 2 Coronary artery disease (4 sudden deaths)
- 3 Myocarditis (5 sudden deaths)
- 9 Wolff-Parkinson-White (2 sudden deaths)
- 13 Arrhythmogenic right ventricular dysplasia (2 sudden deaths)

To sum up our experience, in this subgroup of 53 young competitive athletes, including elite athletes, with cardiac arrest in the field, no cases with HF were documented and ejection fraction was normal in all cases!

What Type of Sports Activity for Patients with HF?

The Italian classification for sports in relation to cardiovascular risk [20, 31] is based on the following parameters: heart rate, cardiac output, and mean arterial pressure. The classification takes into account the level of cardiac risk created by training, practice, and competition and is subdivided into five groups in relation to the degree of cardiovascular demands, from low to high. Four of these categories are typical competitive sports activities requiring possession of a sports eligibility certificate in agreement with the current Italian legislation [20, 21]: all HF patients are excluded from such sports activity. For patients with HF, only participation in noncompetitive sports with minimum to moderate cardiovascular demands, characterized by constant pumping activity, submaximal heart rate, and a decline in peripheral resistance (Table 2) may be considered [31].

Classification of Noncompetitive Sports Activities

There are some limitations to the general classification of sports according the type and intensity of exercise performed [32], and the problem is particularly important for the subcategory of noncompetitive sports activities that are theoretically open to patients with HF. This subcategory includes sports types with differing myocardial oxygen demands (e.g., jogging vs golf), emotional involvement of the subject (e.g., golf and riflery), and exposure to the environment (e.g., trekking, Nordic skiing, swimming) or to air pollution (running or walking on flat ground). Patients with HF must avoid conditions that can induce effort-related arrhythmias or increase myocardial workload related to emotional involvement or environmental exposure such as hot or cold temperatures or high humidity.

The selection of patients with HF to be permitted noncompetitive sports activities must be rigorous and based on a complete clinical and instrumental knowledge (exercise tests, echocardiography, Holter monitoring) of the individual patient, including information about compliance with drug treatment, effort limitations, the presence of both ambient (Holter monitoring) and effort-related arrhythmias, and the effectiveness of protection conferred by drugs or an implanted device during physical activity.

The ideal HF candidate for a noncompetitive sports activity might be someone previously treated with a supervised global approach of exercise training sessions, including sports-specific forms of exercise (e.g., stretching, aerobic exercise, ball games) combined with psychological and psychosocial elements [11].

Conclusions

For a patient with HF, sports activities may be proposed as the last link in the chain of the current therapeutic approach, with physical exertion that is considered to be safe and beneficial following cardiac rehabilitation, supervised exercise training, and home-based training. The clinical implementation of this stimulating therapeutic program must be safety-related for each individual patient. The main limitations are the looming threat of the exercise paradox and the complex problem of devastating cardiac events, which may be related to effort arrhythmias and have been widely documented even in athletes with apparently normal hearts and without HF.

First of all, before participating in sports activity, each patient with HF must be examined carefully, including complete exercise tests, Holter monitoring, and echocardiography to assess contraindications to exercise and sports activity as well individual exercise capacity. The prognostic value of arrhythmias must be estimated, taking into account, as necessary, more extensive evaluations such as microvolt T-wave alternans (mTWA) study, signal-averaged ECG, electrophysiological study etc. Patients with severe HF (NYHA class IV) must be excluded from the sports activity program.

The specific sport *must* be selected from among those classified as "noncompetitive" (see Table 2). A good practical suggestion may be to favor a sports activity that the patient with HF has practiced before. Emotional involvement

Table 2. Classification of non-competitive sports

Running or walking on flat ground	Cross-country skiing
Roadwork	Skating
Jogging	Noncompetitive canoeing
Cycling on flat ground	Trekking (not excessive)
Swimming	Golf
Riflery	

From [31]

and environmental exposure must be foreseen and taken into account. Today, some innovative systems and services in healthcare, such as computer-based clinical guidelines, have been proposed for the management of patients with HF—they are also useful for a more efficient and extensive selection of subjects eligible for sports activity treatment [33, 34].

References

1. Coats AJ, Adamopoulos S, Meyer TE, Conway J, Sleight P (1990) Effects of physical training in chronic heart failure. Lancet 335:803–804
2. Wielenga RF, Huisveld IA, Bol E, Dunselman PH, Erdman RA, Baselier MR, Mosterd WL (1999) Safety and effects of physical training in chronic heart failure. Results of the Chronic Heart Failure and Graded Exercise study (CHANGE). Eur Heart J 20:851–853
3. Hambrecht R, Gielen S, Linke A, Fiehn E, Yu J, Walther C, Schoene N, Schuler G (2000) Effects of exercise training on left ventricular function and peripheral resistance in patients with chronic heart failure: a randomized trial. JAMA 283:3095–3101
4. Keteyian SJ, Brawner CA, Schairer JR, Levine TB, Levine AB, Rogers FJ, Goldstein S (1999) Effects of exercise training on chronotropic incompetence in patients with heart failure. Am Heart J 138(2 Pt 1):233–240
5. McKelvie RS, Teo KK, Roberts R, McCartney N, Humen D, Montague T, Hendrican K, Yusuf S (2002) Effects of exercise training in patients with heart failure: the Exercise Rehabilitation Trial (EXERT). Am Heart J 144:1–4
6. Halle M, Huonker M, Schmidt-Truckssar A, Irmer M, Korsten-Reck U, Durr H, van de Loo G, Keul J, Berg A (1998) Sports in the heart rehabilitation group—experiences with ambulatory rehabilitation at home. Ther Umsch 55:235–239
7. Sturm B, Quittan M, Wiesinger GF, Stanek B, Frey B, Pacher R (1999) Moderate-intensity exercise training with elements of step aerobics patients with severe chronic heart failure. Arch Phys Med Rehabil 80:746–750
8. Maron BJ, Araujo CGS, Thompson PD, Flechter GF, Bayes de Luna A, Fleg JL, Pelliccia A, Balady GJ, Furlanello F, Van Camp SP, Elosua R, Chaitman BR, Bazzarre TL (2001) AHA Science Advisory. Recommendations for Preparticipation screening and the assessment of cardiovascular disease in masters athletes. An advisory for healthcare professionals from the Working Groups of the World Heart Federation, the International Federation Sports Medicine, and the American Heart Association

Committee on Exercise, Cardiac Rehabilitation, and Prevention. Circulation 103:327–334
9. Hambrecht R, Wolf A, Gilien S et al (2000) Effect of exercise on coronary endothelial function in patients with coronary artery disease. N Engl J Med 342:454–460
10. Roberts WC (1984) An agent with lipid-lowering, antihypertensive, positive inotropic, negative chronotropic, vasodilating, diuretic, anorexigenic, weight reducing, cathartic, hypoglycemic, tranquilizing, hypnotic and antidepressive qualities. Am J Cardiol 53:261–262
11. Stampfli U, Wagner D, Dubach P (1999) Cardiovascular diseases and sports. Schweiz Rundsch Med Prax 88:601–608
12. Albert CM, Mittleman MA, Chae CU et al (2000) Triggering of sudden death from cardiac causes by vigorous exertion. N Engl J Med 343:1355–1361
13. Maron BJ (2000) The paradox of exercise. N Engl J Med 343:1409–1411
14. Furlanello F, Bertoldi A, Fernando F, Biffi A (2000) Competitive athletes with arrhythmias. Classification, evaluation and treatment. In: Bayes de Luna A, Furlanello F, Maron BJ, Zipes DP (eds) Arrhythmias and sudden death in athletes. Kluwer Academic, Dordrecht, pp 89–105
15. Mittleman MA, MaclureM, Tofler GH et al (1993) Triggering of acute myocardial infarction by heavy physical exertion: protection against triggering by regular exertion: Determinants of Myocardial Infarction Onset Study Investigators. N Engl J Med 329:1677–1683
16. Willich SN, Lewis M, Lowel H et al (1993) Physical exertion as a trigger of acute myocardial infarction: Triggers and Mechanisms of Myocardial Infarction Study Group. N Engl J Med 329:1684–1690
17. Gibbons LW, Cooper KH Meyer BM et al (1980) The acute cardiac risk of strenous exercise. JAMA 244:1799–1801
18. Ilkka V (1986) The cardiovascular risks of physical activity. Acta Med Scand 711:205–214
19. Al Sheikh T, Zipes D (2000) Guidelines for competitive athletes with arrhythmias. In: Bayes de Luna A, Furlanello F, Maron BJ, Zipes DP (eds) Arrhythmias and sudden death in athletes. Kluwer Academic, Dordrecht, pp 119–151
20. Comitato Organizzativo Cardiologico per l'Idoneità allo Sport (COCIS) (1996) Protocolli cardiologici per il giudizio di idoneità allo sport agonistico 1995. G Ital Cardiol 26:949–983
21. Biffi A, Furlanello F, Caselli G, Bertoldi A, Fernando F (2000) Italian guidelines for competitive athletes with arrhythmias. In: Bayes de Luna A, Furlanello F, Maron BJ, Zipes DP (eds) Arrhythmias and sudden death in athletes. Kluwer Academic, Dordrecht, pp 153–601
22. Maron BJ, Mitchell J (1994) Recommendations for determining eligibility for competition in athletes with cardiovascular abnormalities. J Am Coll Cardiol 24:848–899
23. Corrado D, Basso C, Thiene G (2001) Sudden cardiac death in young people with apparently normal heart. Cardiovasc Res 50:399–408
24. Thiene G, Basso C, Corrado D (2000) Pathology of sudden death in young athletes: European experience. In: Bayes de Luna A, Furlanello F, Maron BJ, Zipes DP (eds) Arrhythmias and sudden death in athletes. Kluwer Academic, Dordrecht, pp 49–69
25. Fletcher GF (1997) How to implement physical activity in primary and secondary prevention: a statement for healthcare professionals from the American Heart Association. Circulation 96:355–357
26. Siscovick DS, Weiss NS, Fletcher RH et al (1984) The incidence of primary cardiac arrest during vigorous exercise. N Engl J Med 311:874–877

27. Furlanello F, Fernando F, Galassi A, Bertoldi A (2001) Ventricular arrhythmias in apparently healthy athletes. In: Malik M (ed) Risk of arrhythmia and sudden death. BMJ Books, London, pp 316–324
28. Furlanello F, Bertoldi A, Galassi A, Dallago M, Fernando F, Biffi A, Inama G, Loricchio ML, Pappone C (1999) Management of severe cardiac arrhythmic events in elite athletes. Pacing Clin Electrophysiol 22:A165
29. Furlanello F, Bertoldi A, Dallago M, Galassi A, Fernando F, Biffi A, Mazzone P, Pappone C, Chierchia S (1998) Atrial fibrillation in elite athletes. J Cardiovasc Electrophysiol 98[Suppl]:563–568
30. Bertoldi A, Furlanello F, Fernando F, Terrasi F, Furlanello C, Dallago M, Inama G, Galassi A, Cappato R (2002) Risk stratification in elite athletes with arrhythmias. In: Furlanello F, Bertoldi A, Cappato R (eds) Proceedings of The New Frontiers of Arrhythmias 2002. GIAC 5 [Suppl 1]:218–219
31. Dal Monte A (2000) The Italian classification of different sports in relation to cardiovascular risk. In: Bayes de Luna A, Furlanello F, Maron BJ, Zipes DP (eds) Arrhythmias and sudden death in athletes. Kluwer Academic, Dordrecht, pp 11–24
32. Mitchell JH, Haskell WL, Raven PB (2000) Classification of sports. In: Bayes de Luna A, Furlanello F, Maron BJ, Zipes DP (eds) Arrhythmias and sudden death in athletes. Kluwer Academic, Dordrecht, pp 25-30
33. Gronda E (2002) Clinical tool for the management of heart failure patients: the Serendipity Projects. In: Furlanello F, Bertoldi A, Cappato R (eds) Proceedings The New Frontiers of Arrhythmias 2002. GIAC 5[Suppl 1]:4–5
34. Gensini GF, Eccher C, Forti S, Graiff A, Sboner A (2002) A guideline-based shared care through a computer-based cooperative system for the management of heart failure. In: Furlanello F, Bertoldi A, Cappato R (eds) Proceedings The New Frontiers of Arrhythmias 2002. GIAC 5[Suppl 1]:5–7

Wireless Home Monitoring in Permanent Cardiac Stimulation: is it Especially Suitable in Congestive Heart Failure Patients?

D. Igidbashian, M. Barbiero, E. Visentin, M. Gemelli

Introduction

Many of the recent developments in the field of implantable pacemakers (PMs) are aimed at improving the documentation of the PM's function, especially regarding the interaction between the device and the cardiovascular system. This includes the relative weight of intrinsic and PM-induced heart beats, heart rate variations, and the incidence of arrhythmias. These data were developed to enable the device to adapt better and more rapidly to the patient's specific clinical situation. However, the use of this enlarged amount of data still depends on direct interrogation of the PM's "memory", to be performed in a PM clinic. Since the standard follow-up scheme of patients with implantable PMs comprises examinations every 3 to 6 or even 12 months, the reaction time to changes in the patient's situation can be quite long. As a possible solution of this limitation, a novel technology denominated "home monitoring" has recently been developed.

Home Monitoring of Pacemaker

Differing completely from what has been called by the same name since the early 1970s, this PM home monitoring (HM) system is a wireless, completely automatic system of long-distance telemetry (though it can also be patient-activated) integrated in a standard PM. It is the result of a telecardiology project carried out by Biotronik GmbH between 1997 and 2000 and consists of the following four components (Fig. 1):

1. The home monitoring pacemaker. A standard dual-chamber rate adaptive pulse generator (PG) equipped with additional unidirectional long-dis-

Cardiology Department, Cardiac Electropysiology and Electrostimulation Unit, Mater Salutis Hospital, Legnago, Italy

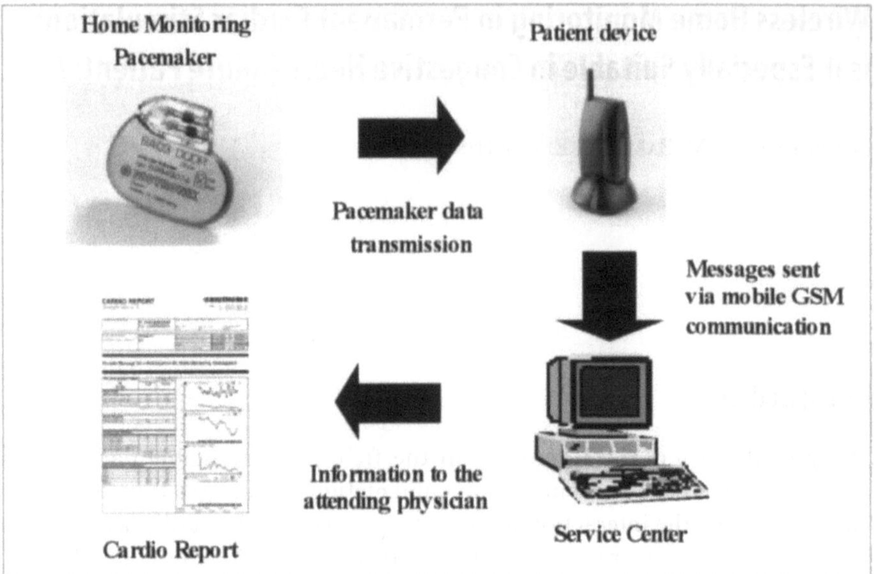

Fig. 1. Components of the home monitoring system

tance telemetry. Using an antenna integrated into the PM's header, it is able to send data over a distance of about 2.5 m to a receiver. The transmitted message contains information from the PM's memory, e.g., trend data, event counters, and histograms. The transmission is automatically initiated once a day, at a time programmed by the physician, which for practical reasons is usually at night. Moreover, the patient can trigger a message at any time by applying a magnet over the PG; besides, in certain risk factors occur, such as a ventricular high rate episode, sensing amplitudes close to the programmed sensitivity, lead failure, or ERI (elective replacement interval), it has the possibility of sending an "event" message. The transmitted parameters are the same for all the different message types. Each message is transmitted seven times within about 1 h in order to increase the probability of reception, in case the patient has momentarily moved out of the GSM (global system of mobile communication) net coverage.

2. Patient device. A customized cellular phone without any other control except an "On/Off" button. The phone comprises a wireless receiver for the long-distance telemetry and a GSM module. The PM messages are relayed through the latter as encrypted short messages via the standard SMS (short message system) protocol.
3. Service center. The service center is the central database where all the messages leaving the PMs are received, automatically decrypted, and subsequently allocated to the physician in charge of the patient. The physician is informed of the medical contents of the messages via the cardio report

(CR) according to his specifications. These relate to the reporting interval, i.e., the interval at which periodic CRs are generated, to the handling of the different event messages that can be produced by the PMs and to the patient-activated messages.

4. Cardio report. This contains data from the PM messages which are displayed in tabular and, for a subset of parameters, in graphic representation mode, together with the long-term average values. This report is currently forwarded to the physician via fax.

Feasibility and Clinical Utility of Home Monitoring

To demonstrate the technical feasibility and clinical utility of this type of wireless information transfer from a PM, allowing the possibility of home monitoring, a European multicenter clinical investigation was started in June 2001 [1, 2]. The patient enrollment phase of this investigation has now been completed. One hundred twenty-two patients with an indication for rate- or non-rate-adaptive dual-chamber pacing had first-generation home monitoring PMs (model BA03 DDDR) implanted. The research protocol provided for the telemetric capability of the device to be activated on hospital discharge and followed for 3 months [1, 2]. During this period, the PM automatically emitted a periodic message once every 24 h, usually programmed to do so during the night. For the first 2 weeks of follow-up, the possibility of patient-triggered messages was also enabled and the patients were asked to manually trigger a message at least once a day during this time interval to test the feasibility of this function. The patients did not have to carry the patient device with them all the time, but were asked to place it on their bedside table. All the messages received in the service center were immediately forwarded to the attending physician as CRs. The reliability and technical feasibility of home monitoring in PM therapy, which was the primary goal of the investigation, was defined as seamless monitoring of the enrolled patients, meaning that any interruptions in the sequence of the home monitoring messages must be rare and brief.

To date, 106/122 of the enrolled patients have finished the study. The mean age of the patients was 70 ± 10 years (range 37-87 years). So far, 7429 periodic CRs (from automatically generated messages) and 996 patient-activated CRs have been created and analyzed, both by the attending physician and by the service center. The preliminary and intermediate results of these have been reported in detail and published [2-4]. In brief, the results indicate that automatic supervision of implantable PMs by home monitoring is technically feasible and reliable, and hence, in accordance with the study protocol, home monitoring enables seamless GSM-net-based supervision of patients with implantable PGs. In particular, the transmissions triggered automatically at night appeared to be quite reliable. This supports the usefulness of the current design of the home monitoring system. On the other hand, the patient-activated messages appeared to be slightly less successful, probably indicating the necessity for a revision in the control mechanisms for the patients.

Regarding the clinical part of the study, the following diagnostic data were reported and analyzed: mean ventricular (V) heart rate (HR); maximal VHR (expression of the shortest V-V interval); percentage of atrial (A)-sensed events (A_S/A_X); percentage of V-sensed events (V_S/V_X); percentage of V-sensed events preceded by A events (A_XV_X/V_X); percentage of intrinsic AV conduction (A_SV_S/A_XV_X); percentage of PM-mediated AV conduction (A_SV_S/A_XV_X and A_PV_S/A_XV_X); maximal ventricular extrasystoles (VES) (V-sensed events not preceded by A-sensed or paced events) frequency per hour; VES couplets, triplets, and runs (i.e., 2, 3, 4, subsequent VES) and ventricular tachycardias (VTs; >8 VES).

The analysis of these data, directed also at assessing possible fields of application, gave interesting insights into the effects of pharmacological therapy. For example the variations in the mean VHR, percentage of A_S/A_X and A_SV_S/A_XV_X yielded information about the effects of drugs such as beta-blockers, digoxin, and certain Ca antagonists; the maximal VHR and the percentage of A_S/A_X gave information about atrial premature events, while the VES hourly frequency and maximal VHR provided data regarding premature V beats, permitting supervision of the efficacy of antiarrhythmic drugs in some of the patients.

Moreover, in addition to the direct detection of rhythm disturbances such as VES, repetitive VES, runs, or VT, of parameters indicating other arrhythmias such as atrial fibrillation (AF), and of data suggesting AV synchrony impairment or sudden changes in HR and A and V sensing, a statistical analysis was performed of combinations of these data with the aim of finding parameters that could automatically identify specific clinical correlations. This permitted automatic identification of all the patients who presented AF, whether paroxysmal or persistent, symptomatic or not, besides identifying a significant number of patients with supra-ventricular tachycardias (SVT) or exit blocks or a high incidence of VES or of VES runs.

Thus, the home monitoring technology, even on the basis of the still incomplete results of the European study, appears to be quite useful already in monitoring dynamic situations which may benefit from closely supervised therapy.

Home Monitoring in Congestive Heart Failure

Among the clinical conditions which might benefit from continuous pacemaker home monitoring, because of its incidence, clinical manifestations, and progression, congestive heart failure (CHF) appears to be particularly indicated. In fact, the incidence of CHF in the average PM patient population aged 65 years and over is approximately 2-5%, increasing to up to 10% in the very elderly aged over 80 [1, 5, 6]. It is the commonest cause of hospitalization in the over 65s and accounts for about 5% of all medical admissions in most countries, absorbing 1.5%-2.5% of the health expenditure in the industrialized countries [5].

CHF is regarded as the result of a dynamic process in which compensatory mechanisms condition an additional disease progression. This compensatory response to an initial cardiac injury, intended to preserve cardiac function, involves activation of the neuroendocrine system, and in time, cardiac remodeling, ventricular dilatation, and fibrosis. Further RAA activation and an increased expression of vasopressin, nitrous oxide, and cytokines contribute to further progression of heart failure.

Ventricular dysfunction is responsible for the majority of CHF manifestations. The progressive deterioration of the dysfunction, generally quantified by an increase in NYHA class, is usually associated with symptoms due to the increase of liquid retention, tachycardia, and particularly, an increased susceptibility to arrhythmias. Among the latter, AF has been demonstrated to increase significantly with the progression of CHF [7]. Moreover, results of recent large randomized mortality trials have shown that of the almost 90% of heart failure patients who die from cardiovascular causes, 50% do so from progressive heart failure while the remainder die suddenly [8, 9]. The studies have also shown a strong relationship between cardiovascular death and NYHA class progression, while sudden death appears to show the opposite behavior [8]. In addition, a significant increase in the PR interval and of the QRS >120 ms has also been associated with progression of NYHA class in CHF patients [7].

Although the current drug therapy based on a combination of ACE inhibitors or AT1 receptor blockade, beta-blockers, diuretics, spironolactone, and digoxin is indisputably useful in CHF patients [6], these agents may also, sometimes, cause severe side effects such as AV conduction disturbances or severe bradychardia with beta-blockers or an increased incidence of arrhythmias with diuretics.

In the clinical setting of CHF in patients needing cardiac pacing, current PM home monitoring technology is capable of remotely monitoring several parameters which can be used to closely monitor many aspects of this usually severe disorder. Among these parameters, the following can be very useful:

- Mean ventricular heart rate
- Atrial intrinsic rhythm, atrial extrasystoles in addition to the number and duration of mode switch activations
- Ventricular intrinsic rhythm
- Frequency of ventricular extrasiystoles, couplets, triplets, and runs
- Number of VTs and their maximum duration
- AV synchrony; AV conduction with spontaneous intrinsic rhythm; AV conduction with atrial pacing, atrio-synchronous ventricular pacing, and dual-chamber stimulation
- Automatically triggered event messages regarding alarming situations such as ventricular runs and VTs

Moreover, the system monitors the atrial and ventricular leads, the amplitudes of the P and R wave, and the battery status, sending event messages in case of lead check failure or P and R wave reduction to less than 50% of the safety margin or ERI parameters.

In CHF patients, the above home monitoring data, in addition to supervision of the incidence of side effects of the medications, can also permit evaluation of several of the desired effects of drugs, such as changes in ventricular heart rate due to beta-blockers and digoxin or a reduction in the incidence of ventricular premature complexes at rest and of arrhythmia under physical load with spironolactone. In brief, it consents real-time control of drug therapy response and prompt correction of undesired effects. Moreover, it makes it possible to monitor the emergence or progression of arrhythmias and the detection of previously non-existent or undetected life-threatening arrhythmias such as VES runs or VTs. Additionally, the possibility of overseeing the heart rate variations and documenting any spontaneous or drug-induced reductions, which seem to be associated with improved survival [10], appears to be quite useful clinically.

Further, early detection of clinical destabilization, on the basis of remote monitoring of determinate parameters such as those above mentioned, may allow it to be corrected early, in the patient's home, before further deterioration of the situation. This sort of intervention could thus reduce the need for hospital admission or repeated readmissions, in line with the recent tendency towards home management of patients with chronic HF [11].

The appraisal of the manifest utility of home monitoring in CHF patients has encouraged the developers and producers of the system, also to apply the home monitoring technology to their triple-chamber PM, which is specifically designed for ventricular resynchronization therapy in CHF patients. The new model in question, denominated Triplos LV-T, was implanted for the first time by us on 30 September 2002 in a patient with severe post-myocardial-infarction CHF, just before this paper was submitted. Because of the very short time since the implant, we have not yet had the opportunity of assessing the utility of the home monitoring feature in this severely compromised patient.

Acknowledgements: The European Study Group on Home Monitoring Technology in Pacemaker Therapy consists of: G. Baumann, Berlin; J. Gill, London; A. Hartmann, Leipzig; D. Igidbashian, Legnago; L. Jordaens, Rotterdam; M. Santini, Rome; M. Schubert, Chemnitz; A. Schuchert, Hamburg; C. Stellbrink, Aachen; E. Wunderlich, Dresden; M. Zabel, Berlin.

References

1. Stellbrink C, Filzmaier K, Mischke K, Löscher S, Hartmann A (2001) Potential applications of home monitoring in pacemaker therapy - a review with emphasis on atrial fibrillation and congestive heart failure. Prog Biomed Res 6:107-114
2. Igidbashian D, Stellbrink C, Hartmann A, Gill JS, Wunderlich E, Santini M (2002) Benefit of permanent pacemaker follow-up with home monitoring. Pacing Clin Electrophysiol 25:534/47 (Abstract)
3. Igidbashian D, Rigatelli G, Zanchetta L (2002) Feasibility of GSM net based pacemaker data transmission using long-range telemetry. Europace 3[Suppl A]:A71, 89/2 (Abstract)

4. Stellbrink C, Hartmann A, Igidbashian D, Gill JS, Wunderlich E, Santini M (2002) Home monitoring for pacemaker therapy: intermediate results of the first European multicenter study. Pacing Clin Electrophysiol 25:686/655 (Abstract)
5. McMurrey JJ, Stewart S (2002) The burden of heart failure. Eur Heart J 4 [Suppl. D]: D50-D58
6. Hunt HA, Baker DW, Chin MH, Cinquegrani MP, Feldman AM, Francis GS et al (2001) ACC/AHA guidelines for the evaluation and measurement of chronic heart failure in the adult: executive summary. Circulation 104:2996-3007
7. Stellbrink C, Auricchio A, Diem B, Briethardt OE, Klass M, Schöndube FA, Klein H, Messmer BJ, Hanrath P (1999) Potential benefit of biventricular pacing in patients with congestive heart failure and ventricular tachyarrhythmia. Am J Cardiol 83:143D-150D
8. Aliot E, de Chillou C, Sadoul N (2002) Ventricular instability and sudden death in patients with heart failure: lessons from clinical trials. Eur Heart J 4 [Suppl D]:D31-D42
9. Ørn S, Dickstein K (2002) How do heart failure patients die? Eur Heart J 4[Suppl D]: D59-D65
10. Lechat P, Hulot JS, Escolano S, Mallet A, Leizerovicz A, Grandjean MW, Pochmaliki G, Dargie H (2001) Heart rate and cardiac rhythm relationships with bisoprolol benefit in chronic heart failure in CIBIS II trial. Circulation 103:1428-1433
11. Ekman I, Swedberg K (2002) Home-based management of patients with chronic heart failure-focus on content not just form. Eur Heart J 23:1323-1325

Electromagnetic Interference in Biventricular and/or ICD Paced Patients

M. Santomauro, L. Ottaviano, D. Da Prato, A. Borrelli, M. Chiariello

Introduction

The potential risk of interaction between electronic systems and implantable cardioverter-defibrillators (ICDs) is well documented and frequently reported on by the scientific press [1–4]. When an electronic medical device is exposed to radiofrequency (RF) signals by electronic systems, the RF energy (Table 1) is absorbed by the electronic circuitry and other components, and functioning may be altered. In a technologically advanced world, radiation from electronic system is omnipresent at home, work, and other everyday environments (Table 2). It is spread by different modes such as electrical leads or cables, electrostatic induction, electromagnetic radiation, intentional transmitters (radar, radio, TV and satellite transmissions, mobile telecommunication systems, scientific equipments), and unintentional transmitters (induction heaters, electrical equipment, car ignition systems, diathermy generators), and constitutes the main source of disturbances to active medical devices equipped with an electrical circuit prone to detect them.

The effects of electromagnetic interference (EMI) on ICDs are based on several physical factors such as the strength of the external signal, the distance between the signal and the ICD, and the frequency range, modulation type,

Table 1. Denominations of electromagnetic radiation frequencies

Denomination	Frequency
Extremely low frequency (ELF)	0-10 kHz
Radio frequency (RF)	30 kHz-300 MHz
Microwave (MW)	300 MHz-300GHz

Department of Cardiology, University Federico II, Naples, Italy

Table 2. Danger scale of electromagnetic interference from electric household appliances

Appliance	Microtesla	Appliance	Microtesla
Ice-cream machine	12	Sewing machine	3
Food grinder	11	Portable radio-tape recorder	2
Washing machine (during spin-drying)	11	Printer	2
Electric typewriter	11	Deep-fryer	2
Electric shaver connected to power line	10	Video tape recorder	2
Carpet cleaner	10	Washing machine (during washing)	2
Vacuum cleaner	10	Hi-fi stereo	2
Personal computer (monitor is the major source of magnetic field)	7-8	Clock radio	1
Air conditioner (single room, movable)	5	Electric knife	1
Hairdryer	4	Desk lamp (halogen lamp)	1
Electric oven	4	Electric grill	0.6
Television set	3	Toaster	0.5

and immunity level of the ICD. The outcome of the effect of EMI on the ICD can be a temporary or permanent malfunction like inhibition of antitachycardia therapy, or a switch from monitor plus therapy to therapy only [5–17] (Table 3).

Table 3. Possible responses to interferences

Inappropriate delivery of shock
Inappropriate delivery of antitachycardia therapy
Inhibition of antitachycardia therapy
Defibrillation therapy inhibition

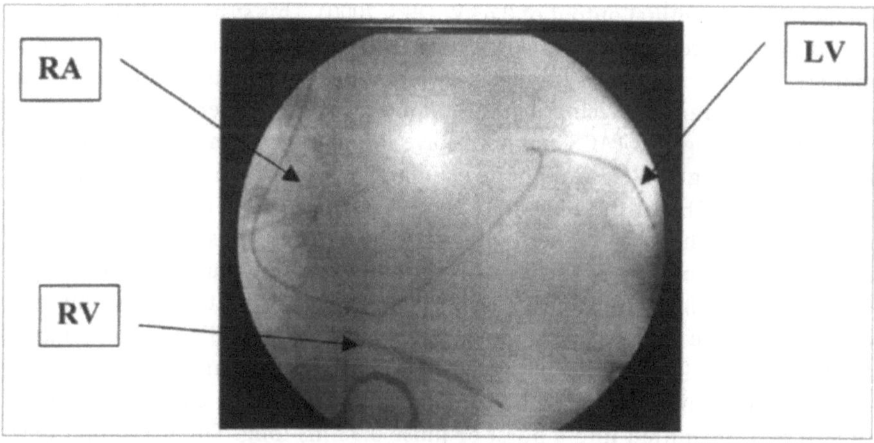

Fig. 1. Biventricular ICD, position of electrocatheter

Left bundle branch block worsens congestive heart failure (CHF) in patients with left ventricular (LV) dysfunction. Asynchronous LV activation produced by right ventricular (RV) apical pacing leads to paradoxical septal motion and inefficient ventricular contraction. Recent studies show improvement in LV function and patient symptoms with biventricular pacing in patients with CHF.

No satisfactory studies on biventricular ICD (BIV-ICD) (Fig. 1) and electronic systems have been reported on.

Cellular Mobile Phones

Cellular phones have become the most recent concern of sources of electromagnetic fields [8–25]. Cellular mobile phone services operate within the frequency ranges 872–960 MHz and 1710–1875 MHz (Table 4). The first cellular system employed was the analog TACS (Total Access Communication System), where the

Table 4. Frequencies of different classes of cellular mobile phone systems

Mobile communication	Frequency range	Higher power level (W)	Medium power level (W)
ETACS	872-950	0.6	0.006
GSM	890-915	2	0.25
DTX 1800	1710-1780	1	0.125
DECT	1880-1900	0.25	0.01
UMTS	1885-2200	n.d.	n.d.

DECT, digital enhanced cordless telecommunication; GSM, global digital phone standard; DTX, discontinuous transmission; UMTS, universal mobile telecommunication system phones have a nominal output of 0.63 W (FEI, 2000). This system is being phased out so that the frequency channels it uses around 900 MHz may be allocated to more recent systems. It uses frequency modulation that results in only very small and essentially random changes in the amplitude of the carrier wave.

Systems using the TACS standard have largely, although not entirely, been replaced by the global digital phone standard (GSM), which mostly operates in either the 900 MHz or the 1800 MHz band. This standard is now widely used in many parts of the world. The digital processing uses phase modulation that again results in only very small and essentially random changes in the amplitude of the carrier wave. To increase the number of users that can communicate with a base station at the same time, a technique called Time Division Multiple Access (TDMA) is employed that allows each channel to be used by eight phones. This is achieved by compressing each 4.6 ms chunk of information to be transmitted into a burst or pulse 0.58 ms long. The maximum powers that GSM mobile phones are permitted to transmit by the present standards are 2 W (900 Hz) and 1 W (1800 Hz). However, because TDMA is used, the average powers transmitted by a phone are never more than one-eighth of these maximum values (0.25 W and 0.125 W, respectively) and are usually further reduced by a significant amount due to the effects of adaptive power control and discontinuous transmission. Adaptive power control (APC) means that the phone continually adjusts the power it transmits to the minimum needed for the base station to receive a clear signal. This can be less than the peak power by a factor of up to a thousand if the phone is near a base station, although the power is likely to be appreciably more than this in most situations. "Discontinuous transmission" (DTX) refers to the fact that the power is switched off when a user stops speaking, either because he/she is listening or because neither user is speaking. So if each person in a conversation is speaking for about half the time, he/she is only exposed to fields from the phone for that half of the conversation. In summary, the largest output from a phone occurs if it is mainly used at large distances from the base station or shielded by buildings, etc. In this situation, the peak powers could approach the values of 2 W (900 Hz) and 1 W (1800 Hz) and the average powers could approach the values of 0.25 W (900 Hz) and 0.125 W (1800 Hz).

A third generation of mobile telecommunications technology has now been agreed and will be introduced in the next few years. In Europe this is called UMTS (Universal Mobile Telecommunication System) and worldwide it is known as IMT-2000 (International Mobile Telecommunications 2000). The frequency bands identified for this system are 1885–2010 MHz and 2110–2200 MHz. The specifications allow some choice in the modulation to be used but it is expected that the main choice will be CDMA (Code Division Multiple Access). The frequency channels will have 5-MHz bandwidths and, as in GSM, each can be used by a number of users at the same time. However, in CDMA, a transmission is "labeled" by a coding scheme that is different for each user. Since all the transmissions occur at the same time, the changes in amplitude of the carrier wave are essentially random (noise-like).

The RF power from a phone is mainly transmitted by the antenna together with circuit elements inside the handset. The antenna is usually a metal helix or a metal rod a few centimetres long extending from the top of the phone. Neither type is strongly directional, although more power is radiated in some directions than others. At points 2.2 cm from an antenna (the distance at which calculations were made), the maximum values of the electric field are calculated to be about 400 V/m for a 2-W, 900-MHz phone and about 200 V/m for a 1-W, 1800-MHz phone, and the maximum magnetic field is calculated to be about 1 μT for both phones. For both 2-W, 900-MHz phones and 1-W, 1800-MHz phones the maximum intensity 2.2 cm from the antenna is very roughly about 200 W/m^2 (this is about one-quarter of the intensity of the sun's radiation on a clear summer day, although the frequency of the emission from a phone is a million or so times smaller). These are the fields and intensities when the antenna is a long way from the head or body. When the antenna is near the body, the radiation penetrates it but the fields inside are significantly less, for the same antenna, than the values outside.

Personal Experience

Our study has evaluated the possible negative effects of environmental electromagnetic radiation on ICDs and bivalvular ICDs (BIV-ICDs), in vitro and in vivo, which increase the possible health risk for patients due to ICD and BIV-ICD malfunction [22–24].

In vitro Tests

In our in vitro study, in collaboration with Ansaldo Trasporti (Naples Research Center) we used an anechoic chamber, in order to facilitate the study of electromagnetic compatibility problems and certify the equipment manufactured by this company. The system has been used to generate electric fields up to a maximum intensity of 40 V/m in the 10 kHz to 1 GHz frequency range. The RF power level needed to generate electric fields of the required intensity is ensured by two amplifiers that deliver 1000 W in the 10 kHz to 220 MHz range, and 100 W in the 100-1000 MHz range, respectively.

We evaluated the effects of a magnetic field with damped wave form motion in the anechoic chamber on 10 single-chamber ICDs (VVI), 15 double-chamber ICDs (DDD), and two BIV-ICDs [22]. ICDs and BIV-ICD were set on standard activity function by a remote control device that monitored before, during and after test, in an anechoic chamber at 1 m above the ground in a horizontal and vertical disposition in order to simulate patient posture.

First, ICD and BIV-ICD were immersed in a magnetic field with damped wave form motion at variable current amplitudes (400 impulse/s, from 10 to 10, then 20 to 30, 40 to 50, and 60 to 80 V/test, current range 100 Å), and then with electromagnetic fields ranging from 30 to 220 MHz and 220 to 1000 MHz.

Susceptibility was demonstrated in the ICDs at 70-80 V/test, we did not observe interference in the BIV-ICDs. The ICD parameters did not change between 200 and 1000 MHz. However, from 30 to 220 MHz we observed temporary malfunctions in 4 of 15 DDD-ICDs tested (particularly between 40.78 and 87.85 MHz), while in 3 ICDs there was an inhibition of antitachycardia therapy.

Our in vitro results show that operating GSM cellular phones can interfere with ICD.

In vivo Tests

In in vivo tests [23, 24] we analyzed 50 ICDs and 6 BIV-ICDs. We tested 21 different models of ICD and 3 different models of BIV-ICD. The tests were performed on patients with implanted ICDs or BIV-ICDs during a standard ambulatory follow-up. The test consisted of positioning cellular phones (ETACS, GSM, and GSM dual-band), during reception of a phone call, at a distance which from 30 cm was gradually reduced to 15, 10, then 5 cm, and at the end was in contact with the patient. The time at which the ICDs and BIV-ICDs were exposed to the electromagnetic field generated by the cellular phones varied from 8 to 10 s for each distance and was for a total of 50 s.

We observed few interference effects caused by the GSM or GSM dual-band cellular phones, only with the antenna on the ICD in 5 ICDs (10%) : inhibition of antitachycardia therapy in two patients, defibrillation therapy inhibition in three. In some cases (PM-dependent patients), the interference was associated with variable symptoms. In no case were symptoms reported when the cellular phone was placed at the ear. Palpitations (8%) were the most commonly reported symptom; light-headedness (3%) or dizziness (3%) and presyncope (0.5%) occurred in a very few cases, syncope was never reported (Table 5). All symptoms stopped when the cellular phone was removed from the ICD.

We observed only one interference effect caused by GSM or GSM dual-band cellular phones on BIV-ICDs, a loss of capture of LV pacing that stopped when the cellular phone was removed from the ICD.

Our results (Fig. 2) show that ICD functioning can rarely be altered by electromagnetic fields generated by cellular phones. The risk of interference is as zero if the cellular phone is placed 15 cm away from the ICD.

Our recommendations are: (1) Keep a distance of at least 15 cm between

Table 5. Side affects seen in in vivo tests of GSM and GSM dual-band cellular phones

Symptoms	% of patients
Palpitations	8
Light-headedness	3
Dizziness	3
Presyncope	0.5
Syncope	0

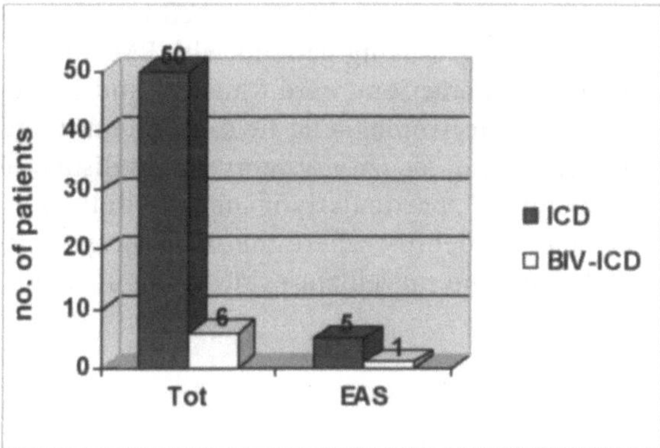

Fig. 2. ICD and BIV-ICD: cellular phone interference results. TOT, total number of ICD and BIV-ICD

the phone and the implantable device; do not carry the phone in the breast-pocket or on the belt if the device is implanted in the chest or abdomen respectively, because digital mobile phones keep emitting signals even though they are in stand-by or receiving mode. (2) Use earphones to keep the phone away from the ear. (3) Switch on the phone only when necessary; if symptoms happen, move away from the source or turn off the transceiver.

Antitheft Electronic Article Surveillance Systems

In respect of antitheft electronic article surveillance (EAS) systems, which are used particularly in supermarkets, shopping centers, and bookstores, interference has been the subject of controversy [26-28, 32–36]. EAS systems typically consist of one or two columns placed opposite each other near entrances and exits; an electromagnetic detection field is produced between the two columns and an alarm sounds if an article with a special tag is carried between the columns (Fig. 3). McIvor [28] has observed inappropriate firing in patients with ICDs in close proximity to a system for controlled access. On some occa-

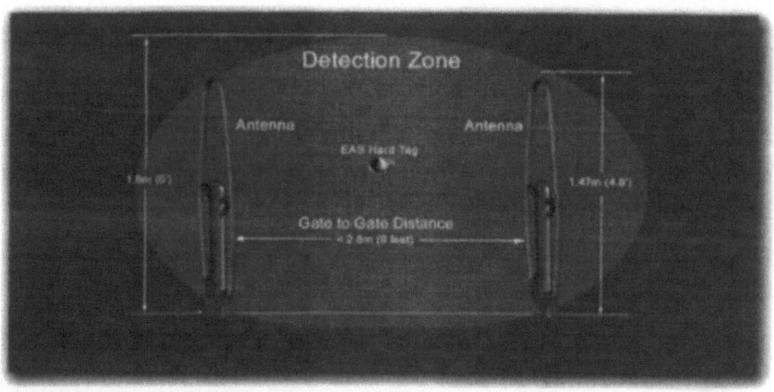

Fig. 3. Anti-theft surveillance system

sions, alarm systems and hand-held metal detectors have resulted in shifts in pacing rate and altered programmed pacing, causing patients with PMs to suffer chest pain and syncope. The device interactions were transient and lasted as long as the patients remained in the electromagnetic field of the antitheft system. It is highly desirable that stores using security systems should display a sign stating "antitheft system in operation", particularly if they are hidden in walls or under the floor. Patients should identify where the security systems are and pass at an ordinary pace through the surveillance gates without standing near or leaning against them.

Personal Experience

Our study was performed in 32 patients with ICDs and with 4 BIV-ICDs followed by our ICD surveillance center. The data from a total of 64 ICD and 8 BIV-ICD patient exposures to EAS were analyzed. The ICDs tested consisted of 21 DDD, and 11 VVI ICDs from five manufacturers and 4 DDD BIV-ICDs. The patients were asked to walk through an antitheft device for up to 30 s, while a six-channel ECG monitored them. Complete interrogation of the ICD and BIV-ICD was performed before and after the exposure of the patients to EAS.

We observed one or more EAS interferences occurring in 5% of the ICDs and 1% of the BIV-ICDs. EAS interference was observed in 4 (18%) of 21 patients with DDD, and 1 (9%) of 4 patients with VVI ICDs. In two case ICDs and one case a BIV-ICD reverted to "monitor only" mode after exposure (Fig. 4).

Our results show that during exposure to EAS, interference with a variety of ICDs was not very common, but in some cases there can be a very high risk to normal functioning of the ICD, particularly if it switches from monitor plus therapy to monitor only. Patients should be advised to not stand unnecessarily in the close proximity of EAS.

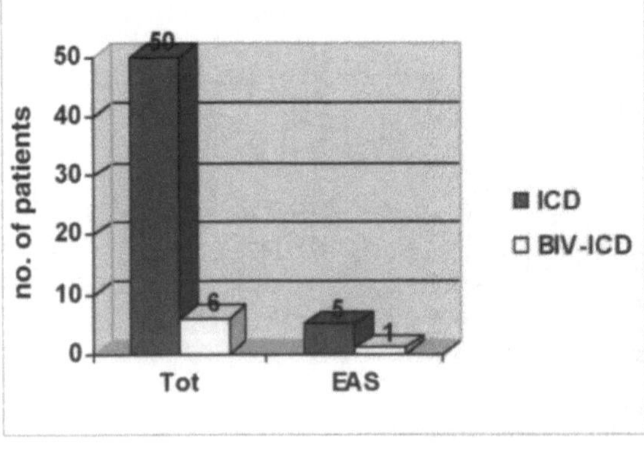

Fig. 4. ICD and BIV-ICD: antitheft surveillance system interference results. TOT, see Fig. 2

Magnetic Resonance Imaging

Magnetic resonance imaging is a widely used techique during which the patient is exposed to strong electromagnetic fields. Patients carrying implanted ICDs and BIV-ICDs should not undergo MRI investigation. In ICD patients, magnetic resonance imaging must be avoided because of it is high risk of damaging the ICD circuit and causing the ICD to malfunction or break.

Conclusions

Electromagnetic interference is a well-known and long recognized problem that can interfere with implanted electronic medical devices. Patients with ICDs can have, with just a little caution, a low risk of interference from electromagnetic fields. However, the development of electronic and new technological systems that can generate electromagnetic fields that can interfere with the normal functioning of ICDs requires continuous monitoring. About BIV-ICDs there is not enough information to evaluate the risks. More studies on electromagnetic interference and BIV-ICDs should be done.

References

1. Irnich W (1984) Interference in pacemakers. Pacing Clin Electrophysiol 7:1021-1048
2. Barbaro V, Bartolini P (1999) External electromagnetic interference with implantable cardiac pacemakers and defibrillators. MESPE J 1:128-133
3. Barbaro V, Bartolini P, Tarricone L (1991) Evaluation of static magnetic field levels interfering with pacemakers. Physiol Med 7(2):73-76
4. Toivonen L, Valjus J, Hongisto M, Mesto R (1991) The influence of elevated 50 Hz electric and magnetic fields on implanted cardiac pacemakers: the role of the lead configuration and programming of sensitivy. Pacing Clin Electrophysiol 14:2114-2122
5. Belott P, Sands S et al (1984) Resetting of DDD pacemakers due to EMI. Pacing Clin Electrophysiol 7:169
6. Hayes D (1992) EMI update. 9th Annual National Symposium on Pacing and Arrhythmia Control, February
7. Telectronics Technical Note (1996) Electromagnetic Interference and the pacemaker patient: an update
8. Barbaro V, Bartolini P, Andrea D et al (1995) Do European GSM mobile cellular phones pose a potential risk to pacemaker patients? Pacing Clin Electrophysiol 18:1218-1224
9. Naegeli B, Osswald S, Deola M, Burkart F (1996) Intermittent pacemaker disfunction caused by digital mobile phones. J Am Coll Cardiol 27:1471-1477
10. Barbaro V, Bartolini P, Bellocci F et al (1998) Electromagnetic interference of digital and analog cellular telephones with implantable cardioverter defibrillators: in vitro and vivo studies. Pacing Clin Electrophysiol 22:626-634
11. Ehles C, Andresen D, Bruggemann T, Thormann L, Wehner H (1995) Functional pacemaker intereference by mobile telephones (abstract). Circulation 92[Suppl 1]:(1)738

12. Meisei E, Kopscek H, Klinghammer L, Daniel WG (1995) Intereference of mobile phones with function of implanted pacemakers - how significant is the risk? (abstract). Circulation 92 [Suppl 1]:(1)738
13. Hayes DL, Von Feldt LK, Neubauer SA, Christiansen JR, Rasmussen MI (1995) Effect of digital cellular phones on permanent pacemaker. Pacing Clin Electrophysiol 18:863-871
14. Nowak B, Rosocha S, Zeuerhoff C et al (1996) Is there a risk for interactions between mobile phones and single-lead VDD pacemakers? (abstract). J Am Coll Cardiol 27 [Suppl A]:236A
15. Carillo R, Williams DB, Traad EA, Schor JS (1996) Electromagnetic filters impede adverse interference of pacemakers by digital telephones (abstract). J Am Coll Cardiol 27 [Suppl A]:15
16. Ellenbogen KH, Wood MH (1996) Chiamata urgente o numero sbagliato? J Am Coll Cardiol 27(6):1478-1479
17. Barbaro V, Bartolini P, Donato A, Militiello C (1996) Interferenze tra telefoni cellulari e pacemaker. Stato dell'arte al 1995. Cardiostimolazione 14:10-19
18. Barbaro V, Bartolini P, Donato A, Militello C, Santini F (1995) GSM and TACS cellular phones can alter pacemaker function. BEMS Abstract Book: Seventeeth Annual Meeting. Boston, Mass, 18-22 June pp 24-26
19. Barbaro V, Bartolini P, Donato A, Militello C (1996) Electromagnetic interference of analog cellular telephones with pacemaker. Pacing Clin Electrophysiol 19:1410-1418
20. Tofani S (1996) Stazioni radio base per la telefonia cellulare e sanità pubblica. AIRM – XIV Atti Congresso Nazionale Caserta, 1-3 1996 July
21. Carrillo R (1995) Preliminary observations on cellular telephones and pacemaker. Pacing Clin Electrophysiol 18:863
22. Santomauro M, Amendolara A, Costanzo A, Damiano M, Noverino P, Russo F, Amendolara M, Chiariello M (1997) Cellular phones and pacemakers: how do they interact? In: Raviele A (ed) Cardiac Arrhythmias 1997. Spinger-Verlag Italia, Milan, pp 514- 521
23. Santomauro M, D'Ascia C, Costanzo A, Ottaviano L, Cresta R, Donnici G, Chiariello M (2000) Interferenze elettromagnetiche nei portatori di device impiantabili: rischi potenziali o reali? Cardiologia 2000: 34° Convegno Internazionale, pp 410-414
24. Santomauro M, D'Ascia C, Costanzo A, Ottaviano L, Cresta R, Donnici G, Chiariello M (2000) How risk mobile telephones for patients with pacemaker or ICD? Cardiac Arrhythmias: Cento 2000 Fifth International Symposium pp 58-63
25. Barbaro V, Bartolini P, Donato A et al (1981) GSM cellular phones interferences with implantable pacemakers: in vitro observations. Proceedings of the V International Symposium on Biomedical Engineering, Santiago de Compostela, pp 275-276
26. Barbaro V, Bartolini P, Donato A, Militello C (1996) Sistema Telepass: analisi dei rischi di interferenza elettromagnetica con pacemaker. Rome, Istituto Superiore di Sanità (Rapporti ISTISAN 96/42) p 56
27. Barbaro V, Bartolini P, Donato A, Militello C, Polichetti A, Vecchia P (1996) Sistemi automatizzati per il controllo degli accessi: analisi dei rischi sanitari. Rome, Istituto Superiore di Sanità (Rapporti ISTISAN 96/2), p 52
28. McIvor ME (1995) Environmental electromagnetic interference from electronic article surveillance devices. Pacing Clin Electrophysiol 18:2229-2230
29. Barbaro V, Bartolini P, Battisti S et al (1991) Esposizione al campo elettromagnetico e corretto funzionamento dei pacemaker: il caso del treno ad alta velocità ETR450. 54° Congresso Nazionale della Società Italiana di Medicina del Lavoro e Igiene Industriale. L'Aquila, 9-12 October 1991, pp 1147-1150

30. Bartolini P (1994) Interazione dei campi elettromagnetici prodotti da una risonanza magnetica con protesi e materiali ferromagnetici. Ann Ist Super Sanità 30:51-70
31. Gimbel JR, Johnson D et al (1996) Sicurezza d'impiego della tecnica di imaging con risonanza magnetica in cinque pazienti con pacemaker cardiaci permanenti. Pacing Clin Electrophysiol 19:913-919
32. Dodinot B, Godenir J et al (1993) Electronic article surveillance: a possible danger for pacemaker patients. Pacing Clin Electrophysiol 16:46-53
33. Lévy S, FESC (1999) ESC Statement on possible interference between electronic article surveillance system & implanted pacemakers or defibrillators. Newsletter, vol 8, no 2.
34. Mugica J, Henry L, Podeur H (2000) Study of interactions between permanent pacemakers and electronic antitheft surveillance systems. Pacing Clin Electrophysiol 23(3):333-337
35. Groh WJ, Boschee SA, Engelstein ED (1999) Interaction between electronic article surveillance systems and implantable cardioverter-defibrillators. Circulation 100:387-392
36. McIvor ME, Reddinger J, Floden E (1998) Study of pacemaker and implantable cardioverter defibrillator triggering by electronic article surveillance devices. Pacing Clin Electrophysiol 21:1847-1861

Organizational and Economic Aspects of the Management of Congestive Heart Failure

R.F.E. Pedretti

Congestive heart failure (CHF) is a major public health problem; in the United States nearly 5 million patients are affected by CHF, and nearly 500,000 patients are diagnosed with CHF for the first time each year [1]. This disorder is the underlying reason for a million office visits and hospital days each year; moreover, nearly 300,000 patients die of CHF as a primary or contributory cause each year, and the number of deaths has increased steadily despite advances in treatment [1].

CHF is primarily a disease of the elderly: approximately 6%-10% of people older than 65 years have CHF, and approximately 80% of patients hospitalized with CHF are more than 65 years old. CHF is the most common Medicare diagnosis-related group (DRG), and more Medicare dollars are spent for the diagnosis and treatment of CHF than for any other diagnosis [1].

Advances in the treatment of CHF and early intervention to prevent decompensation may delay disease progression and improve survival. After the initial evaluation, further diagnostic testing, and the implementation of standard medical therapy, outpatient management strategies focus on maintenance of patient stability. The purpose of the present report is to examine current CHF management strategies and programs [2].

Education and Counseling

Education and counseling of the patient with CHF are essential aspects of patient care that promote clinical stability. The fundamental aspects of education and counseling on positive outcomes for patients with CHF were underscored in a recent study by Serxner et al. [3]. In an intervention notable for lack of contact with a healthcare provider, these investigators tested the impact

Divisione di Cardiologia, IRCCS Fondazione Salvatore Maugeri, Istituto Scientifico di Tradate, Italy

of serial mailings of education materials on readmission rates, compliance, and costs. The educational materials were personalized; self-care was emphasized, and recommended health behaviors were promoted. The materials were mailed to patients in the intervention group four times at 3-week intervals for a total of 12 weeks. Compared with the usual-care control group, patients who received the mailed materials demonstrated a 51% reduction in total admissions and reduced costs and reported better compliance with weighing and following a low-salt diet. A clear and organized plan of patient education and counseling is critical to the achievement of optimal outcomes. Physicians, advanced practice nurses, home health nurses, dietitians, and pharmacists all play important roles in this process [2].

An important place to begin teaching is a clear, understandable, and simple explanation of the pathophysiology and a clarification of the expected symptoms of CHF and symptoms of worsening failure. Patients must understand that progressive dyspnea on exertion or a sudden change in orthopnea or paroxysmal nocturnal dyspnea is not expected. In two investigations, inability of CHF patients to recognize early signs of worsening heart failure delayed their seeking and obtaining appropriate medical therapy [4, 5]. One goal of self-management is to have patients understand the role of fluid retention in worsening symptoms and be able to seek care early, thereby avoiding hospitalization [2]. Initially, close communication between the patient and healthcare provider about dosage adjustments is essential if self-management is to be effective. If patients or their families are unable or unwilling to assume this degree of responsibility, alternatives include home visits by a nurse to administer a diuretic or "drop-in" visits by the patient to a heart failure clinic or physician's office. Patients should also be encouraged to follow dietary recommendations as well as activity and exercise prescriptions. The goals of education and counseling are to assist patients in complying with the therapeutic regimen, to maintain clinical stability and function, and to improve their quality of life. These goals are best achieved when the patient and family are knowledgeable about every aspect of the condition and treatment and are active participants in the plan of care.

Hospital Discharge and Outpatient Heart Failure Management Programs

The facilitation of a CHF patient's successful transition into the outpatient setting begins in the hospital with the implementation of a discharge plan. A successful transition can be achieved through a focused, comprehensive, multidisciplinary discharge plan that begins immediately after admission and is re-evaluated several times during the patient's hospital stay. The patient and family are important members of the multidisciplinary discharge planning team.

There is considerable diversity among outpatient heart failure management programs. These programs were designed and implemented primarily to reduce hospitalization rates and associated costs. In most programs, an improvement in quality of life also was a major goal. Although there is some overlap, the programs studied can be classified as follows:

1. Specialty heart failure clinics
2. Specialty heart failure care outside the clinical setting that involves community outreach
3. Increased access to primary care

Specialty Heart Failure Clinics

In the heart failure clinic model, care is delivered in an outpatient setting by practitioners with heart failure expertise to patients who attend the clinic. In some cases, one or more members of the program team deliver care while the patient is still in the hospital, but the primary site of care delivery is an outpatient clinic. In nurse-coordinated or nurse-facilitated models, the nurse assists cardiologists in coordinating or facilitating care. In nurse-managed or nurse-directed care, a nurse- usually an advanced practise nurse - has primary responsibility for the day-to-day care of patients.

Community Outreach

In specialty heart failure care outside the clinic setting that involves community outreach, care is delivered primarily in patients' homes. Patients do not routinely go to a clinic or other outpatient setting to receive care; rather, the healthcare provider calls on the telephone or comes to the home.

Increased Access to Primary Care

Weinberger et al. [6] studied the impact of intensive primary care on outcomes in 1396 patients (100% were men, 504 with heart failure) who were veterans who had been discharged from the General Medical Service of Veterans Affairs Medical Centers with a diagnosis of diabetes, chronic obstructive pulmonary disease, or heart failure. Using a randomized controlled clinical trial, these investigators assigned enrolled patients to either usual care or a program of increased access to primary care. The intensive primary care program included care directed by teams of primary care physicians and nurses. Care consisted of (1) assessment by a primary care nurse before patient discharge of postdischarge needs, provision of relevant educational materials, and assignment of a primary care physician with a card given to the patient that contained the names and numbers of the primary care team; (2) a visit by the primary care physician before discharge to discuss the postdischarge regimen; (3) a clinic appointment within 1 week of discharge; (4) a telephone call from the primary care nurse within 2 days of discharge to assess problems; and (5) revision of the therapeutic plan by the physician and nurse at clinic visits. Outcomes included significantly greater numbers of rehospitalizations, hospital days, and multiple admissions in heart failure patients randomized to the program of increased access to primary care compared with the usual-care group. There was no difference in quality of life between the groups, but patients in the intervention group reported greater satisfaction with care.

Conclusions

The incidence of heart failure is increasing. It is therefore incumbent on healthcare providers to evaluate their heart failure practices and to incorporate the most current knowledge of the pathophysiology, assessment, and treatment modalities for heart failure into their patient care. Current practice guidelines provide a basis for the treatment of patients with heart failure. Critical to the success of heart failure management is the discharge planning process and follow-up in the outpatient setting. Integration of medical care and patient education with close communication between inpatient and outpatient care providers is essential. Monitoring and enhancement of patient compliance are the responsibility of both in-hospital and outpatient heart failure team members. An integrated and innovative approach to the management of heart failure patients based on consensus recommendations can contribute to improved patient outcomes, including reduced morbidity rates, improved functional status and quality of life, enhanced compliance, reduced rates of rehospitalization, reduced costs, and prolonged survival.

References

1. Hunt Sa, Baker DW, Chin MH, Cinquegrani MP et al (2001) ACC/AHA Guidelines for the evaluation and management of chronic heart failure in the adult. Circulation 104:2996-3007
2. Grady KL, Dracup K, Kennedy G et al (2000) Team management of patients with heart failure. A statement for healthcare professionals from the Cardiovascular Nursing Council of the American Heart Association. Circulation 102:2433-2456
3. Serxner S, Miyaii M, Jeffords J (1998) Congestive heart failure disease management: a patient education intervention. Congestive Heart Failure 4:23-28
4. Friedmann MM (1997) Older adults' symptoms and their duration before hospitalization for heart failure. Heart Lung 26:169-176
5. Francio G (1998) Approach to the patient with severe heart failure. In: Rose E, Stevenson L (eds.) Management of end-stage heart disease. Lippincott-Raven, Philadelphia pp 39-52
6. Weinberger et al

CURRENT TRENDS AND TREATMENTS OF ATRIAL FIBRILLATION AND FLUTTER

Atrial Fibrillation: New Insights into Electrophysiologic Mechanisms

E.N. Prystowsky, B.J. Padanilam

Introduction

Anyone who considers the mechanism(s) of a tachyarrhythmia in humans must address both potential arrhythmia triggers as well as anatomic substrate. The anatomic substrate includes not only alterations in the myocardial architecture (for example fibrosis), but also ion channel disturbances. Arrhythmia triggers are protean and typically multiple in a given individual. For example, it is common for a patient with atrial fibrillation (AF) to relate onset of their arrhythmia on one occasion during sleep but on another occasion during activity. Further, while a patient may be susceptible to a specific trigger (for example alcohol or caffeine) it is very uncommon for the ingestion of such substances consistently to initiate their tachycardia. The diversity and complexity of arrhythmia triggers for a specific patient make it very difficult to target suppression of the triggers as the therapeutic pharmacologic goal.

Disturbances in ion channels or myocardial architecture are clearly arrhythmogenic, as evidenced by a wealth of data accumulated over many decades. Classic examples include the propensity for sustained ventricular tachycardia and ventricular fibrillation in a patient after myocardial infarction, reentry using an accessory pathway as part of the tachycardia circuit, and polymorphic ventricular tachycardia and ventricular fibrillation in the long QT syndrome [1]. Pathology studies of patients with long-standing (AF) demonstrate changes consistent with the promotion of reentrant circuits, but it is not clear whether the anatomic changes cause or are the consequence of AF [2, 3].

Suppression of an arrhythmia with an antiarrhythmic drug often gives few clues as to the relative importance of substrate versus trigger for that patient. For example, in patients with atrioventricular (AV) reentry in whom the antiarrhythmic drug clearly blocks conduction over the accessory pathway a modification of the anatomic substrate is likely the major cause for suppres-

The Care Group, LLC, Indianapolis, Indiana, USA

sion of tachycardia [4]. In other patients with AV reentry, antiarrhythmic drugs that do not block conduction over the accessory pathway and, in fact, allow tachycardia induction at electrophysiologic study can still prevent tachycardia recurrence, possibly by suppressing triggers of the arrhythmia [5]. This distinction in AV reentry can be postulated by evaluating drug effects on a critical part of the tachycardia circuit, which is not possible in AF. The fact that a drug alters atrial conduction or refractoriness may have no relevance to the clinical outcome for a patient with AF. Nonpharmacologic approaches including surgery and catheter ablation present a better understanding of how the treatment prevents the arrhythmia. Examples include catheter ablation of accessory pathways to prevent AV reentry or the cavotricuspid isthmus to prevent atrial flutter. Isolation of the pulmonary veins to prevent AF, discussed in detail below, is a good example of an apparent isolation of the triggers for this arrhythmia. In reality, for many arrhythmias both the substrate and trigger are important, as clearly demonstrated in patients who undergo successful ablation of AV and AV node reentry, who typically have ectopy after the procedure that once resulted in sustained tachycardia.

The remainder of this paper will deal with experimental and clinical observations in patients with AF that need to be considered when deciding the relative importance of the atrial substrate and triggers for initiation and maintenance of AF. These factors include epidemiology, pathology, experimental models, and results of surgery and catheter ablation to cure AF.

Epidemiology of AF

AF is primarily a disease associated with aging. The prevalence appears to be less than 1% in those under 60 years of age but above 6% in patients 80 years or older [6]. In the recent Anticoagulation and Risk Factors in Atrial Fibrillation study, the prevalence of AF was 0.95% among 1.9 million patients evaluated in a large community practice [7]. As in other studies, prevalence increased markedly with age, and for men it was over 10% in those 80 years or older. Why is it that AF increases so dramatically with age? One potential answer relates to the changes in the atria that occur with aging [8]. Alterations in atrial tissue begin in the first year of life, and by the fourth and fifth decades there are small fat spots appearing in the right atrium in the region of the AV node and septum [8]. In the left atrium the endocardial thickening is diffuse and increases with age. By the sixth decade there is an increase in sclerotic changes associated with hypertrophy and collagen replacement. Eventually there is loss of myocardial fibers and an increase in fatty metamorphosis. These anatomic abnormalities that occur with aging clearly support an anatomic substrate as a key component for the mechanism of AF.

Davies and Pomerance [3] performed pathologic studies of the atria in patients with AF who died. They subgrouped patients into those in whom AF lasted for less than 2 weeks before death and those who had AF for more than 1 month before death. In nearly 75% of cases of prolonged AF there was loss of sinus node and internodal tract muscle as well as atrial dilatation. Importantly, these authors offered an alternative explanation for the pathologic changes seen and wondered whether the fibrotic changes were the cause or consequence of the arrhythmia. This observation directly addresses the notion that AF begets AF. More recent studies in patients with lone AF have analyzed atrial biopsies and have shown histologic changes consistent with myocarditis [9]; in some patients there have been high serum levels of antibodies against myosin heavy chains [10], the significance of which is not clear. In our opinion, the significance of atrial anatomic changes in patients with lone AF requires more investigation.

Lone AF occurs more frequently than previously reported and accounted for 35% and 29% of all patients with AF in two large populations studies [11, 12]. In these patients it seems reasonable to consider triggers of primary importance, although it is impossible to rule out substrate abnormalities that are subtle, for example, extended distribution of prolonged and fractionated atrial electrograms [13].

Hypertension is a condition very frequently associated with AF [11, 12]. AF is also relatively common in patients with congestive heart failure. Are there any clues to the relative importance of substrate and triggers as the cause of AF in these two conditions? Patients with congestive heart failure likely have diseased atria in association with ventricular dysfunction, and anatomic abnormalities of the atria are to be expected. This could lead to alterations in atrial conduction and refractoriness, allowing the milieu for reentry. This might also be true in some patients with hypertension. Alternatively, it is equally possible that the increased atrial volume and pressure that may occur with these pathologic states could lead to increased atrial triggers. Stretch-induced currents in the atrium are mediated through stretch-activated channels [14]. Many studies in ventricular tissue have shown that mechanical stretch can alter changes in ventricular refractoriness but also results in stretch-induced depolarizations that lead to ectopy. Contraction-excitation feedback has also been demonstrated in atrial tissue [14]. In the atrial experiments there was a marked increase in inducibility of AF, but it is feasible that in humans increased atrial volume and pressure could result in increased automaticity, for example, from the pulmonary veins. This remains to be tested. One other common association with AF is coronary artery disease. While not proved, it seems reasonable that this would lead to changes in atrial substrate more commonly than in atrial triggers.

In summary, the above analysis of epidemiologic factors associated with AF leaves one with more questions than answers regarding the mechanism of AF. It is tempting to dichotomize the primacy of triggers to those younger patients with lone AF and the primacy of substrate for reentry to elderly individuals, but this is obviously too simplistic. More likely, there is a delicate balance between these two mechanisms in many patients that is necessary to result in persistent AF. One should not assume that mere atrial changes with aging result in a marked susceptibility to AF. We have performed atrial and ventricular programmed electrical stimulation in thousands of patients with ventricular arrhythmias who are over 60 years old and it is decidedly uncommon to initiate AF in these individuals. Even the recent results of the trial of the angiotensin-converting enzyme inhibitor irbesartan to lower the rate of AF recurrence in patients also treated with amiodarone can be explained by a salutary effect to alter atrial remodeling or a hemodynamic effect to reduce triggered activity by interfering with contraction-excitation feedback mechanisms [15].

Experimental Data

Reentry

The multiple wavelet hypothesis was proposed by Moe et al. [16, 17] as the mechanism of AF. In this theory, the larger the number of wavelets present, the more likely it is that AF will sustain. The wavelet number depends on the atrial mass, refractoriness, and conduction velocity in various areas of the atria. In essence, the most favorable situation for AF to sustain would be a large atrial mass with short refractory periods associated with conduction delay. Allessie et al. [18] validated the multiple wavelet hypothesis of Moe. Reentry may not require a significant mass of tissue, as suggested by the work of Spach and associates [19, 20], who demonstrated the concept of anisotropic reentry in small pieces of atrial tissue. More recently, stable microreentrant sources have been described as the mechanism of AF in contrast to the multiple larger wavelet hypothesis [21].

In summary, there are substantial data in animal models for the occurrence of multiple reentrant circuits as the cause of AF and more recently for single or few microreentrant circuits to provide fibrillatory conduction.

Ectopic Focus Theory

Scherf and colleagues [22, 23] advanced the concept of a rapidly firing ectopic focus as the cause of AF. Topical application of aconitine to the atria yielded observations that supported the focal mechanism theory for AF. In essence, these experiments confirmed that a single rapidly firing focus could lead to fibrillatory conduction, and when the focus was suppressed the AF terminated. This theory was overwhelmed by the preponderance of data on reentry and remained dormant for many years. It was recently rekindled by the important observations of Haïssaguerre and colleagues [24, 25], who demonstrated the ability to prevent AF with discrete applications of energy given to various sites around the pulmonary veins (PVs) in the left atrium. The PV foci likely come from the myocardial sleeves described by Nathan and Eliakim [26]. Cheung [27] demonstrated PV ectopic foci and conduction block to the left atrium in an experimental model. Focal atrial discharges as the putative cause of AF have also been demonstrated in right atrial sites [28] and possibly from the ligament of Marshall [29].

Without a doubt, electrophysiologic investigations into the mechanism and cure of AF involving PV focal discharges have become the research du jour for the electrophysiologic community. Chen et al. [30] analyzed PV cardiomyocytes from dogs undergoing an experimental protocol of rapid atrial pacing. Compared with control, the PV cardiomyocytes from the rapid pacing model had faster beating rates and shorter action potential durations. Further, the cardiomyocytes with pacemaker activity had a higher incidence of delayed or early afterdepolarization.

Studies of the electrophysiologic properties of human PVs have also been done [31, 32]. In patients with frequent episodes of paroxysmal AF, the distal PV has the shortest effective refractory period. Ectopic beats from the PVs were suppressed with propranolol, verapamil, and procainamide [31]. A comparison of PV electrophysiologic properties was performed in patients with and without paroxysmal AF [32]. In patients with AF the PV effective refractory period was shorter than that of the left atrium, whereas the reverse was true in the control patients. The PV effective refractory periods and functional refractory periods in patients with AF were shorter than those observed in control patients, but left atrial effective refractory periods were not significantly different. Decremental conduction was more frequently observed in PVs in patients with AF.

In summary, there are now robust data from experimental models as well as humans confirming various venous structures in the heart, most commonly the PVs, to be a potential source of a rapidly firing foci that could clearly lead to fibrillatory conduction or merely periods of short bursts of rapid atrial tachycardia.

Results from Surgery and Radiofrequency Catheter Ablation to Cure Atrial Fibrillation

Surgical Approaches

Cox et al. [33] through a series of modifications over time developed the maze surgical procedure to cure AF. This successful operation has not been widely adopted by clinicians. The original concept of the procedure was based on a reentry model of AF and attempted to create a series of lines throughout the right and left atria that would prevent maintenance of reentrant wavelets. Importantly, a key part of this surgical procedure is isolation of the PVs from the left atrium. Surgical modifications of this approach targeted primarily at isolating the PVs effectively prevent recurrent AF [34, 35]. Kottkamp et al. [36] recently reported a video-assisted minimally invasive surgical technique to create contiguous lesion lines involving the PV orifices and the mitral annulus using radiofrequency energy. During follow-up of over 1 year more than 90% of patients were free of AF. The above, more limited surgical approaches that primarily prevent PV-to-left-atrium conduction certainly support the concept that the area in and around the PVs of the heart is critically important in a substantial number of patients to AF initiation, maintenance, or both.

Radiofrequency Catheter Ablation

Over the past several years several right atrial, left atrial, and combined atrial catheter ablation approaches have been investigated in an attempt to cure AF. At present, the most successful approach appears to be electrical isolation of all the PVs, not only PVs demonstrating ectopic activity. Success, defined by no recurrence of clinical AF in the absence of antiarrhythmic drugs, ranges from 62% to 85% [37-40]. Most investigators have used entrance block to the PVs as a measure of success (Fig. 1). A recent publication that evaluated a combined PV exit and entrance block strategy as a measure of success did not appear to show an advantage over other approaches [40]. It is noteworthy that a substantial number of patients in AF at the time of ablation have restoration of sinus rhythm during the ablation [38, 41]. While it is tempting to implicate a rapidly discharging automatic focus as the cause of AF in these patients [27, 30],

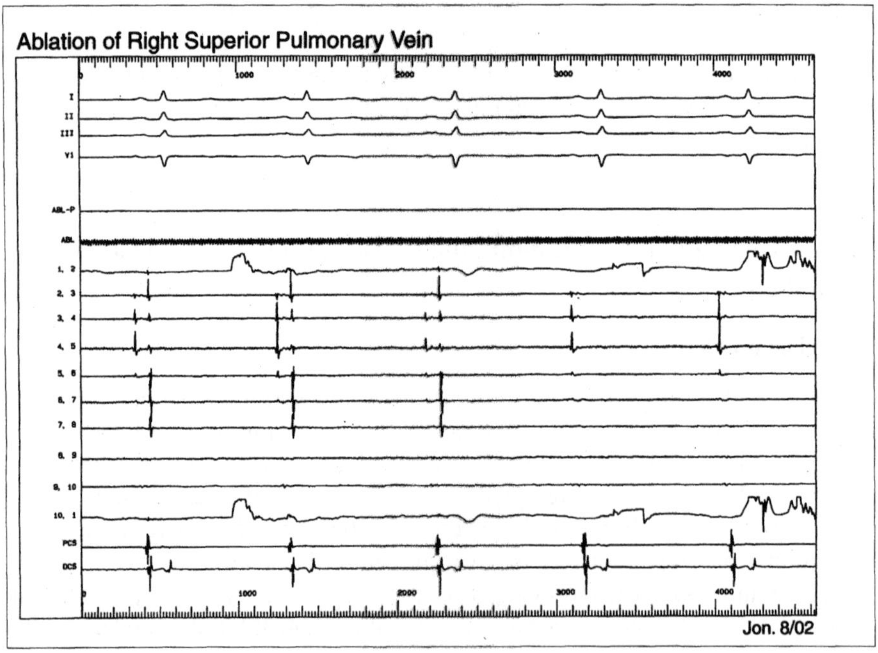

Fig. 1. Entrance block into the right superior pulmonary vein demonstrated during application of radiofrequency energy

experimental data in canine PVs have demonstrated the electrophysiologic substrate for reentry to occur within the PV [42]. Thus, either mechanism could theoretically be possible in this situation.

Summary

There are epidemiologic, pathologic, and experimental data to support reentry as the cause of AF in humans. Alternatively, there are also substantial data to support the primacy of triggers, most likely from the PVs or other venous structures as the mechanism of AF in humans. It may be that triggers are far more important for paroxysmal AF, especially in younger patients without demonstrable heart disease, and reentry remains very important for the development of persistent AF, especially in those individuals with underlying heart disease. Future investigations will likely elucidate the delicate balance between these two mechanisms in various patient subgroups. For the present, regardless of which is the more important mechanism in a patient with AF, if the trigger for AF can be eliminated then a good clinical outcome can be anticipated.

References

1. Prystowsky EN, Klein GJ (1994) Cardiac arrhythmias: an integrated approach for the clinician. McGraw-Hill, New York
2. Prystowsky EN, Katz A (2002) Atrial fibrillation. In: Topol EJ (ed) Textbook of cardiovascular medicine, 2nd edn. Lippincott Williams & Wilkins, Philadelphia
3. Davies MJ, Pomerance A (1972) Pathology of atrial fibrillation in man. Br Heart J 34:520-525
4. Prystowsky EN, Klein GJ, Rinkenberger RL, Heger JJ, Naccarelli GV, Zipes DP (1984) Clinical efficacy and electrophysiologic effects of encainide in patients with the Wolff-Parkinson-White syndrome. Circulation 69:278-287
5. Kerr CR, Prystowsky EN, Smith WM, Cook L, Gallagher JJ (1982) Electrophysiological effects of disopyramide phosphate in patients with Wolff-Parkinson-White syndrome. Circulation 65:869-878
6. Fuster V, Ryden LE, Asinger RW et al (2001) ACC/AHA/ESC guidelines for the management of patients with atrial fibrillation: a report of the American College of Cardiology/American Heart Association Task Force on Practice Guidelines and the European Society of Cardiology Committee for Practice Guidelines and Policy Conferences (Committee to Develop Guidelines for the Management of Patients with Atrial Fibrillation). J Am Coll Cardiol 38:1266i-lxx
7. Go AS, Hylek EM, Phillips KA et al (2001) Prevalence of diagnosed atrial fibrillation in adults: national implications for rhythm management and stroke prevention: the anticoagulation and risk factors in atrial fibrillation (ATRIA) study. JAMA 285:2370-2375
8. Bharati S, Lev M (1992) Histology of the normal and diseased atrium. In: Falk RH, Podrid PJ (eds) Atrial fibrillation: mechanisms and management. Raven Press, New York

9. Frustaci A, Chimenti C, Bellocci F et al (1997) Histological substrate of atrial biopsies in patients with lone atrial fibrillation. Circulation 96:1180-1184
10. Maixent JM, Paganelli F, Scaglione J et al (1998) Antibodies against myosin in sera of patients with idopathic paroxysmal atrial fibrillation. J Cardiovasc Electrophysiol 9:612-617
11. Prystowsky EN, Margiotti R, Fogel RI et al (1996) Atrial fibrillation with and without heart disease: clinical characteristics and proarrhythmia risk. Circulation 94:I-191
12. Levy S, Maarek M, Coumel P et al, for the College of French Cardiologists (1999) Characterization of different subsets of atrial fibrillation in general practice in France: The ALFA study. Circulation 99:3028-3035
13. Nakao K, Seto S, Ueyama C et al (2002) Extended distribution of prolonged and fractionated right atrial electrograms predicts development of chronic atrial fibrillation in patients with idiopathic paroxysmal atrial fibrillation. J Cardiovasc Electrophysiol 13:996-1002
14. Reiter MJ (2000) Contraction-excitation feedback. In: Zipes DP, Jalife J (eds) Cardiac electrophysiology: from cell to bedside. Sauders, Philadelphia, pp 249-255
15. Madrid AH, Bueno MG, Rebollo JMG et al (2002) Use of irbesartan to maintain sinus rhythm in patients with long-lasting persistent atrial fibrillation: a prospective and randomized study. Circulation 106:331-336
16. Moe GK, Abildskov JA (1959) Atrial fibrilltion as a self-sustaining arrhythmia independent of focal discharge. Am Heart J 58:59-70
17. Moe GK, Rheinboldt WC, Abildskov JA (1964) A computer model of atrial fibrillation. Am Heart J 67:200-220
18. Allessie MA, Lammers WJEP, Bonke FIM et al (1985) Experimental evaluation of Moe's multiple wavelet hypothesis of atrial fibrillation. In: Zipes DP, Jalife J (eds) Cardiac arrhythmias. Grune & Stratton, New York, pp 265-276
19. Spach MS, Boineau JP (1997) Microfibrosis produces electrical load variations due to loss of side-to-side cell connections: a major mechanism of structural heart disease arrhythmias. Pacing Clin Electrophysiol 20[Pt II]:397-413
20. Spach MS, Dolber PC, Heidlage JF (1988) Influence of the passive anisotropic properties on directional differences in propagation following modification of the sodium conductance in human atrial muscle: a model of reentry based on anisotropic discontinuous propagation. Circ Res 62:811-832
21. Ravi M, Allan S, Chen J, Berenfeld O, Jalife J (2000) Stable microreentrant sources as a mechanism of atrial fibrillation in the isolated sheep heart. Circulation 101:194-208
22. Scherf D, Romano FJ, Terranova R (1948) Experimental studies on auricular flutter and auricular fibrillation. Am Heart J 36:241
23. Scherf D, Schaffer AI, Blumenfeld S (1953) Mechanism of flutter and fibrillation. Arch Intern Med 91:333-352
24. Jais P, Haïssaguerre M, Shah DC (1997) A focal source of atrial fibrillation treated by discrete radiofrequency ablation. Circulation 95:572-576
25. Haïssaguerre M, Jais P, Shah DC et al (1998) Spontaneous initiation of atrial fibrillation by ectopic beats originating in the pulmonary veins. N Engl J Med 339:659-666
26. Nathan H, Eliakim M (1966) The junction between the left atrium and the pulmonary veins: an anatomic study of human hearts. Circulation 34:412-422
27. Cheung DW (1981) Pulmonary vein as an ectopic focus in digitalis-induced arrhythmias. Nature 294:582-584
28. Chen SA, Tai CT, Yu WC et al (1999) Right atrial focal atrial fibrillation: electrophysiologic characteristics and radiofrequency catheter ablation. J Cardiovasc Electrophysiol 10:328-335

29. Hwang C, Karageuzian HS, Chen PS (1999) Idiopathic paroxysmal atrial fibrillation induced by a focal discharge mechanism in the left superior pulmonary vein: possible roles of the ligament of Marshall. J Cardiovasc Electrophysiol 10:636-648
30. Chen YJ, Chen SH, Chen YC et al (2001) Effects of rapid atrial pacing on the arrhythmogenic activity of single cardiomyocytes from pulmonary veins: implication in initiation of atrial fibrillation. Circulation 104:2849-2854
31. Chen SA, Hsieh MH, Tai CT et al (1999) Initiation of atrial fibrillation by ectopic beats originating from the pulmonary veins: electrophysiological characteristics, pharmacological responses, and effects of radiofrequency ablation. Circulation 100:1879-1886
32. Jais P, Hocini M, Macle L et al (2002) Distinctive electrophysiological properties of pulmonary veins in patients with atrial fibrillation. Circulation 106:2479-2485
33. Cox JL, Schuessler RB, D'Agostino JH Jr et al (1991) The surgical treatment of atrial fibrillation, III: development of a definitive surgical procedure. J Thorac Cardiovasc Surg 101:569-583
34. Hioki M, Ikeshita M, Iedokoro Y et al (1993) Successful combined operation for mitral stenosis and atrial fibrillation. Ann Thorac Surg 55:776-778
35. Melo J, Adragao P, Neves J et al (1999) Surgery for atrial fibrillation using radiofrequency catheter ablation: assessment of results at one year. Eur J Cardiothorac Surg 15:851-854
36. Kottkamp H, Hindricks G, Autschbach RR et al (2002) Specific linear left atrial lesions in atrial fibrillation. Intraoperative radiofrequency ablation using minimally invasive surgical techniques. J Am Coll Card 40(3):475-480
37. Haïssaguerre M, Shah DC, Jais P et al (2000) Electrophysiological breakthroughs from the left atrium to the pulmonary veins. Circulation 102:2463-2465
38. Pappone C, Rosanio S, Oreto G et al (2000) Circumferential radiofrequency ablation of pulmonary vein ostia: a new anatomic approach for curing atrial fibrillation. Circulation 102:2619-2628
39. Marrouche NF, Dresing T, Cole C et al (2002) Circular mapping and ablation of the pulmonary vein for treatment of atrial fibrillation. Impact of different catheter technologies. J Am Coll Card 40(3):464-474
40. Gerstenfeld EOP, Dixit S, Callans D et al (2002) Utility of exit block for identifying electrical isolation of the pulmonary veins. J Cardiovasc Electrophysiol 13:972-979
41. Oral H, Knight BP, Ozaydin M et al (2002) Segmental ostial ablation to isolate the pulmonary veins during atrial fibrillation: feasibility and mechanistic insights. Circulation 106:1256-1262
42. Hocini M, Ho SY, Kawara T et al (2002) Electrical conduction in canine pulmonary veins: electrophysiological and anatomic correlation. Circulation 105:2442-2448

Pharmacological Therapy of Atrial Fibrillation and Flutter: Advances and Limitations of Specific Antiarrhythmic Drugs

P. Alboni

A problem that has long been debated is whether in patients with atrial fibrillation (AF) we should try to maintain as far as possible the normal sinus rhythm (SR) by utilizing antiarrhythmic drugs and cardioversion in case of relapses, or only to control the heart rate with drugs that slow atrioventricular nodal conduction (digoxin, β-blockers, calcium channel blockers). The presumed benefits of maintaining SR include the following: better exercise tolerance and a reduction of symptoms, a reduction in the risk of cerebrovascular accidents, improvement of quality of life, and prolonged survival. In fact, however, these possible advantages have never been investigated in large prospective studies. The AFFIRM trial was presented at the last Congress of the American College of Cardiology, but has not been published up to now.

The aim of this trial was to compare the two therapeutic strategies of rhythm control and rate control. The inclusion criteria were the following: an episode of AF documented on electrocardiogram within the last 6 weeks; duration of AF ≥ 6 h and < 6 months; patients aged ≥ 65 years or < 65 years plus ≥ 1 clinical risk factor for stroke (hypertension, diabetes, heart failure, prior stroke or transient ischemic attack, left atrium > 50 mm, left ventricular ejection fraction < 40%). There were no exclusion criteria but, obviously, patients aged less than 65 years without heart disease or risk factors for stroke were not included. During the recruitment period, 4060 patients were randomized to the two arms of the study: (1) rate control and anticoagulation and (2) rhythm control and anticoagulation. The mean age of the patients was 70±9 years, 71% had hypertension, 38% ischemic heart disease, 23% a history of heart failure, and 24% left ventricular ejection fraction (EF) < 40%. The most used antiarrhythmic drugs were amiodarone, sotalol, and propafenone. At 5-year follow-up there was a high prevalence of normal SR (38%) in the rate control arm, despite the fact that these patients did not receive therapy to obtain this effect, and 60% in the rhythm control arm were in normal SR. The primary endpoint, total mortality at 5-year follow-up, was similar in the rate control and rhythm

Divisione di Cardiologia e Centro Aritmologico, Ospedale Civile, Cento (FE), Italy control arms, 26% and 27% respectively. A secondary endpoint, ischemic stroke, occurred in 5.7% of rate control patients and 7.3% of the rhythm control ones (NS). The prevalence of major bleeding was similar in the two arms (2% and 2.1%). Scores on all quality of life measures were similar in the two groups at all time points, and changes with time were similar in both groups. These results demonstrate that in patients with AF and a risk factor for stroke, therapy to control heart rate is at least as effective as therapy to keep the patients in SR with the aim of preventing clinical events.

Another trial (PIAF) with the same study design was recently published [1]. In this study, 252 patients with AF were randomized to rate control and rhythm control strategies and the primary endpoints were symptoms (palpitations, dyspnea, and dizziness) and quality of life after 1-year follow-up. At the end of the observation period, 10% of the rate control patients were in normal SR, versus 56% of the rhythm control patients ($p<0.001$). The results were similar to those of the AFFIRM study. Symptomatic improvement was reported in a similar percentage of patients of both arms. There were no significant differences in terms of the primary endpoint between the two groups at any point during the course of the trial.

What are the clinical implications of these two recent trials? Maintenance of SR with the available therapeutic means does not prevent cardiovascular events and does not reduce mortality; consequently, the choice of therapeutic strategy should be mainly symptom-based. When AF is responsible for severe palpitations, dyspnea, or other symptoms, we should try to maintain SR as far as possible; if the AF-induced symptoms are only slight, there is no indication to force maintenance of SR.

When we choose the rhythm control strategy, the antiarrhythmic agents most used in Europe are the class IA drugs disopyramide and quinidine, the class IC drugs flecainide and propafenone, and the class III drugs amiodarone and sotalol. β-blockers are generally not included in the antiarrhythmic agents; however, metoprolol has been shown to be more effective than placebo [2] and can be considered in some clinical situations.

Class I Antiarrhythmic Drugs

All class I antiarrhythmic drugs have been shown to be superior to placebo, but there are contrasting data on their efficacy, mainly because they were often tested in small patient populations with different clinical characteristics. On the whole, they seem to be effective in preventing symptomatic AF recurrences in about 40%-50% of the patients after 1-year follow-up.

Proarrhythmias and Other Relevant Adverse Effects

Class I antiarrhythmic drugs have a negative inotropic effect and can precipitate heart failure in patients with left ventricular dysfunction.

It is well known that quinidine can induce torsade de pointes (TdP), generally associated with significant QT prolongation. TdP typically occurs early during quinidine therapy, but cases occurring late have also been reported [3]. Risk factors include QT prolongation, sinus bradycardia, hypokalemia, and concomitant therapy with other QT prolonging agents. Disopyramide has also been implicated in TdP.

Safety has been an extremely important concern with class I agents, given the results of the CAST study [4]. Flecainide- and propafenone-induced proarrhythmia is primarily of two types: monomorphic ventricular tachycardia (VT) unrelated to QT prolongation and "slow" atrial tachycardia/flutter with 1:1 atrioventricular conduction. VT appears to occur primarily in patients with ischemic heart disease, left ventricular dysfunction, or other structural heart diseases. Ischemia-induced ventricular proarrhythmia has been postulated as the mechanism of excess mortality in the CAST trial. Overviews of the flecainide experience for supraventricular tachycardias and AF estimates the risk of proarrhythmia at about 4%, equally divided between ventricular and atrial tachyarrhythmias [5]. Overall, cardiotoxicity, including proarrhythmia with flecainide and propafenone, occurs more commonly in patients with a structural heart disease than in patients with normal heart [6]. Both these drugs have proved to be safe in patients with AF without structural heart disease [6, 7].

Class III Antiarrhythmic Drugs

Sotalol and amiodarone are currently the most frequently used class III drugs for maintaining SR in patients with AF. There are contrasting data on the efficacy of sotalol on the maintenance of SR, but it seems to be similar to that of class I drugs. The ventricular rate during AF recurrences is substantially attenuated and, as a consequence, the hemodynamic pattern of AF recurrences is better after sotalol treatment than without treatment [8].

Amiodarone is the most effective antiarrhythmic agent. A large randomized trial (CTAF) was carried out in order to compare the effects of low-dose amiodarone (200 mg daily) with conventional therapy (propafenone and sotalol) in maintenance of SR [9]. After 1 year, 70% of the patients assigned to amiodarone had no symptomatic recurrences of AF and the drug efficacy was superior to that of propafenone and sotalol. In the randomized CHF-STAT trial [10], in which amiodarone was used in order to investigate the effects on mortality in patients with heart failure, the drug showed a significant potential to convert patients in AF to SR (amiodarone 30%, placebo 7%, p=0.002). Moreover, the drug prevented the development of new-onset AF and significantly reduced the ventricular rate in those with permanent AF.

Proarrhythmias and Other Relevant Adverse Effects

Sotalol can induce TdP and the risk increases directly with the dose, the degree of QT prolongation, and the presence of relevant ventricular enlargement [11]. In patients with a history of VT, receiving 160 and 320 mg daily, TdP occurred in 0.6% and 1.6%, respectively; at 480 mg daily the rate increased markedly to 4.4% [11]. The incidence is lower in patients receiving sotalol for AF rather than VT. As with quinidine, TdP may be precipitated by hypokalemia, bradycardia, and other medications inducing QT prolongation. Bradycardia is of particular concern with sotalol therapy, given the β-blocker inherent in the formulation.

The prevalence of TdP is lower with amiodarone; in fact the risk of this proarrhythmia appears to be less than 1% despite frequently marked QT prolongations. However, the use of amiodarone is limited by other side effects. In the Chun series [12], the actuarial rates of withdrawal due to adverse effects were 8%, 22%, and 30% at 1, 3, and 5 years, respectively. The most frequent toxicities were skin discoloration (4.5%), pulmonary fibrosis (3.6%), and thyroid abnormalities (2.7%); none of the cases of pulmonary fibrosis was fatal. The CHF-STAT, EMIAT, and CAMIAT trials, which examined a prophylactic role for low-dose amiodarone in high-risk patients, did not show excess mortality in amiodarone-treated patients, and the GESICA trial evidenced a significant reduction in total mortality. These data are very important, since other antiarrhythmic drugs showed excess mortality.

First Choice of Antiarrhythmic Drug

In choosing from the available antiarrhythmic drugs, several guidelines have been proposed to help maximize the likelihood of clinical success, but there is little consensus on the best approach. In essence, there is no "one size fits all" antiarrhythmic drug to maintain SR, and it is difficult to predict before starting therapy which agent will be the most effective. For this reason, all antiarrhythmic drugs are selected on a safety-first basis and tailored to the underlying clinical situation. In general, in patients with no or minimal structural heart disease, class I agents or sotalol appear the first-line choice. These drugs are not highly effective (about 50% of patients without AF recurrences at 1 year), but the risk of proarrhythmia appears very low in these patients (0%-1%) [13-15]. The risk is increased in the presence of electrolyte disturbances, reduced creatinine clearance, bradycardia, and long QT interval.

In patients with hypertension without or with minimal left ventricular hypertrophy, sotalol or other β-blockers could represent the first-line choice since they are effective in the prevention of AF recurrences and reduce blood pressure; in this clinical situation class IC drugs can be used well. In patients with a high resting sinus rate, sotalol or other β-blockers should be considered as first-choice treatment.

In the presence of severe left ventricular hypertrophy or valvular heart disease, the first-line choice is amiodarone. The risk of ventricular proarrhythmia with class I agents or sotalol is uncertain in patients with this condition, but all serious proarrhythmias with these drugs seem to occur in persons with structural heart disease [13, 14]. In patients with very frequent AF recurrences, with large right or left atria, or with a long AF history, amiodarone also represents the first-choice treatment.

In the presence of ischemic heart disease, class I antiarrhythmic drugs should be avoided and sotalol becomes the first-line choice; amiodarone represents the second choice.

In patients with left ventricular dysfunction, with or without heart failure, amiodarone is the antiarrhythmic drug of choice as the risk of other agents appears unacceptably high.

In patients with adrenergically mediated AF, first-line choices are sotalol or other β-blockers, while in those with vagally mediated AF, the use of drugs with vagolytic action such as flecainide and disopyramide is suggested, although large prospective studies are lacking. It must be emphasized that in some clinical situations there is no indication for any antiarrhythmic drug or any other treatment. These situations can be summarized as follows [15]:

- After the first episode of AF, unless there is significant hemodynamic impairment;
- Patients with well-tolerated, short-lasting, and self-limited episodes of AF;
- Patients with an episode of AF during acute myocardial infarction or other acute affections, unless there is a history of previous AF attacks;
- Patients with an episode of AF just after cardiac surgery, unless there is a history of previous AF attacks.

References

1. Hohnloser SH, Kuck KH, Lilienthal J (2000) Rhythm or rate control in atrial fibrillation. Pharmacological intervention in atrial fibrillation (PIAF): a randomized trial. Lancet 356:1789-1794
2. Kühlkamp V, Schirdewan A, Stangl K, Homberg M, Plock M, Beck OA (2000) Use of metoprolol CR/XL to maintain sinus rhythm after conversion from persistent atrial fibrillation. A randomized, double-blind, placebo-controlled study. J Am Coll Cardiol 36:139–146
3. Roden DM, Woosley RL, Primm RK (1986) Incidence and clinical features of the quinidine associated long QT syndrome. Implications for patient care. Am Heart J 111:1088–1093
4. CAST Investigators (1989) Effect of encainide and flecainide on mortality in a randomized trial of arrhythmia suppression after myocardial infarction. N Engl J Med 321:406–412
5. Hohnloser SH, Zabel M (1992) Short- and long-term efficacy and safety of flecainide acetate for supraventricular arrhythmias. Am J Cardiol 70:3A–10A
6. Podrid PJ, Anderson JL (1996) Safety and tolerability of long-term propafenone for supraventricular tachyarrhythmias. Am J Cardiol 78:430–434
7. Chimienti M, Cullen MT, Casaderi G et al (1996) Safety of long-term flecainide and propafenone in the management of patients with symptomatic paroxysmal atrial fibrillation: report from the flecainide and propafenone Italian study investigators. Am J Cardiol 77:60A–65A

8. Alboni P, Razzolini R, Scarfò S et al (1993) Hemodynamic effects of oral sotalol during both sinus rhythm and atrial fibrillation. J Am Coll Cardiol 22:1373–1377
9. Roy D, Talajic M, Dorian P et al (2000) Amiodarone to prevent recurrence of atrial fibrillation. N Engl J Med 342:913–920
10. Deedwania PC, Singh BN, Ellenbogen K et al (1998) Spontaneous conversion and maintenance of sinus rhythm by amiodarone in patients with heart failure and atrial fibrillation. Observations from the Veterans Affairs Congestive Heart Failure Survival Trial of Antiarrhythmic Therapy (CHF-STAT). Circulation 98:2574–2579
11. Betapace package insert. Berlex Laboratories, 1994
12. Chun SH, Sager PT, Stevenson WG et al (1995) Long-term efficacy of amiodarone for the maintenance of normal sinus rhythm in patients with refractory atrial fibrillation or flutter. Am J Cardiol 76:47–50
13. Hughes MM, Trohman RG, Simmons TV et al (1992) Flecainide therapy in patients treated for supraventricular tachycardia with near normal left ventricular function. Am Heart J 123:408–412
14. Prystowsky EN (1994) Inpatient versus outpatient initiation of antiarrhythmic drug therapy for patients with supraventricular tachycardia. Clin Cardiol 17:II:7–10
15. Alboni P (1999) Quando non prescrivere un trattamento cronico al paziente con fibrillazione atriale. G Ital Cardiol 1999;29:824–827

Rhythm Control Versus Rate Control: Unresolved Riddle in Daily Clinical Practice

F. Gaita, S. Grossi, R. Riccardi, C. Giustetto, E. Caruzzo, F. Bianchi, L. Vivalda, E. Richiardi, G. Pistis

Atrial fibrillation (AF) is the most common supraventricular arrhythmia: the prevalence is 1% over the age of 60 years and above 5% over the age of 70 [1]. In the past 10 years various studies have suggested a worse outcome in patients affected by AF. From the analysis of the Framingham study population, AF seems related to excessive mortality, irrespective of underlying structural heart disease, age, diabetes, smoking, hypertension, or stroke, with an odds ratio of 1.5 in men and of 1.9 in women [2]. Other studies have shown an increased risk of death in patients with AF, between 1.3 and 2.6 with respect to those in sinus rhythm [3, 4]. In patients with dilated cardiomyopathy AF has been shown as an independent predictor of sudden death when the ejection fraction is less than 50% [5]. AF is thought to increase the risk of death mainly through thromboembolic complications and their hemodynamic consequences. The risk of cerebral thromboembolism in patients with nonvalvular AF is increased by a factor of 5-7, with a probability of ischemic stroke of 5% per year; the risk increases in presence of hypertension, diabetes, previous ischemic events, recent heart failure, and age over 65 years (in the 50% of cases cerebral events occur in patients older than 75 years). Even in patients with lone AF the risk of stroke is increased four times compared to age-matched controls in sinus rhythm [6]; counting transient ischemic attacks and asymptomatic stroke, the incidence rises to 7% per year [7, 8]. The hemodynamic consequences of AF are related to the rapid and irregular ventricular response and to the lack of atrial contribution to ventricular filling. They are more evident in patients with reduced left ventricular function, and the loss of atrial kick may reduce cardiac output by up to 20% in patients with impaired diastolic function [9]. The persistence of a rapid ventricular rate for more than 6 months may induce the development of a reversible form of tachy-cardiomyopathy [10]. However, the real impact of AF on prognosis has been questioned more recently, and critical attention must be paid to the actual role of AF in

Divisione di Cardiologia, Ospedale Mauriziano Umberto I, Turin, Italy

the clinical outcome of affected patients. Its hemodynamic and thromboembolic consequences can be limited by the use of anticoagulant therapy and drugs that slow the heart rate. Does the prognostic value of AF go beyond that? Even in patients at high risk, such as those with heart failure, the proposition that AF has independent prognostic significance is controversial, following from some studies but not from others [11].

Moreover, the negative influence of AF may be related to inappropriate therapy: comparing two groups of patients with heart failure in two different periods (1985-1989 and 1990-1993), the abolition of the use of class I antiarrhythmic drugs in patients with impaired left ventricular function and the use of anticoagulant therapy improved total mortality and eliminated the negative contribution of coexisting AF on outcome [12]. The bulk of these data introduce the suspicion that rhythm is not the main determinant of prognosis in heart disease. When correctly treated, the prognosis of AF seems to be linked to that of the underlying heart disease.

In this context, for many clinicians the initial therapy for AF has to be directed at the maintenance of sinus rhythm by both cardioversion and antiarrhythmic drugs, with the rationale of improving exercise tolerance, quality of life, and survival, reducing symptoms and the risk of stroke with possible discontinuation of anticoagulant therapy. However, the responsiveness of AF to the drug therapy does not exceed the 50% and comes at a cost in adverse effects that can sometimes be serious. On the other hand, an alternative may simply consist in the rate control strategy, in which the ventricular response is slowed by nodal blocking agents or by atrioventricular junction ablation in conjunction with anticoagulation. Recently the results of two different prospective randomized trials comparing the two different approaches have been published.

In the AFFIRM study [13] 4060 patients with a mean age of 70±9 years and a history of AF likely to be recurrent, likely to cause illness or death, eligible for both the treatment strategies and with at least one other risk factor for stroke and/or death were enrolled. Patients were randomized to undergo rate control or rhythm control. Baseline characteristics did not differ between the two groups. In the rate-control group β-blockers, calcium channel blockers, and digoxin, alone or in association, were used, whereas in the rhythm control group electrical cardioversion and antiarrhythmic drugs were chosen by the treating physician. The primary endpoint was overall mortality. The composite secondary endpoint comprised death, disabling stroke, major bleeding, disabling anoxic encephalopathy, and cardiac arrest. After a mean follow-up of 3.5 years 80% of patients in the rate control group had adequate control of ventricular response and 34.6% were in sinus rhythm; 248 patients crossed over to the rhythm control group, most commonly for uncontrolled symptoms and congestive heart failure. The prevalence of sinus rhythm in rhythm control group was 62.6%. Five hundred ninety-four patients crossed over to the other group, mostly because of inability to maintain sinus rhythm and drug intolerance. In this group more than two-thirds of patients started therapy with amiodarone or sotalol, and at the end of the study two-thirds had undergone at least one trial of amiodarone. The primary endpoint (overall mortality) occurred in 26.7 % in the rhythm control group and in 25.9% in the rate control group: the difference is not statistically different, the composite secondary endpoint either. A nonsignificant trend in favor of the rate control group was evident. Proarrhythmias such torsade de pointes and bradycardiac arrest, although uncommon in the study, and hospitalization were more frequent in the rhythm control group. The incidence of stroke was low in both groups, about 1%, and was related to discontinuation or reduced effect of anticoagulation therapy. In this study of patients with AF and other risk factors for stroke the strategy aimed at rhythm control had no clear advantages but showed a nonsignificant trend toward increased mortality. In a substudy presented by Waldo at the 23rd session of NASPE, patients of 80 centers in the rhythm control group were randomized to receive amiodarone, sotalol, or a class I antiarrhythmic drug. The endpoint was 1 year of sinus rhythm maintenance. Amiodarone was the most effective, with a success rate of about 60% versus 34%-39% for sotalol and 23% for the class I drug, with no differences in side effects.

The RACE trial [14] enrolled 522 patients with persistent AF or flutter who had undergone one or two previous electrical cardioversion procedures. The mean age was 68±9 years and in 90% or the patients one or more risk factors for stroke were present. Two hundred sixty-six patients randomized to rhythm control underwent serial cardioversion and received antiarrhythmic drugs, the sequence of which was strictly indicated in the protocol and included amiodarone as the last choice. Two hundred fifty-six patients in the rate control group were treated with calcium channel blockers, β-blockers, and digitalis alone or in combination. Baseline characteristics did not differ between the two groups. The primary endpoint was a composite of death from cardiovascular causes, heart failure, thromboembolic complications, bleeding, implantation of a pacemaker, and severe adverse effects of drugs. After a mean follow-up of 2.3±0.6 years 39% of the rhythm control group had sinus rhythm as compared with 10% in the rate control group. The primary end point occurred in 17.2% of the rate control group and in 22.6% of the rhythm control group, giving a nonsignificant trend in favor of the rate control group.

The distribution of the various components of the primary endpoint was similar in the two groups except in respect of thromboembolism, which was more frequent in the rhythm control group. The investigators concluded that rate control is not inferior to rhythm control for the prevention of death and morbidity from cardiovascular causes in patients with persistent AF after electrical cardioversion.

The results of the two studies indicate that in older patients with persistent or recurrent AF and risk factors for stroke and death, maintenance of sinus rhythm is not superior to rate control in terms of survival, stroke, bleeding, and cardiac arrest, with a nonsignificant trend in favor of rate control, particularly in hypertensive patients and in women. However, a word of comment is needed. The comparison between rate and rhythm control in terms of mortality in patients with AF could hardly ever not have been in favor of the former. As described above, the prognostic impact of AF, even in groups of patients in worst conditions, mainly depends on uncontrolled rate and thromboembolic events. Once rate control and effective anticoagulation treatment are established, AF should have no prognostic significance in the majority of cases. In addition, in the AFFIRM study patients with frequent or severe symptoms might have been considered unsuitable for the rate control strategy and therefore may not have been enrolled by some investigators. The incidence of stroke in both studies was greater in patients in whom anticoagulation therapy was discontinued or subtherapeutic. However, in the AFFIRM study patients in rhythm control with stroke had discontinued or subtherapeutic anticoagulation therapy more often than those in rate control with stroke. Continuation and a better effectiveness of anticoagulation therapy would have had a positive impact on the prognosis in the rhythm control group and might well have improved this group's results. The timing of the discontinuation of anticoagulant therapy is not clear, but these results suggest that caution must be used.

Furthermore, the difference in the presence of sinus rhythm between the rhythm and rate control approaches in both studies is not striking: 62.6% versus 34.6% in the AFFIRM study and 39% versus 10% in the RACE study. The lack of any more significant difference may be due to the presence of patients with paroxysmal AF in the rate control group in the AFFIRM study and to the limited effectiveness of antiarrhythmic drugs, amiodarone included, on the maintenance of sinus rhythm in the rhythm control group. Pharmacological therapy is indeed far from being considered ideal: its effectiveness in maintaining sinus rhythm does not exceed 50%, with a significant burden of side effects such as proarrhythmia and negative inotropic effects.

The different subgroups of patient must be taken into account. In patients aged less than 65 years, in the presence of heart failure, in the AFFIRM study, and in male and in normotensive patients in the RACE study, the trend is in favor of rhythm control. In clinical practice these subgroups include on the one hand younger patients with structurally normal hearts and paroxysmal arrhythmia without risk factors for stroke and often symptoms refractory to rate control and on the other patients who are more ill who need the hemodynamic benefit of atrial contractility. In the AFFIRM study these two groups of patients, frequently crossed over from the rate control to the rhythm control strategy. In this setting the goal still remains the maintenance of sinus rhythm. On the other hand, a statistically significant excess of mortality is evident in women in the rhythm control group in the RACE study. In the Framingham study women had a greater relative risk of death and were more prone to drug induced QT interval prolongation; female sex was also a risk factor for stroke among older patients with AF [15]. Hypertension was also a marker of a worse outcome in the rhythm control group in both studies. It is the most common cause of left ventricular hypertrophy, which is associated with an increased risk of drug-related arrhythmic events [16].

The attempt to maintain sinus rhythm is not deemed imperative especially in older, hypertensive patients, in women, and in the presence of persistent or recurrent AF. A balance between risks and benefits should be carefully considered in each patient.

Further progress in the pharmacological and nonpharmacological therapy of AF is needed in order to improve the success rate of the rhythm control strategy while limiting its adverse effects.

References

1. The National Heart, Lung and Blood Institute Working Group on Atrial Fibrillation (1993) Atrial fibrillation: current understandings and research imperatives. J Am Coll Cardiol 22:1830
2. Benjamin EJ, Wolf PA, D'Agostino RB (1998) Impact of atrial fibrillation on the risk of death - The Framingham Heart Study. Circulation 98:946-952
3. Kannel WB, Abbott RD, Savage DD, McNamara PM (1982) Epidemiological features of chronic atrial fibrillation. The Framingham Study. N Engl J Med 306:1018-1022
4. Levy S, Maarek M, Coumel P el al (1999) Characterization of different subset of atrial fibrillation in general practice in France: the Alfa study. Circulation 20:1592-1599
5. Hoffman T, Meinertz T, Kasper W et al (1988) Mode of death in idiopathic dilated cardiomyopathy: a multivariate analysis of prognostic determinants. Am Heart J 116:1455-1463
6. Brand FN, Abbott RD, Kannel WB, Wolf PA (1985) Characteristics and prognosis of lone atrial fibrillation: 30 year follow-up in the Framingham study. JAMA 245:3449-3453
7. Wolf PA, Abbot RD, Kannel WB (1991) Atrial fibrillation as an independent risk factor for stroke: the Framingham study. Stroke 22:983-988
8. Atrial Fibrillation Investigators (1994) Risk factors for stroke and efficacy of antithrombotic therapy in atrial fibrillation: analysis of pooled data from randomised controlled trials. Arch Intern Med 154:1499-1457
9. Upshaw CB Jr (1997) Hemodynamic changes after cardioversion of chronic atrial fibrillation. Arch Intern Med 157:1070-1076
10. Grogan M, Smith HC, Gersh BJ, Wood DL (1992) Left ventricular dysfunction due to atrial fibrillation in patients initially believed to have idiopathic dilated cardiomyopathy. Am J Cardiol 69:1570-1573
11. Ehrlich JR, Nattel S, Hohnloser SH (2002) Atrial fibrillation and congestive heart failure. J Cardiovasc Electrophysiol 13:399-405
12. Stevenson WG, Stevenson LW, Middlekauff HR (1996) Improving survival for patients with atrial fibrillation and advanced heart failure. J Am Coll Cardiol 28:1458-146
13. The Atrial Fibrillation Follow Up Investigation of Rhythm Management (AFFIRM) Investigators (2002) A comparison of rate control and rhythm control in patients with atrial fibrillation. N Engl J Med 347:1825-1833
14. Van Gelder IC, Hagens VE, Bosker HA et al, for the Rate Control versus Electrical Cardioversion for Persistent Atrial Fibrillation Study Group (2002) A comparison of rate control and rhythm control in patients with recurrent persistent atrial fibrillation. N Engl J Med 347:1834-1840

15. Hart RG, Pearce LA, McBride R et al (1999) Factors associated with ischemic stroke during aspirin therapy in atrial fibrillation: analysis of 2012 participants in the SPAF I-III clinical trials. Stroke 30:1223
16. Reiffel JA (1998) Impact of structural heart disease on the selection of class III antiarrhythmics in the prevention of atrial fibrillation and flutter. Am Heart J 135:551-556

The AFFIRM Study and Its Implications for the Pharmacological Treatment of Atrial Fibrillation

A. CAPUCCI, G.Q. VILLANI

Introduction

Thromboembolism is the major complication in atrial fibrillation (AF), and its prevention constitutes a major challenge in the modern treatment of this common arrhythmia. The embolic risk is not equal in all subgroups of AF patients but relates to the underlying heart condition: while nonrheumatic AF carries a 5.6-fold embolic risk, arrhythmia of rheumatic origin carries a 17.6-fold risk in comparison with healthy controls. However, nonrheumatic AF is responsible for the larger percentage of strokes (15%-20% of cerebrovascular accidents of ischemic origin). Another important factor affecting the risk of thromboembolism is age: cerebrovascular accidents associated with AF represent 6.7% of the total number of cerebrovascular accidents in the 50- to 59-year-old group and 36.2% in the over 80-year-old group [1, 2].

In the past decade there has been widespread of oral anticoagulation treatment (warfarin) in preference to antiplatelet treatment (aspirin/indoprofen) to reduce the risk of cardiovascular mortality and morbidity in patients with rheumatic and nonrheumatic AF. This treatment has been based on evidence from randomized control trials that compared long-term anticoagulation and antiplatelet treatments with placebo .

In addition, many therapeutic efforts have been concentrated on maintaining sinus rhythm in order to reduce the clinical implications of frequently recurrent or permanent AF (reduced global cardiac function and exercise tolerance). In particular, it is possible that persistent sinus rhythm in the AF patient population may be the best prophylaxis of embolic events. Recently two trials evaluated the effects of the rhythm control versus rate control strategy on clinical endpoints in AF patients. One of these was the AFFIRM study.

Cardiology Department, Guglielmo da Saliceto Hospital, Piacenza, Italy

The AFFIRM Study

The Atrial Fibrillation Follow-up Investigation of Rhythm Management (AFFIRM) study, conducted at 213 centers in the US and Canada, randomized a total of 4060 patients to receive rate control therapy or rhythm control therapy [3]. Eligible patients had documented AF with 6 h or more of AF in the previous 6 months. The qualifying episode had occurred within the previous 12 weeks and was no more than 6 months in duration. To be eligible, patients needed to be able to take at least two drugs in each treatment arm, have the ability to take anticoagulants, and be able to undergo any long-term therapy which was thought to be needed. In addition, they had one or more risk factors for stroke or death, which included:

- Age ≥ 65 years
- Hypertension
- Diabetes
- Congestive heart failure
- Prior stroke or transient ischemic attack
- Left atrial dimension ≥ 50 mm as determined by echocardiography
- Left ventricular shortening fraction ≤ 25% as determined by echocardiography
- Left ventricular ejection fraction ≤ 40% as determined by any technique

In the rhythm control arm the study protocol permitted anticoagulation therapy after normal rhythm had been achieved and maintained for 1 month. The crossover rate in the rate control arm was 12%, compared with 37% in the rhythm control arm.

After an average 3.5-year follow-up period 85%-90% of the rate control group remained on warfarin therapy versus 70% of the rhythm control group. An INR below 2 was detected in 33% of the rate control and in 58% of rhythm control arm. At follow-up, 60% of patients in the rhythm control arm were in normal sinus rhythm, while successful rate control was achieved in 80% of the rate control patients. All-cause mortality was not significantly different between the two groups and no differences were shown in several components of the secondary endpoint. In particular, ischemic stroke appeared in 5.7% of rate control and 7.3% of rhythm control patients, while the incidence of bleeding complication was 2% in the rate control versus 2.1% in the rhythm control arm. Adverse events are reported in Table 1.

This recent study suggests that:

1 In a population of patients with persistent AF, antiarrhythmic therapy is able to maintain sinus rhythm only in 40%-60% patients between.
2 In these AF patients, the lack of longer-term anticoagulation therapy may account for the higher stroke rate.
3 At present, in patients with persistent/paroxysmal AF anticoagulation therapy must be considered mandatory even during periods of sinus rhythm.
4 Rate control may be an acceptable primary therapy in patients with AF.

Table 1. Adverse events in the AFFIRM study

	Rate control arm (% of patients)	Rhythm control arm (% of patients)	p
Death	26	27	0.058
Torsade de pointes	0.2	0.8	0.004
VT/VF	1.7	1.2	NS
Cardiac arrest	0.1	0.8	0.004
Bleed	2	2.1	NS
Ischemic stroke	5.7	7.34	NS

References

1. Feinberg WM, Blackshear JL, Laupacis A et al (1995) Prevalence, age distribution and gender of patients with atrial fibrillation. Arch Intern Med 155:469-473
2. Wolf PA, Abbor RD, Konnel WB et al (1991) Atrial fibrillation as an independent risk factor for stroke: the Framingham study. Stroke 22:983-988
3. Wyse G, on the behalf of the Atrial Fibrillation Follow-up Investigation of Rhythm Management (AFFIRM) trial. Communication of American College of Cardiology 51st Annual Scientific session, 2002

Amiodarone in the Treatment of Atrial Fibrillation: New Perspectives from Clinical Trials

G.M. De Ferrari, B. Petracci

Atrial fibrillation (AF) is the most common sustained cardiac arrhythmia and both its incidence and the burden it lays on the health system are steadily increasing, primarily because of the increase in the elderly proportion of the population [1-3]. Among the diverse pharmacological agents potentially useful in restoring and maintaining sinus rhythm, amiodarone is characterized by both a multiplicity of sites of action and high efficacy. Several studies have supported the use of this compound [4]. Trials evaluating intravenous use of amiodarone have recently been reviewed in detail [5]. The present paper will briefly evaluate a small number of recent clinical studies supporting the use of oral amiodarone in preventing recurrent episodes of AF in the general population and in selected clinical settings.

Roy and colleagues conducted a large prospective randomized trial (the Canadian Trial of Atrial Fibrillation, CTAF) comparing low-dose amiodarone to sotalol or propafenone in the prevention of AF recurrences [6]. Eligible patients had had at least one episode of symptomatic, documented AF lasting more than 10 min in the previous 6 months for which long-term antiarrhythmic therapy was planned. A total of 403 patients were enrolled: 201 received amiodarone while 202 were assigned to either sotalol or propafenone (with 101 patients on each). Amiodarone was given at a loading dose of 10 mg per kilogram body weight each day for 14 days, followed by 300 mg/day for 4 weeks and then a maintenance dose of 200 mg/day.

After a mean of 16 months of follow-up, 35% of the patients assigned to amiodarone treatment had a recurrence of AF, as compared with 63% of the patients assigned to treatment with sotalol or propafenone ($p<0.001$, Fig. 1). The results thus indicate that amiodarone was about twice as effective as two commonly used antiarrhythmic drugs in preventing AF recurrences. The trial also suggests the overall safety of low doses of amiodarone, since this agent was well tolerated and serious adverse events were uncommon. No proarrhyth-

Department of Cardiology, IRCCS Policlinico San Matteo, Pavia, Italy

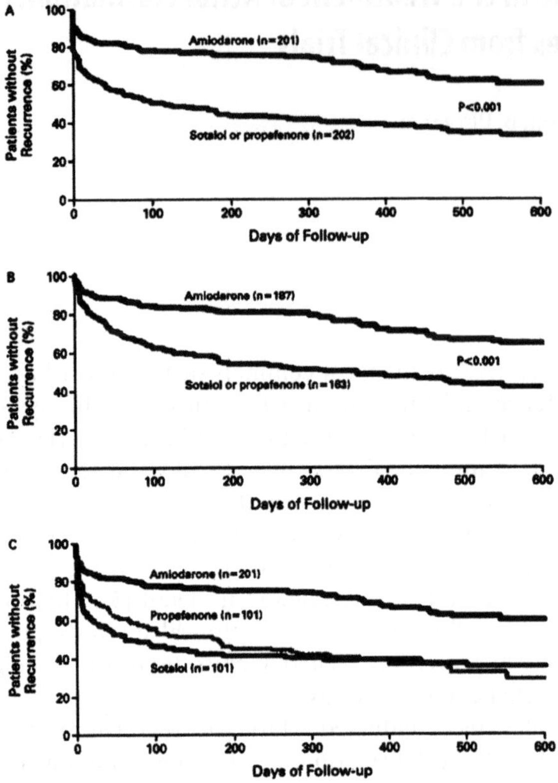

Fig. 1. Kaplan-Meyer estimates of the percentage of patients remaining free of recurrences of AF in the CTAF study. (From [6], reproduced with permission)

mic effect was observed, and side effects related to amiodarone therapy occurred in a small proportion of patients: hypothyroidism occurred in 1% of patients, hyperthyroidism in 0.5%, and suspect pulmonary toxicity in 2% of the patients. No patient died as a result of pulmonary toxicity.

The impact of the different treatment options available in the CTAF study on hospital costs has been recently evaluated by Lumer et al [7]. Patients in the amiodarone group had fewer electrical cardioversions (65 vs 109 for patients in the sotalol/propafenone group) and pacemaker insertions (4 vs 11). The average patient receiving amiodarone spent fewer days in hospital (0.47 vs 0.97) and incurred lower costs for admissions where AF was the admitting diagnosis ($532 vs $898, p=0.03). Thus, amiodarone appears preferable to sotalol or propafenone from an economic point of view as well.

The preliminary results of the pharmacological substudy of the AFFIRM trial [8] are in good agreement with the finding that amiodarone is superior to the other antiarrhythmic agents. The substudy consisted in the randomized assignment of patients in the rhythm control group to receive amiodarone, sotalol, or class I drugs. The primary endpoint was "success" of the drug at 1 year, based on whether the patient survived, was in sinus rhythm, had not required cardioversion, and was still taking the drug. In the amiodarone vs class I comparison, amiodarone was successful in 62% of the patients, while class I agents were successful in 23% ($p<0.001$), and in the amiodarone vs sotalol comparison, amiodarone was successful in 60% of the patients while sotalol was successful in 39% ($p=0.001$). No difference was found between sotalol and class I agents (success rates of 34% and 23%, respectively, $p=0.16$).

Despite the suggested higher efficacy of amiodarone compared with other antiarrhythmic agents, recurrences of AF, particularly in the first days after cardioversion, are still rather high. Thus, the search for either new compounds or agents that could act synergistically with amiodarone appears worth pursuing.

A recent trial evaluated the efficacy of combining an angiotensin I type 1 blocker with amiodarone in the prevention of the recurrences of AF [9]. The study aimed at experimental demonstration of a role of angiotensin II inhibitors in the prevention of atrial electrical remodeling [10], a major factor in the high incidence of early recurrences of AF after sinus rhythm restoration [11]. A previous analysis of the TRACE study had suggested that the ACE inhibitor trandolapril reduced the incidence of new onset of AF among patients with a recent myocardial infarction and left ventricular dysfunction [12]. Madrid et al. randomized 154 patients with an episode of persistent AF lasting more than 7 days (median 6 months) to irbesartan or placebo in addition to amiodarone 400 mg/day for 2 months and thereafter 200 mg/day. Mean age was 66 years, average left ventricular ejection fraction was 66%, and average left atrial inferosuperior dimension 45 mm. After 2 months 85% of the patients taking both irbesartan and amiodarone were in sinus rhythm as compared with 63% of patients taking amiodarone alone ($p=0.008$). The event-free survival curves appeared to proceed parallel thereafter, so that the difference was maintained at 1 year (79% and 56% of patients in sinus rhythm in the amiodarone ± irbesartan and in the amiodarone only groups, respectively). This consideration, in addition to the finding that no patient in the amiodarone ± irbesartan group had a recurrence within 1 h after electrical cardioversion (as compared with 4 out of 46 in the amiodarone-only group) is in agreement with the hypothesis that remodeling has a role in the early recurrences after cardioversion and that angiotensin is a significant contributor to this process. The study also confirms good efficacy and tolerability of this dosage of amiodarone in the prevention of AF recurrences.

A different area of increasing interest is in the prevention of AF after open heart surgery. Postoperative AF occurs in 25%-40% of patients and is associated with a greater likelihood of hypotension, heart failure, ventricular arrhythmias, need for a pace-maker, and a three-fold increase in the risk of stroke or transient ischemic attack [13, 14]. The incidence of postoperative AF increases markedly with age and is significantly reduced by treatment with β-blockers

[15]. Few studies have addressed the effect of oral amiodarone in the prevention of postoperative AF. Daoud et al. [16] found that amiodarone lowered the incidence of fibrillation by 53%. Preoperative loading time was relatively long (13 days) and the use of β-blockers was rather low, probably accounting for the high incidence in the placebo arm (53%). Redle et al. [17] used a 1- to 4-day preoperative loading time (2 g amiodarone) and a daily dose of 400 mg for 7 days postoperatively. They observed a nonsignificant 25% reduction in the incidence of AF in a population averaging 64 years of age.

Giri et al. [18] enrolled 220 patients aged 60 years or older undergoing open heart surgery in the AFIST study. Patients enrolled less than 5 days before surgery received 6 g amiodarone or matching placebo over 5 days, beginning on preoperative day 1 (400 mg four times daily for 1 day, 600 mg twice daily on the day of surgery, and 400 mg twice daily on postoperative days 1-4). Patients enrolled at least 5 days before surgery received 7 g amiodarone or matching placebo over 10 days, beginning on preoperative day 5 (200 mg three times daily for 5 days before surgery, 400 mg twice daily on the day of surgery, and 400 mg twice daily on postoperative days 1-4). Approximately 90% of patients were treated with β-blockers in both groups with an average preoperative daily dose of metoprolol, the most used compound, of 140 mg. β-Blocker dosage was reduced after surgery in one out of four patients and had to be discontinued for at least two doses in one out of five patients. Patients assigned to amiodarone treatment had a lower incidence of AF (22.5% vs 38%, p=0.01, Fig. 2), and a markedly lower incidence of symptomatic AF (4.2 vs 18%, p=0.001). This latter

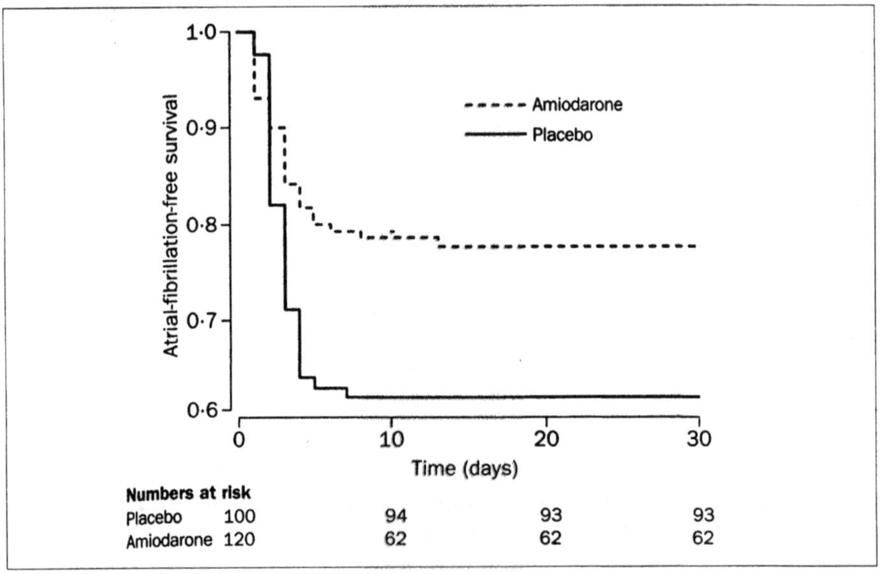

Fig. 2. Kaplan-Meyer analysis for 30 days AF-free survival. (From [18], reproduced with permission)

finding is likely to be related to the lower mean ventricular response during AF in the amiodarone group (106 vs 137 bpm) as well as to the shorter average duration of the arrhythmia episodes (9 vs 23 h). Additionally, a difference was found in the incidence of cerebrovascular accident (1.7 vs 7.0, p=0.04) and of postoperative ventricular tachycardia (1.7 vs 7.0, p=0.04). Interestingly, there was no increase in the incidence of side effects potentially related to the vasodilating and negative inotropic and chronotropic effects of amiodarone: i.e. no increase in hypotension, symptomatic bradycardia, or heart block, while a trend toward more nausea in the active compound group was noted. Mortality was also similar in the two groups. Subgroup analysis suggests that the effect of amiodarone on the occurrence of AF was less obvious in patients with heart failure, those aged less than 70 years, with prior AF, with an enlarged left atrium, and in those taking β-blockers (Fig. 3). Despite the limited number of patients in each subgroup, these findings may suggest that the antiadrenergic activity of amiodarone has played a significant role in the beneficial effect observed, and that a longer duration of treatment may be necessary to significantly affect the altered substrate present among patients with a history of AF and an enlarged left atrium. At any rate, it should be pointed out that the study did not have enough power to assess whether amiodarone was synergistic with β-blockade, and that the interaction between these two agents has been extensively investigated in a different clinical setting, namely that of prevention of sudden death in patients with left ventricular dysfunction after myocardial infarction. Analysis of thousands of patients indicates that amiodarone was actually more effective in reducing malignant arrhythmias among patients treated with β-blockers than in patients not so treated, indicating a synergistic effect [19]. This apparent discrepancy may be due to the different clinical conditions or to the fact that treatment was chronic rather than short-lasting.

An additional aspect that deserves attention is that of AF in the setting of heart failure. The association between AF and heart failure is well documented, but the impact of AF on survival remains controversial, as is the best approach to follow in these patients. From a pathophysiological point of view it appears likely that AF may contribute to the progression of heart failure [20], and that an attempt at restoration of sinus rhythm may be particularly warranted in the population with dilated heart failure with the goal of preserving atrial transport function, of limiting atrial enlargement, and, potentially, of lowering embolic risk.

In contrast to these theoretical considerations, several drawbacks of an aggressive approach against AF in patients with heart failure exist. First, although electrical external cardioversion is generally effective in the restoration of sinus rhythm in the overall population, the success rate of this procedure is reduced in patients with heart failure, particularly in those with a long duration of the arrhythmia. Second, the recurrence rate is believed to be very high, since the presence of both left atrial enlargement and left ventricular dysfunction are considered to be powerful predictors of the recurrence rate. Finally, there is no demonstration that among patients with heart failure,

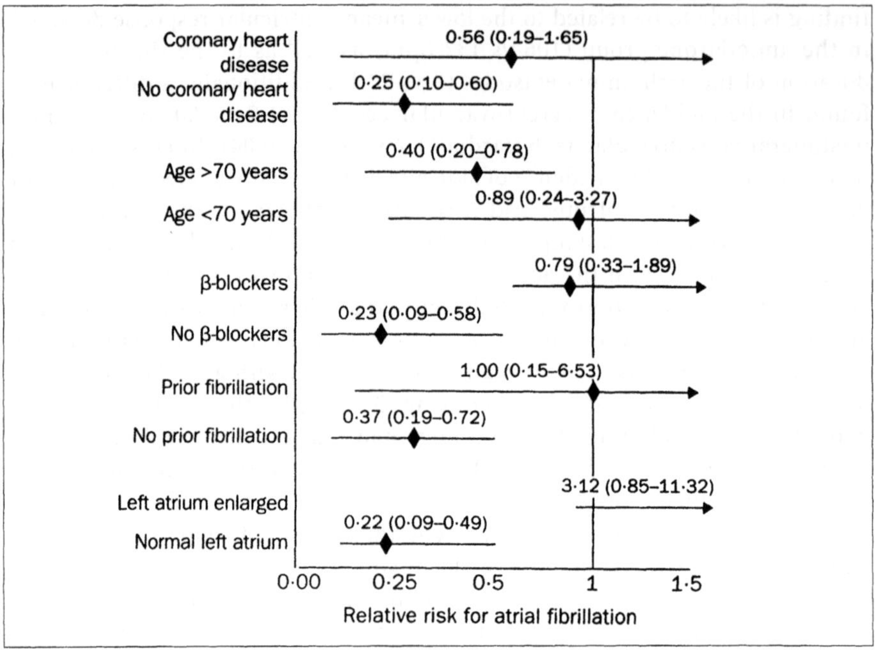

Fig. 3. Risk-adjusted relative risk for developing postoperative AF on amiodarone in various subgroups. (From [18], reproduced with permission)

restoration and maintenance of sinus rhythm is associated with improvement in left ventricular function and quality of life.

We assessed the effects of a combined strategy of internal cardioversion and chronic amiodarone treatment on the maintenance of sinus rhythm and on quality of life and left ventricular function during follow-up in forty patients (39 males and 1 female, mean age 56 ± 7years), with dilated cardiomyopathy and advanced heart failure (mean NYHA class 2.8± 0.6) evaluated as candidates for heart transplantation [21]. All patients had a history of permanent AF (duration 3 months to 10 years) with a previous failed external cardioversion. The patients had a very dilated and hypokinetic left ventricle, with a mean end-diastolic volume of 282 ± 94 ml and a mean ejection fraction of 28 ± 7%, a dilated left atrium (mean diameter 52 ± 7 mm), and a reduced left appendage flow velocity (24 ± 12 cm/s). The patients were given amiodarone 400 mg/day beginning 4 weeks before the procedure and 200 or 300 mg/day after the procedure, in addition to oral warfarin to keep INR values between 2 and 3.5, and to the optimal medical treatment for heart failure.

Internal cardioversion was acutely effective in 100% of patients. A recurrence of AF was observed within a few minutes in two patients (5%), and within the following 24 h in one additional patient (2%). Thus, 24 h after the procedure 37 out of 40 patients were discharged in sinus rhythm. One year after internal cardioversion, 74% of the patients (95% CI: 56%-91%) were in sinus rhythm. No significant side effect was associated with the use of amiodarone.

Overall, a statistically significant improvement was observed during follow-up in both clinical conditions and indexes of left ventricular function. Figure 4 shows the comparison between baseline conditions and the conditions 6 months after the procedure in NYHA class and left ventricular ejection fraction. Thanks to the marked improvement, two patients were removed from the active heart transplant list.

These considerations underline the need for a controlled randomized trial to determine the potential long-term benefits of sinus rhythm maintenance in patients with heart failure. The primary aim of the Atrial Fibrillation and Congestive Heart Failure (AF-CHF) trial is to determine whether restoring and maintaining sinus rhythm significantly reduces cardiovascular mortality compared with a rate control strategy in patients with congestive heart failure with a left ventricular ejection fraction of 35% or less and AF. Enrolment will be concluded in May 2003 with a minimum follow-up of 2 years. This trial should provide definitive information about two widely applicable treatment strategies for AF in patients with heart failure.

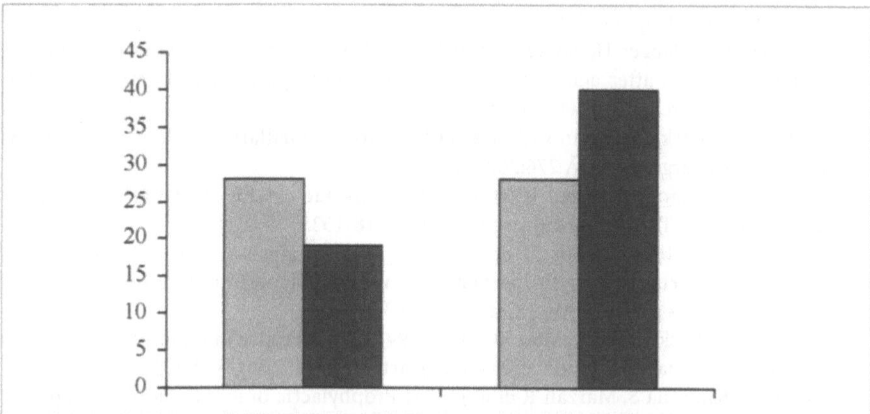

Fig. 4. Comparison between baseline and 6-month follow-up after cardioversion in the clinical conditions and in indexes of left ventricular function. To use the same y-axis as used for left ventricular ejection fraction, the value relative to the NYHA class should be divided by a factor of 10. A significant improvement after cardioversion was observed in this group of 40 patients

References

1. Kannel WB, Abbott RD, Savage DD et al (1982) Epidemiologic features of chronic atrial fibrillation: the Framingham Study. N Engl J Med 306:1018-1022
2. Feinberg WM, Blackshear JL, Laupacis A et al (1995) Prevalence, age, distribution, and gender of patients with atrial fibrillation: analysis and implications. Arch Intern Med 155: 469-473
3. Stewart S, MacIntyre K, MacLeod MMC et al (2001) Trends in hospital activity, morbidity and case fatality related to atrial fibrillation in Scotland, 1986-1996. Eur Heart J 22:693-701

4. Nichol G, McAlister F, Pham B et al (2002) Meta-analysis of randomised controlled trials of the effectiveness of antiarrhythmic agents at promoting sinus rhythm in patients with atrial fibrillation. Heart 87:535-543
5. Hilleman DE, Spinler SA (2002) Conversion of recent onset atrial fibrillation with intravenous amiodarone: a meta-analysis of randomized controlled trials. Pharmacotherapy 22:66-74
6. Roy D, Talajc M, Dorian P et al (2000) Amiodarone to prevent recurrence of atrial fibrillation. N Engl J Med 342:913-920
7. Lumer GB, Roy D, Talajc M et al (2002) Amiodarone reduces procedures and costs related to atrial fibrillation in a controlled clinical trial. Eur Heart J 23:1050-1056
8. Waldo A (2000) Presentation at the late breaking session, 23rd Annual Scientific Session of the North American Society of Pacing and Electrophysiology, San Diego, May 2002
9. Madrid AH, Bueno MG, Rebollo JMG et al (2002) Use of irbesartan to maintain sinus rhythm in patients with long-lasting persistent atrial fibrillation. A prospective and randomized study. Circulation 106:331-336
10. Nakashima H, Kumagai K, Urata H et al (2000) Angiotensin II antagonist prevents electrical remodeling in atrial fibrillation. Circulation 101:2612-2617
11. Alessie MA (1998) Atrial electrophysiological remodeling: another vicious circle? J Cardiovasc Electrophysiol 9:1378-1393
12. Pedersen OD, Bagger H, Kober L et al (1999) Trandolapril reduces the incidence of atrial fibrillation after acute myocardial infarction in patients with left ventricular dysfunction. Circulation 100:376-380
13. Mathew JP, Parks R, Savino JS et al (1996) Atrial fibrillation following coronary bypass graft surgery. JAMA 276:300-306
14. Lynn GM, Stefanko K, Reed JF et al (1992) Risk factors for stroke after coronary artery bypass. J Thorac Cardiovasc Surg 104:1518-1523
15. Kowey PR, Taylor JE, Rials SJ et al (1992) Meta-analysis of the effectiveness of prophylactic drug therapy in preventing supraventricular arrhythmia early after coronary bypass grafting. Am J Cardiol 69:963-965
16. Daoud EG, Strickberger A, Man KC et al (1997) Preoperative amiodarone as prophylaxis against atrial fibrillation after open heart surgery. N Engl J Med 337:1785-1791
17. Redle JD, Khurana S, Marzan R et al (1999) Prophylactic oral amiodarone compared with placebo for prevention of atrial fibrillation after coronary bypass surgery. Am Heart J 138:144-150
18. Giri S, White CM, Dunn AB et al (2001) Oral amiodarone for prevention of atrial fibrillation after open heart surgery, the Atrial Fibrillation Suppression Trial (AFIST): a randomised placebo-controlled trial. Lancet 357:830-836
19. Janse MJ, Malik M, Camm AJ, Julian DG, Frangin GA, Schwartz PJ on behalf of the EMIAT Investigators 1 (1998) Identification of post acute myocardial infarction patients with potential benefit from prophylactic treatment with amiodarone. A substudy of EMIAT (the European Myocardial Infarct Amiodarone trial). Eur Heart J 19:85-95
20. De Ferrari GM, Tavazzi L (1999) The role of arrhythmias in the progression of heart failure. Eur J Heart Fail 1:35-40
21. De Ferrari GM, Landolina M, Casella M et al (2001) Internal cardioversion of permanent atrial fibrillation in patient with severe heart failure: 1 year follow-up. Eur Heart J 22:562 (Abstract)

Drugs as Pretreatment before Electrical Cardioversion

G. L. Botto, M. Luzi, A. Sagone

Introduction

Atrial fibrillation (AF) is the most common arrhythmia found in clinical practice [1] and is associated with a doubling of overall morbidity and mortality from cardiovascular disease compared to healthy population [2]. While electrical cardioversion (CV) is a widely used and potentially definitive treatment for AF, it is not always successful. Even when sinus rhythm (SR) is achieved, the arrhythmia often recurs. Antiarrhythmic drugs may potentially augment electrical CV efficacy, and may facilitate maintenance of SR. However, use of these agents is not without risk.

Antiarrhythmic Drugs to Facilitate Electrical Cardioversion

The majority of patients will be successfully cardioverted with DC shock alone. The procedure itself may restore SR in up to 95% of patients with persistent AF, using external biphasic shock [3]. While the standard of practice dictates that DC shock alone be attempted before antiarhythmic agents are added, empiric pretreatment with drugs is becoming more common. Studies looking at administration of antiarrhythmic agents before the application of electrical CV are typically small, and rarely placebo-controlled.

Recently, Oral et al. [4] examined ibutilide in facilitating transthoracic CV. DC shock successfully cardioverted 100% of the patients who underwent pretreatment with ibutilide, compared to 72% of those who did not receive the agent. Those who failed to achieve SR with electrical CV alone were later successfully cardioverted when ibutilide was added before the electrical procedure. Two patients (3%) who received ibutilide suffered from polymorphic ventricular tachycardia (in neither case did this lead to death).

Department of Cardiology, S. Anna Hospital, Como, Italy

The use of class IC drugs or amiodarone as pretreatment before electrical CV will be discussed further below.

Time Course of Recurrences of Atrial Fibrillation

The most relevant clinical problem after successful CV is the risk of recurrences, which is particularly high in the first minutes to hours following electrical CV, by either internal [5] or external methods[6]. The phenomenon has only recently been described, acquiring a new set of acronyms: recurrence may occur in a very early phase (minutes) after electrical shock (IRAF, immediate recurrence of atrial fibrillation), in a subacute phase (first 24-48 h or up to 7-14 days) (ERAF, early recurrence of atrial fibrillation), or in the weeks or months following the successful procedure (LRAF, late recurrence of atrial fibrillation) [1].

Immediate and Early Recurrences of Atrial Fibrillation

The phenomena of IRAF and ERAF are difficult to characterize; however, two important concepts are implicated and may strongly interact. First, a growing number of patients have AF initiated, and possibly maintained, by an ectopic focus of repetitive atrial activity [7]. Secondly, AF itself causes changes in the cellular electrophysiology that have the effect of further increasing the tendency to fibrillation [8], and there is a reversal of this electrophysiological remodeling after a certain period of SR [9]. The first of these two concepts relates to the triggers for initiation of the AF and the second to the substrate predisposing the subject to and maintaining the arrhythmia.

The most important atrial parameter of AF-induced electrical remodeling is the refractory period. During control, early premature beats did not induce any arrhythmia. After few hours of AF, the atrial refractory period was shortened and a premature stimulus was followed by a short run of rapid atrial responses. Twenty-four hours of AF further shortened the atrial refractory period, and now early premature beats triggered paroxysms of AF [8]. Some studies have tested the efficacy of drug treatment before CV in preventing AF relapse, reducing atrial refractoriness maladaptation, or preventing premature supraventricular beats.

Calcium-Blocker Agents in Preventing Early Recurrences of Atrial Fibrillation

Intracellular calcium overload is the most important mechanism sustaining electrophysiological remodeling. Animal experiments have shown that verapamil infusion before short episodes of artificially induced AF [10] significantly reduced the electrical changes of the atria. If electrical remodeling in humans is also related to intracellular calcium overload, the frequency of relapse might be lowered by drugs that lower the intracellular calcium concentration.

Tieleman et al. [11], using transtelephonic monitoring, studied 61 patients cardioverted for persistent AF. Being on intracellular calcium-lowering medication preceding the CV was the only significant variable related to maintenance of SR.

De Simone et al. [12] were the first to demonstrate in a randomized fashion the beneficial effect of oral pretreatment with verapamil, associated with an antiarrhythmic drug, in reducing the incidence of ERAF after external or internal electrical CV. They found a higher incidence of AF recurrences in patients who received propafenone alone, before electrical CV than in patients who received propafenone combined with verapamil, suggesting that intracellular calcium-lowering drugs reduce electrical remodeling, which may in turn lead to a more rapid recovery after CV.

More recently, the final result of the VERAF Study [13] clearly demonstrated that verapamil alone, in patients who were not taking antiarrhythmic agents at the time of CV, is highly effective in reducing IRAF and ERAF after successful CV, but is ineffective in preventing arrhythmia recurrences in the long run.

Antiarrhythmic Drugs to Prevent Recurrences of Atrial Fibrillation

There is a clear evidence that any tendency to atrial ectopic activity is exaggerated in the early period following CV. Bianconi et al. [6] tested the efficacy of propafenone in a placebo-controlled study involving 100 patients, comparing two different strategies: pretreatment with oral propafenone or propafenone only after CV. Pharmacological conversion before DC shock was obtained in 6% of the subjects. Propafenone did not exert any significant effect on the success rate of the procedure. Arrhythmia recurrence was significantly reduced within 10 min after CV (0% vs 17% in the placebo group) and also within 24 h and 48 h. After CV the incidence of supraventricular ectopic beats was higher in the placebo patients.

Oral amiodarone is more effective than propafenone or sotalol in the long-term maintenance of SR [14]. However, its use around electrical CV of AF may be difficult because amiodarone loading requires al least 4-6 weeks to reach therapeutic plasma levels, and during the first weeks of treatment patients may be at risk of recurrences. Capucci et al. [15] randomized 92 patients with persistent AF and organic heart disease to pretreatment with oral amiodarone 400 mg/day 1 month before and 200 mg/day 2 months after CV or oral diltiazem 180 mg/day 1 month before and 2 months after CV. In the amiodarone group 25% of patients reverted to SR before the procedure, and amiodarone pretreatment increased CV efficacy. ERAF was similar in the different groups, while at 2 months the recurrence rate was lower in amiodarone-treated patients (32% vs 52-56%). It is possible to suppose the beneficial effect of amiodarone to be either on the prolongation of the atrial refractoriness and/or of the reduction in intracellular calcium concentration. Both these mechanisms may have affected the atrial remodeling phenomenon.

Conclusions

Antiarrhythmic pharmacotherapy may effectively supplement electrical CV of AF in two ways. After DC CV alone has failed, antiarrhythmic agents may be given before CV to facilitate the procedure. Ibutilide and amiodarone have proven most effective in this regard.

If AF recurs, antiarrhythmic drugs may be given, after a second CV attempt, to improve maintenance of SR. The mechanism underlying early recurrence of AF is unclear for the majority of patients, but is likely to be multifactorial. Contributing factors may include electrophysiological remodeling, which strongly interacts with triggering factors such as atrial ectopic beats, and both are probably modulated by the autonomic nervous system.

The administration of class IC and class III antiarrhythmic drugs has a favorable effect in reducing early recurrences, mainly by reducing the incidence of atrial ectopic beats, which is counterbalanced by the possibility of post-CV bradyarrhythmias. An alternative approach could be pretreatment with verapamil, alone or together with antiarrhythmic drugs, to reduce maladaptation of electrophysiological parameters induced by AF itself.

Amiodarone is the most effective agent in the maintenance of SR in the long run, but the benefit gained may not outweigh the threat of associated side effects.

References

1. ACC/AHA/ESC guidelines for the management of patients with atrial fibrillation. (2001) J Am Coll Cardiol 38:1266i-ixx
2. Kannel WB, Wolf PA (1992) Epidemiology of atrial fibrillation. In: Falk RH, Podrid PJ (eds) Atrial fibrillation mechanisms and management. Raven, New York, pp 81-92
3. Mittal S, Ayati S, Stein KM et al (2000) Transthoracic cardioversion of atrial fibrillation. Comparison of rectilinear biphasic versus damped sine wave monophasic shocks. Circulation 101:1282-1287
4. Oral H, Souza JJ, Michaud GF et al (1999) Facilitating transthoracic cardioversion of atrial fibrillation with ibutilide pretreatment. N Engl J Med 340:1849-1854
5. Timmermans C, Rodriguez LM, Smeets JLRM et al (1998) Immediate reinitiation of atrial fibrillation following internal defibrillation. J Cardiovasc Electrophysiol 9:122-128

6. Bianconi L, Mennuni M, Lukic V et al (1996) Effects of oral propafenone administration before electrical cardioversion of chronic atrial fibrillation: a placebo-controlled study. J Am Coll Cardiol 28:700-706
7. Jais P, Haissaguerre M, Shah DC et al (1997) A focal source of atrial fibrillation treated by discrete radiofrequency ablation. Circulation 95:572-576
8. Wijffels MCEF, Kirchhof CJHJ, Dorland R et al (1995) Atrial fibrillation begets atrial fibrillation: a study in awake chronically instrumented goats. Circulation 92:1954-1968
9. Yu WC, Lee SH, Tai CT et al (1999) Reversal of atrial electrical remodeling following cardioversion of long standing atrial fibrillation in man. Cardiovasc Res 42:470-476
10. Tieleman RG, De Langen CDJ, Van Gelder IC et al (1997) Verapamil reduces tachycardia-induced electrical remodeling of the atria. Circulation 95:1945-1953
11. Tieleman RG, Van Gelder IC, Crijins HJGM et al (1998) Early recurrence of atrial fibrillation after electrical cardioversion: a result of fibrillation-induced electrical remodeling of the atria? J Am Coll Cardiol 31:167-173
12. De Simone A, Stabile G, Vitale DF et al (1999) Pre-treatment with verapamil in patients with persistent or chronic atrial fibrillation who underwent electrical cardioversion. J Am Coll Cardiol 34:810-814
13. Botto GL, Belotti G, Cirò A et al, on behalf of the VERAF study group (2002) Verapamil in prevention of early recurrence of atrial fibrillation: final results of the VERAF study. Eur Heart J 23:660
14. Roy D, Talajic M, Dorian P et al, for the Canadian Trial of Atrial Fibrillation Investigators (2000) N Engl J Med 342:913-920
15. Capucci A, Villani GQ, Aschieri D et al (2000) Oral amiodarone increases the efficacy of DC cardioversion in restoration of sinus rhythm in patients with chronic atrial fibrillation. Eur Heart J 21:66-73

Atrial Fibrillation and Flutter: the Latest from the Planet of Right Radiofrequency Catheter Ablation

M. Lunati, G. Magenta, G. Cattafi, R. Vecchi, M. Paolucci, T. Di Camillo

Atrial Fibrillation

The creation of an interventional procedure effective in curing atrial fibrillation (AF) started with the surgical Maze procedure conceived and proposed by Cox in 1991 [1]. Electrophysiologists have tried since then to replicate the partitioning of the atria, performed by the surgeon with linear incisions, using a less invasive catheter-based technique, radiofrequency catheter ablation (RFCA) to achieve atrial compartmentalization [2, 3].

Right Atrial Linear Ablation Procedures

Limiting the linear ablative approach to the right atrium (RA) has the advantages of giving an easier, shorter, and less complicated procedure than a left atrial or a biatrial approach. The ablative lines are generally two: an intercaval line created along the posterior aspect of the RA from the superior vena cava to the inferior vena cava and a septal line from the superior vena cava across the fossa ovalis down to the coronary sinus.

The success rate for abolition of AF without drugs ranges from 0% to 30%; with concomitant drugs favorable outcomes can range from 10% to 50%. The overall success of the largest series published to date [3-6] gives these results: complete elimination without drugs 12%, control with drug therapy 21%. The high recurrence rate is partly due to the incomplete line generated by point-to-point application of RF energy and the consequent persistence of gaps. Recent studies have aimed to eliminate these discontinuities with the help of non conventional mapping systems [noncontact or Carto, Biosense Websters)] with promising results [5].

Another approach, recently introduced, is based on the use of multipolar ablative catheters to create a complete line, without gaps, delivering energy

U.O. di Elettrofisiologia, Dipartimento Cardiotoracovascolare A. De Gasperis, A.O. Niguarda Cà Granda, Milan, Italy

from each successive electrode without moving the catheter. In the Right Atria Microcatheter Ablation study, with an initial European experience followed by a US experience, the creation of a line was easily achieved and verified through the decrease of the local electrogram amplitude. The success rate of this approach, which is a hybrid approach to AF (linear ablation ± drugs), is approximately 40%.

We can report some interesting data concerning the RALL (Right Atrial Linear Lesions), study an Italian multicenter prospective study designed to investigate the clinical benefits of a right endocardial Maze procedure performed with a steerable catheter equipped with six coil electrodes, each 7 mm long, and with a thermocouple temperature control system (Medtronic Amazr). Ninety-five patients (52 male, 43 female; mean age 60±10 years) with paroxysmal AF refractory to one or more antiarrhythmic drugs and without clear evidence of focal origin were enrolled in the study. Structural heart disease was present in 52% and no evidence of heart disease in 48%. RFCA was performed in sinus rhythm with three lines (posterolateral, septal, and cavotricuspid isthmus). Procedure time was 104.2±40 min and X-ray exposure 29.4±15 min. No procedure-related complications occurred. After RFCA antiarrhythmic drug therapy was left unchanged in 85% of the study group, while 15% of the patients were off drugs. After a mean follow-up of 374±121 days, 59 patients (62%) had a 75% reduction in AF, 21 patients (22%) had a reduction in 50% of AF, and 15 patients (16%) had no benefit. A clinical improvement, assessed by a semiquantitative evaluation of quality of life, was achieved in 80% of the patients. These preliminary data show that a right atrial linear ablation procedure associated with previously ineffective drugs can significantly reduce episodes of symptomatic AF and improve quality of life in a selected patient population.

The exact role of linear ablation to treat drug-refractory AF is still debatable but is nevertheless increasing due to the difficulties of eliminating AF with pure focal ablation. Compartmentalization of the right atrium (with the aid of new mapping and ablative utilities) combined with additional pharmacological therapy may well still have a place.

Atrial Flutter

The electrophysiological demonstration of cavotricuspid isthmus block is a confirmed end-point of an ablative procedure for recurrent common atrial flutter, but in some cases, because of anatomical problems, this can be difficult to achieve or demonstrate, and some adaptation, either in mapping or in ablative strategy must be planned [7].

Ablative Tools

The linear ablation of the critical area should be an anatomically directed procedure, performed in sinus rhythm, and aimed at blocking of the electrical conduction between the tricuspid anulus and the inferior vena cava. Sometimes, because of local conditions (length of the isthmus and thickness of the myocardium, or prominence of a fibrous eustachian ridge), the conventional 4-mm-tip electrode cannot produce a stable block. In these cases (approximately 10%-15 % of all the procedures) one can now turn to other tools: (1) the 8-mm-long-tip electrode which allows longer and larger lesions, (2) the cooled-tip-electrode, which allows deeper penetration of the RF energy. The theorical risk of complications can cause some fear, but, surprisingly, the rate of problems reported to date for both conventional and nonconventional ablation of flutter continues to be extremely low [8-10].

Ablation End-Point

The use of multiple simultaneous recordings by means of multipolar (10-20) catheters and, more recently, the use of nonfluoroscopic mapping systems [non-contact, Carto, Localisa (Medtronic), real-time position management (RPM), etc.] has made easier the mapping, comprehension of the atrial sequence, and identification of the vulnerable area. The end-point of stable (persisting for 30 min after RFCA) bidirectional isthmus block can now be demonstrated in several ways [11-13]:

1. Pacing at the low septal right atrium (inside the coronary sinus) and at the low lateral righ atrium and analysis of the activation sequence can clearly show whether an isthmus block has been achieved.
2. The so called "differential pacing" technique can validate double potentials, recorded on the ablation line, as a sign of isthmus block.
3. Pacing the posterior wall detects conduction through a permeable terminal crest, which can mimic persistence of isthmus conduction after an otherwise effective procedure.
4. The use of unipolar electrograms which change from biphasic to positive morphology during conduction block.
5. The analysis of change of the P wave morphology during RA pacing after an effective block can give important clues on this matter.
6. The recording of double potentials separated by an isoelectric constant interval along the extent of the isthmus after the ablation confirm the block.

Right Atrial Atypical Flutters

Finally, the criteria for the diagnosis of atypical flutter, non-cavotricuspid-isthmus-dependent, have been defined [14]. The circuits (clockwise or counterclockwise) of supraventricular tachyarrhythmias, which occur after surgical repair of congenital heart disease (so-called scar-related or incisional reentrant flutters), can be peritricuspid, periatriotomy or based on a dual loop reentry. The assessment of the most convenient and safest segment of the circuit as the target of choice of the ablative procedure is greatly facilitated by three-dimensional mapping (Carto, Localisa).

References

1. Cox J (1991) The surgical treatment of atrial fibrillation. IV. Surgical technique. J Thorac Cardiovasc Surg 101:584-592
2. Swartz JP, Perrelsels G, Silvers J et al (1994) A catheter based curative approach to atrial fibrillation in humans. Circulation 90 [Suppl 1]:I-335
3. Haissaguerre M, Gencel L, Fischer B et al (1994) Successful catheter ablation of atrial fibrillation. J Cardiovasc Electrophysiol 5:1045-1052
4. Gaita F, Riccardi R, Calo' L et al (1998) Atrial mapping and radiofrequency catheter abaltion in patients with atrial fibrillation. Electrophysiological findings and ablation results. Circulation 97:2136-2145
5. Packer DL, Asirvatham S, Stenens CL et al (2000) Utility of non contact mapping for identifying gaps in long linear lesions in patients with atrial fibrillation. Pacing Clin Electrophysiol 23:673
6. Natale A, Leonelli F, Beheiry S et al (2000) Catheter ablation approach on the right side only for paroxysmal atrial fibrillation therapy: long term results. Pacing Clin Electrophysiol 23:224-233
7. Poty H, Saoudi N, Abdel Aziz A (1995) Radiofrequency ablation of type 1 atrial flutter. Prediction of late success by electrophysiological criteria. Circulation 92:1389-1392
8. Shah DC, Haissaguerre M, Jais P et al (1997) Simplified electrophysiologically directed catheter ablation of recurrent common atrial flutter. Circulation 96:2505-2509
9. Rodriguez LM, Nabar A, Timmermans C et al (2000) Comparison of results of an 8 mm split-tip versus a 4 mm tip ablation catheter to perform radiofrequency ablation of type I atrial flutter. Am J Cardiol 85:110-111
10. Jais P, Shah DC, Haïssaguerre M et al (2000) Prospective randomized comparison of irrigated tip versus conventional tip catheters for ablation of common flutter. Circulation 85:772-776
11. Shah D, Haïssaguerre M, Takahashi A et (2000) Differential pacing for distinguishing block from persistent conduction through an ablation line. Circulation 102:1517-1522
12. Villacastin J, Almendral J, Arenal A et al (2000) Usefulness of unipolar electrograms to detect isthmus block after radiofrequency ablation of typical atrial flutter. Circulation 102:3080-3085
13. Tada H, Oral H, Sticherling C et al (2001) Elecrogram polarity and cavotricuspid isthmus block during ablation of typical atrial flutter. J Cardiovasc Electrophysiol 12:393-399
14. Shah DC, Jais P, Hocini M et al (2002) Catheter ablation of atypical right atrial flutter. In: Zipes DP Haïssaguerre M (eds) Catheter ablation of arrhythmias, 2nd edn. Futura, Armonk, NY

Impact of LocaLisa on Ablation Management

F. Atienza, J. Almendral, A. Arenal, E.G. Torrecilla, J. Jiménez, M. Ortiz

Conventional Catheter Techniques: Current Practice and Limitations

The vast majority of conventional mapping techniques currently used involve the recording of electrical events from electrodes positioned at various intracardiac locations. This process requires catheter movement through multiple sites within the heart to obtain activation mapping and entrainment data at these places. Insight into the electrophysiological behavior of the heart is obtained by combining the information from the electrogram recording with anatomical information gathered from fluoroscopic images. Therefore, optimal positioning of catheters for electrophysiological studies and interventional procedures requires integration of a knowledge of cardiac anatomy and radiographic correlates of the main anatomic landmarks with their intracardiac electrograms [1]. But cardiac chambers and the catheters positioned inside them are three-dimensional structures represented by fluoroscopy in two-dimensional planes, and thereby we frequently misjudge the spatial relationships between them. By using sequential fluoroscopic views, we can try to determine more precisely the relative position of the catheters inside the heart chambers. Nevertheless, the processing of data to form an electrospatial representation of cardiac activation is a cumbersome task, highly dependent on the mental agility and memory of the operator.

Recent pathophysiological and technical progress has made ablation a valid treatment option for complex arrhythmogenic substrates, such as focal and persistent atrial fibrillation, atypical atrial flutter, incisional atrial tachycardias, and some complex forms of ventricular tachycardia [2-4]. However, appropriate diagnosis and treatment of the underlying electrophysiological mechanisms require the assessment of numerous potential sites for ablation

Electrophysiology Laboratory, Cardiology Department, Hospital General Universitario Gregorio Marañón, Madrid, Spain

and the ability to navigate to the site of choice. In this context, traditional techniques can be lengthy and inaccurate if lesions are to be deployed in a predicted close proximity to previous lesions, e.g., linear ablation procedures, exposing the patient and staff to extensive radiation [5].

The LocaLisa Mapping System

Several advanced mapping techniques have been developed to overcome the challenges seen with traditional electrophysiological methods. The LocaLisa system is a nonfluoroscopic navigation system with the ability to track multiple intracardiac electrodes. The system uses three pairs of skin electrode, positioned in *x*, *y*, *z* directions around the heart, sending three low-power (1 mA), high-frequency (30 kHz) currents. When an electrical current is applied externally through the thorax, a voltage drop occurs across internal organs like the heart. Therefore, these transthoracic currents generate three orthogonal electrical fields in the heart, creating a voltage gradient along their axis. By measuring the voltage of these signals via standard catheter electrodes, the position of an intracardiac electrode is calculated relative to a stationary reference electrode. Finally, the computer generates a three-dimensional picture of the electrodes' positions. Further technical details of the system can be found elsewhere [6].

The feasibility and accuracy of the system have already been demonstrated [6]. All electrode positions are identifiable with an error of 1-2 mm, with an optimal reproducibility and stability during long-lasting procedures, remaining unaffected by the cyclical variations due to cardiac movement. Moreover, the externally applied electrical fields do not interfere with intracardiac electrogram recordings. The method does not require specially designed catheters, allowing catheter exchange during the procedure and freedom of catheter choice, including complex catheter designs, such as multielectrode catheters or irrigated-tip catheters.

Potential Advantages of New Mapping Technologies

The LocaLisa system has the ability to accurately localize catheter position in three dimensions, allowing catheter movement in the absence of fluoroscopy. The system provides real-time simultaneous visualization of the position of the ablation catheter and other reference diagnostic catheters within the heart, and up to a maximum of ten electrodes can be displayed in a three-dimensional plot. Intracardiac catheters can be tracked, and various points of interest can be tagged throughout the procedure. This ability to annotate the anatomical sites associated with previously recorded electrogram events gives us the possibility to return the catheter to its previous location. Additionally, it allows measurement of the distance from the catheter to a specific target position. However, the system does not combine advanced mapping and conventional recording system capabilities in a single package, and lacks the possibility of obtaining activation or voltage maps. Thus, it still needs two separate systems that do not fully communicate with one another.

Clinical Benefits of the LocaLisa System

Despite its recent introduction in the market, the LocaLisa mapping system has already demonstrated significant clinical benefits over conventional techniques for the treatment of several types of arrhythmias. It can improve approaches to mapping and ablation procedures of arrhythmias that are currently effectively treated with conventional systems by reducing fluoroscopy and procedure times. When compared with a properly matched control group, LocaLisa reduced procedure-related exposure to ionizing radiation by 35% during ablation of supraventricular tachycardias, regardless of the arrhythmia substrate [7]. The technique has also been helpful for an anatomically guided approach to atrioventricular nodal reentrant tachycardia, avoiding repeated ablations at the same location and in close proximity to the proximal His bundle, and reducing the number of radiofrequency pulses and fluoroscopy time [8]. In patients with atrial flutter, the system can be used to delineate the area of interest (by identifying His, coronary sinus ostium, and tricuspid annulus), allowing the creation of a linear lesion in the right atrial isthmus, with a significant reduction of radiation exposure [6, 9]. Thus, this electrospatial mapping system has shown a potential to partially replace fluoroscopy during catheter ablation, reducing patient and operator exposure to radiation.

Additionally, LocaLisa could also facilitate ablation of complex arrhythmia ablation by reducing the limitations of conventional techniques. Incisional atrial tachycardias due to reentry around surgical scars can be safely and effectively treated with the assistance of this system [10]. Scars and critical isthmuses for the tachycardia were identified using conventional methods (by demonstrating split potentials and concealed entrainment), and were marked on the LocaLisa image. With this system support, lines of block closing the critical isthmuses were created. During pulmonary vein disconnection, it is often difficult to determine the exact position of the ablation catheter relative to the Lasso catheter. Continuous 3D monitoring of ablation and mapping catheters reduced fluoroscopy and pulmonary vein disconnection times [11, 12]. Finally, ventricular tachycardia ablation can also be facilitated using this system, which enables repeated applications closely around an apparently successful ablation site to ensure elimination of the arrhythmogenic area [13].

In conclusion, real-time 3D continuous monitoring using the LocaLisa system results in a significant reduction of fluoroscopy times in virtually all ablation procedures and facilitates the approach to complex arrhythmia substrates.

References

1. Singer I (1999) Catheterization and electrogram recordings. In: Singer I (ed) Interventio-nal electrophysiology. Williams & Wilkins, Baltimore, pp 27-59
2. Haïssaguerre M, Jaïs P, Shah DC et al (1998) Spontaneous initiation of atrial fibrillation by ectopic beats originating in the pulmonary veins. N Engl J Med 339:659-666
3. Nakagawa H, Shah N, Matsudaira K et al (2001) Characterization of reentrant circuit in macroreentrant right atrial tachycardia after surgical repair of congenital heart disease: isolated channels between scars allow "focal" ablation. Circulation 103:699-709
4. Marchlinski FE, Callans DJ, Gottlieb CD, Zado E (2000) Linear ablation lesions for control of unmappable ventricular tachycardia in patients with ischemic and nonischemic cardiomyopathy. Circulation 101:1288-1296
5. Rosenthal LS, Mahesh M, Beck TJ et al (1998) Predictors of fluoroscopy time and estimated radiation exposure during radiofrequency catheter ablation procedures. Am J Cardiol 82:451-458
6. Wittkampf FHM, Wever EFD, Derksen R et al (1999) LocaLisa. New technique for real-time 3-dimensional localization of regular intracardiac electrodes. Circulation 99:1312-1317
7. Kirchhoh P, Loh P, Eckardt L et al (2002) A novel nonfluoroscopic catheter visualization system (LocaLisa) to reduce radiation exposure during catheter ablation of supraventricular tachycardias. Am J Cardiol 90:340-344
8. Senatore G, Carreras G, Taglieri C et al (2002) Catheter ablation of nodal re-entrant tachycardia with LocaLisa navigation system. Europace 3[Suppl A]:A239
9. Senatore G, Carreras G, Taglieri C et al (2002) Catheter ablation of atrial flutter with LocaLisa navigation system. Europace 3[Suppl A]:A240
10. Molenschot M, Ramanna H, Hoorntje T et al (2001) Catheter ablation of incisional atrial tachycardia using a novel mapping system: LocaLisa. Pacing Clin Electrophysiol 24:1616-1622
11. Wittkampf F, Loh P, Derksen R et al (2002) Real-time, three dimensional, non-fluoroscopic localization of the Lasso catheter. J Cardiovasc Electrophysiol 13:630
12. Macle L, Jaïs P, Shah D et al (2000) Pulmonary vein disconnection guided by the LocaLisa system. Circulation 102[Suppl 5]:560
13. Wever EFD, Elvan A, Ramanna H et al (1999) Catheter ablation of ventricular tachycardia in patients with structural heart disease using a nonfluoroscopic localization system (Localisa). Pacing Clin Electrophysiol 22, 4-II:P734

Pacing in Atrial Fibrillation: Therapies for Rhythm Control

A. CARBONI

Introduction

For atrial fibrillation (AF) to occur, certain conditions such as triggers, initiators, and perpetuators are required: a trigger to start the arrhythmia; spatial inhomogeneity in the refractory period; a region of unidirectional conduction block; and short wavelength to allow reentry through the region of functional block; a sufficient atrial tissue mass to sustain a critical number of wavelets [1].

The retrospective design of previous trials on the role of pacing in preventing chronic AF has introduced a selection bias with a negative impact on the outcome measured [2]. Atrial pacing for prevention of AF was first proposed some years ago; the majority of the studies were conducted in patients with brady-tachy syndrome, and to date all that has been demonstrated is that DDD mode is superior to VVI mode in preventing the development of chronic AF [3-5].

Over a period of 4 years the Holter functions were used in a study by Garrigue et al. [6] to monitor the occurrence of atrial arrhythmias (AA) in 213 chronically DDD-paced patients. It was found that 48.5% of the patients experienced AA that they noticed during follow-up. AA duration was less than 24 h in 31.1% asymptomatic patients (81.5% of the episodes), between 24 h and 8 days in 10.3% and permanent in only 7.5%; 67 patients out of 154 without AA prior to implantation presented at least one episode of AA within 207±203 days after implantation; in 37 patients out of 59 who had AA before implantation, AA recurred much earlier (within 127±113 days). These results suggest a high prevalence of AA in patients on long-term pacemaker therapy, most episodes being asymptomatic.

Other studies have focused on the correlation between the coupling interval of premature beats and the subsequent development of AF: neither vagal or sympathetic prevalence seems to influence significantly the beginning of the arrhythmia, whereas the coupling interval of the atrial premature beats plays a critical role in the inducibility of atrial flutter or fibrillation [7].

Department of Cardiology, Az. Ospedaliera Parma, Italy

Pacing Therapies for Prevention of AF

Dual-Site Right Atrial Pacing

This therapy was first proposed by Saksena et al. [8, 9]. The pacemaker can be a single-chamber or a dual-chamber device, with two leads in the right atrium. To guarantee continuous atrial capture, the basal rate of the implanted pacemaker has to be programmed in the range of 80-90 bpm. If the patient does not tolerate this relatively high pacing rate, or a high pacing percentage is not achieved, drug treatment must be used to lower the intrinsic rhythm of the patient.

Biatrial Stimulation

This technique, proposed by Daubert, showed good results in the pilot study that were not confirmed by the prospective, randomized study [10, 11]. Apart from the effectiveness of this pacing modality, it does not affect the quality of life of patients because the algorithm used is in effect a triggered pulse to abolish the interatrial conduction delay.

Automatic Atrial Overdrive

This algorithm guarantees a pacing percentage of about 100%. Vitatron first implemented it 10 years ago in a dual-chamber pacemaker (Harmony). This algorithm necessarily increases the mean heart rate of patients, so it should be applied in patients without angina, which could be a consequent symptom.

Interatrial Septum Pacing

This pacing mode was proposed some years ago [12]. A bipolar screw-in lead is required with a short dipole (<10 mm) to avoid malfunctions due to the detection of ventricular far field in the atrial channel. To have the interatrial septum constantly paced, specific algorithms are needed to automatically ensure about 100% pacing. Automatic atrial overdrive and algorithms related to premature atrial contraction (PAC) are indicated.

PAC-Related Algorithm

Algorithms directly related to the ectopic atrial activity are designed to avoid the post-PAC pause (Fig. 1) and other PACs that are possible triggers for AF. The post-PAC pause suppression paces the atrium only for one or two cycles after the PAC, and this action is unlikely to cause any important symptom to the patient. The suppression of PAC activity (Fig. 2) is based on a time-limited atrial overdrive similar to the standard atrial overdrive, but only for a few minutes. There is no reason to expect particular symptoms related to these algorithms.

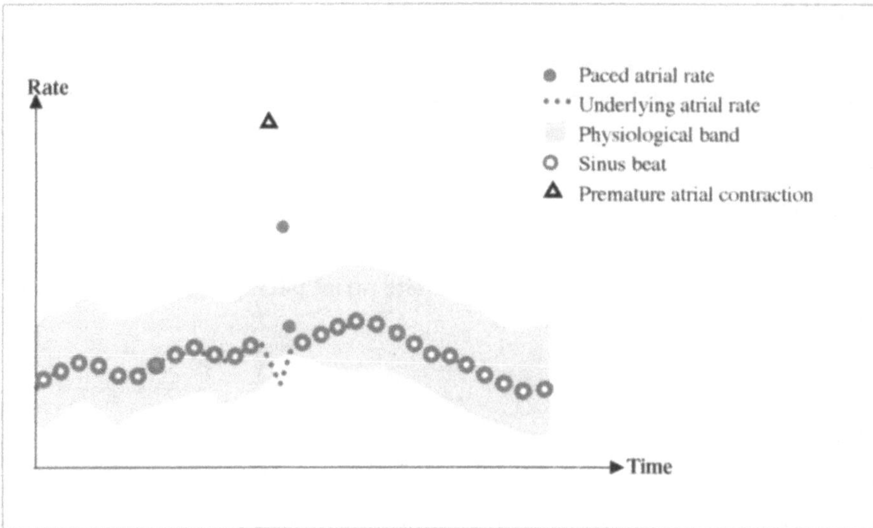

Fig. 1. Post PAC response

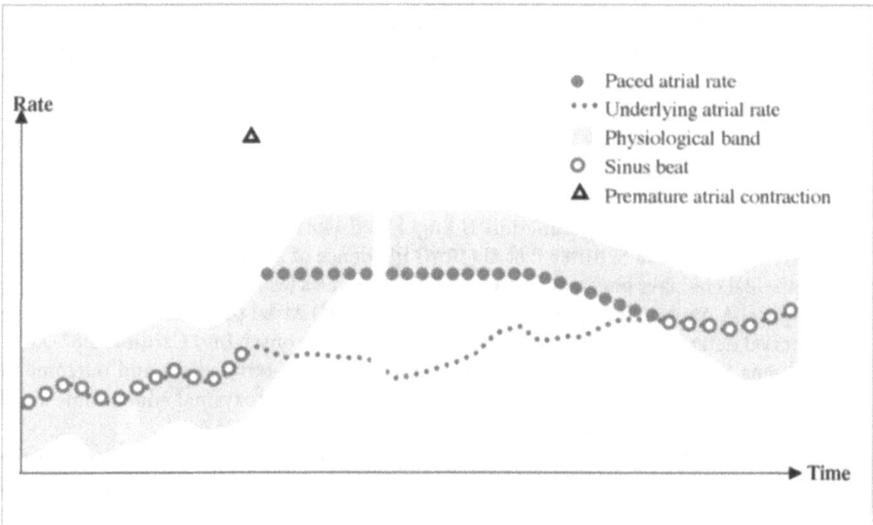

Fig. 2. PAC suppression

Post-Exercise Rate Control

This algorithm never increases the heart rate, but simply avoids an abrupt decrease in it after physical exercise. The intervention rate is computed as a function of the spontaneous heart rate previously reached by the patient during effort, and of the duration of effort.

Post-AF Response

This algorithm prevents early recurrences of AF immediately after cessation of an AF episode by increasing the pacing rate for a certain period at the end of the episode.

Rate Soothing

This algorithm paces the atrium at a rate slightly higher than the spontaneous rate (3 bpm) to induce a kind of dual-site atrial pacing involving the sinus node and the implanted electrode.

References

1. Rensma PL, Allessie MA, Lammers WJ et al (1988) Length of excitation wave and susceptibility to reentrant atrial arrhythmias in normal conscious dogs. Circ Res 62:395-410
2. Santini M, Alexidou G, Ansalone G et al (1990) Relation of prognosis in sick sinus syndrome to age, conduction defects and modes of permanent cardiac pacing. Am J Cardiol 65:729-735
3. Andersen HR, Nielsen JC, Thomsen PEB et al (1997) Long-term follow-up of patients from a randomised trial of atrial versus ventricular pacing for sick-sinus syndrome. Lancet 350:1210-1216
4. Connolly SJ, Kerr CR, Gent M et al (2000) Effects of physiologic pacing versus ventricular pacing on the risk of stroke and death due to cardiovascular causes. N Engl J Med 342:1385-1391
5. Lamas GA, Lee KL, Sweeney MO et al (2002) Ventricular pacing or dual-chamber pacing for sinus-node dysfunction. N Engl J Med 346:1854-1862
6. Garrigue S, Cazeau S, Ritter P et al (1996) Incidence of atrial arrhythmias in patients with dual chamber pacemakers. Arch Mal Coeur Vaiss 89:873-881
7. Capucci A, Santarelli A, Boriani G, Magnani B (1992) Atrial premature beats coupling interval determines lone paroxysmal atrial fibrillation onset. Int J Cardiol 36:87-93
8. Saksena S, Prakash A, Boccadamo R et al (2000) Long-term safety and outcome of dual site right atrial pacing in patients with refractory paroxysmal and chronic atrial fibrillation. Pacing Clin Electrophysiol 23:235
9. Boccadamo R, Mammacari A, Di Belardino N et al (2001) Differences between the algorithms and influence on quality of life. Atrial Fibrillation. IV International Meeting, Proceedings
10. Revault G, Mabo P, Daubert JC (2000) Long term effects of biatrial synchronous pacing to prevent drug-refractory atrial tachyarrhythmia: a nine year experience. J Cardiovasc Electrophysiol 11:1081-1091
11. Mabo P, Daubert JC (1999) Symbiapace study. Pacing Clin Electrophysiol 22:755, abstract 221
12. Bailin SJ et al (2001) Pacing from Bachmann's bundle prevents CAF: final results from a prospective randomized trial. Pacing Clin Electrophysiol 24:595, abstract 227

Pacing in Atrial Fibrillation: Therapies for Rate Control

A. SCHUCHERT

Atrial fibrillation is the most common atrial arrhythmia in Western Europe. It is associated with a poor prognosis and increasing costs for the health care system [1].

There are two approaches to treating patients with atrial fibrillation. Paroxysmal or persistent atrial fibrillation can be terminated using medical or electrical cardioversion. This approach is described as rhythm control. With the second approach, rate control, the patients remain in persistent or permanent atrial fibrillation or with recurrent episodes of paroxysmal atrial fibrillation, and only the ventricular rate and the irregularity of subsequent ventricular beats are controlled. This second approach is usually combined with long-term oral anticoagulation. Both the AFFIRM and the RACE trials compared the prognostic impact of rhythm control with that of the rate control strategy [2, 3]. The two studies demonstrated that the two strategies have a similar outcome with regard to death and stroke. The ventricular rate was higher in the rate control group than in the rhythm control group, and this is assumed to represent a compensatory rate increase due to the loss of atrial filling. This paper aims to review the value of pacing therapy for efficient rate control in patients with atrial fibrillation.

First, the ventricular rate must be assessed separately at rest and during exercise. Appropriate methods for measuring the ventricular rate at rest are surface ECG, the Holter ECG, and, in pacemaker patients, the diagnostic pacemaker counters. Heart rate during exercise can be determined with a surface ECG during an exercise test, with 24-h Holter ECG, and with extended pacemaker counters. Some more recent diagnostic pacemaker counters additionally allow the ventricular rate to be analyzed immediately after the onset of an episode of paroxysmal atrial fibrillation. Extended ECG and rate recording enable the ventricular rate to be registered during not only symptomatic, but also asymptomatic atrial fibrillation.

Medical Clinic III, Hamburg-Eppendorf University Hospital, Hamburg, Germany

The ventricular rate of patients with atrial fibrillation may be within the optimal range or it may be either too slow or too fast. Ventricular rates between 60 and 80 bpm at rest and (220 minus age in years) bpm during maximal exercise are assumed as optimal for most patients. The heart rate in patients with ventricular rates above 100 bpm at rest and 150 bpm during moderate exercise is too high. In addition to symptoms such as palpitations, the latter group can develop tachycardia-induced cardiomyopathy. On the other hand, a ventricular rate below 50 bpm at rest and 90 bpm during maximal exercise is too low; this is also known as chronotropic incompetence. Typical symptoms in patients whose heart rate is too low can be dizziness, syncope, and an impaired capacity for exercise.

Drug administration, pacemaker therapy, and in selected cases interventional procedures in combination with pacemaker implantation are treatments to lower ventricular rate and rate irregularity in patients with ventricular rates that are too fast. Medical treatment is the first approach in most patients. The oldest rate control drug is digitalis, which reduces fast ventricular rates at rest but has limited effect in reducing fast rates during exercise. More effective rate control during both rest and exercise has been shown for calcium antagonists and β-blockers. The limitation of both these drugs seems to be in patients with heart failure due to impaired systolic function: calcium antagonists are not indicated in these patients [4]. β-Blocker therapy with bisoprolol had no beneficial effects on mortality and frequency of hospitalization among patients with heart failure and atrial fibrillation, in contrast to patients with sinus rhythm [5]. Amiodarone is very efficient for rhythm control, and also very effective in reducing mean ventricular heart rate in patients with persistent atrial fibrillation [6]. The limitation of long-term amiodarone administration is the frequent occurrence of serious noncardiac side effects.

At present, the need to control ventricular rates that are too high is not generally accepted as an indication for permanent cardiac pacing. Pacemaker therapy can be indicated in patients who need the above-mentioned drugs for effective rate control and develop intermittent slow ventricular rates in combination with symptoms. Wittkampf et al. analyzed the effects of ventricular pacing on beat-to-beat rate variation in patients with permanent atrial fibrillation [7]. As expected, ventricular pacing at a constant rate prevented the occurrence of long RR intervals (i.e., slow ventricular rates). Their new finding was that constant pacing at the same time reduced the frequency of short RR intervals (i.e., fast ventricular rates). As a consequence, the average ventricular rate remained unchanged. However, higher pacing rates were necessary in many patients to achieve more or less complete suppression of shorter RR intervals.

The most recent solution is the invention of pacing algorithms such as the flywheel and ventricular rate stabilization algorithms to stabilize the ventricular rate without the need to adjust the lower pacing rate to a higher value. The flywheel algorithm paces the ventricle with a dynamic adaptation of the escape interval, resulting in pacing if the rate after a spontaneous beat drops by more than 15 bpm. The algorithm was assessed in the RASTAF study in a randomized cross-over study design for 1 month [8]. In patients with infrequent pacing in the control phase, the flywheel improved quality of life and exercise capacity. The recently invented ventricular rate stabilization algorithm starts to pace the ventricle earlier that means instead of –15 bpm with flywhell as soon as the time interval exceeds –3 bpm. Its efficacy has been demonstrated during an acute study [9]. The clinical impact is being assessed in the ongoing RASTAF II study.

The most frequent interventional approach for rate control is ablation of the atrioventricular (AV) node followed by implantation of a pacemaker ("ablate and pace") [10, 11]. At present, patients undergoing this treatment receive the pacemaker, and then the pacemaker settings have to be tailored to the patient by activating the rate-stabilizing algorithms. As symptomatic bradycardia can no longer occur, the patients can receive the maximum dose of digitalis, β-blocker, and in selected cases also a calcium antagonist in combination [12]. Patients with permanent atrial fibrillation receive a single-chamber rate response pacemaker. In cases of chronotropic incompetence, dual-sensor systems, e.g., combining a physiologic with an activity sensor, allow broader rate flexibility during daily life and better patient-tailored programming in the few patients who report symptoms with the standard rate response setting. Patients with paroxysmal atrial fibrillation should receive a dual-chamber pacemaker offering a fast beat-to-beat mode switch, since such a system will avoid pacemaker-triggered ventricular tachyarrhythmia in the event of an episode of paroxysmal atrial fibrillation. After atrial fibrillation has ceased, the pacemaker returns immediately to AV synchronous pacing. AV node ablation should be restricted to patients who remain highly symptomatic or who have fast ventricular rates. In these patients the pacemaker restores the constant and regular ventricular rate at rest and the rate response increases the ventricular rate during exercise.

Pacemaker therapy is already an accepted indication for patients with atrial fibrillation and too slow ventricular rates. This is an indication in the German guidelines for pacing therapy [13]. The indication to pace is definite in patients with slow ventricular rates or long pauses in combination with symptoms of impaired cerebral perfusion or heart failure. Patients with slow ventricular rates (<40 bpm) or long pauses (>3–4 s) and an assumed cause of their clinical symptoms constitute a relative indication. Pace making is not indicated in patients without symptoms even if the ventricular rate is slower than 40 bpm or if some RR intervals are longer than 3 s [13]. In Germany, slow ventricular rates in combination with atrial fibrillation are the reason for implantation in 24% of all patients who receive a pacemaker [14]. The American guidelines have not yet mentioned this indication.

During the past 10 years very few studies have assessed the effects of pacemaker therapy in this patient group, which is well known to have a worse prognosis than other groups. In an analysis of 318 patients, patients with bradyarrhythmia had a 1-year mortality of 15%, which was higher than those of patients with dual-nodal disease (13%), advanced AV block (7%), and sick sinus syndrome (5%) [15]. Pacemaker therapy improved the bradycardia-related symptoms such as syncope, dizziness, or impaired exercise tolerance in these patients. So far no studies have been performed indicating that pacemaker therapy prolongs survival in these patients.

Conclusions

The optimal range for the ventricular rate in patients with atrial fibrillation is between 60 and 90 bpm at rest. Ventricular rates below 50 bpm at rest and 90 bpm during exercise are too slow. Symptomatic patients improve with implantation of a single-chamber ventricular pacemaker and activation of the rate response (VVIR).

Ventricular rates above 100 bpm at rest and 150 bpm during moderate exercise are too fast. Rate control is mandatory in both symptomatic and asymptomatic patients. The primary approach is drug therapy, which can have some limitations. New improved pacing functions mean that "ablate and pace" should be replaced by "pace and ablate." Patients with drug-refractory atrial fibrillation could receive pacemaker therapy with pacemakers offering new pacing algorithms for rate stabilization. Ventricular pacing allows more aggressive medical rate control because intermittent inadvertent bradycardia cannot occur. AV node ablation is a very effective treatment for the few patients who still remain highly symptomatic.

References

1. Chugh SS, Blackshear JL, Shen W-K, Hammill SC, Gersh BJ (2001) Epidemiology and natural history of atrial fibrillation: clinical implications. J Am Coll Cardiol 37:371–378
2. Wyse DG on behalf of the AFFIRM Investigators (2002) Survival in patients presenting with atrial fibrillation: the Atrial Fibrillation Follow-up Investigation of Rhythm Management (AFFIRM) Study. Late breaking trials, ACC 2002
3. Crijns HJ, van Gelder IC, Tijssen JG, Hagens VE, Bosker HA, Kamp O, Kingma T, Kingma JH (2002) Rate-control versus electrical cardioversion for persistent atrial fibrillation. A randomized comparison of two treatment strategies concerning mortality and morbidity: the RACE Study. Late breaking trials, ACC 2002
4. Remme WJ, Swedberg K, Task Force for the Diagnosis and Treatment of Chronic Heart Failure, European Society of Cardiology (2001) Guidelines for the diagnosis and treatment of chronic heart failure. Eur Heart J 22:1527–1560
5. Lechat P, Hulot J-S, Escolano S, Mallet A, Leizorovicz A, Werhlen-Grandjean M, Pochmalicki G, Dargie H, on behalf of the CIBIS II Investigators (2001) Heart rate and cardiac rhythm relationships with bisoprolol benefit in chronic heart failure in CIBIS II trial. Circulation 103:1428–1433
6. Deedwania PC, Singh BN, Ellenbogen K, Fisher S, Fletcher R, Singh SN, for the Department of Veterans Affairs CHF-STAT Investigators (1998) Spontaneous conver-

sion and maintenance of sinus rhythm by amiodarone in patients with heart failure and atrial fibrillation. Circulation 98:2574–2579
7. Wittkampf FH, de Jongste MJ, Lie HI, Meijler FL (1988) Effect of right ventricular pacing on ventricular rhythm during atrial fibrillation. J Am Coll Cardiol 11:539–545
8. Labonte RE (2000) Symptom reduction through ventricular rate stabilization in patients with conducted chronic atrial fibrillation. Europace Suppl D 1:10/4
9. Lee J (1999) Acute testing of the rate-smoothed pacing algorithm for ventricular rate stabilization. Pacing Clin Electrophysiol 22:554-561
10. Wood MA, Brown-Mahoney C, Kay GN, Ellenbogen KA (2000) Clinical outcomes after ablation and pacing therapy for atrial fibrillation. Circulation 101:1138–1144
11. Ozcan C (2001) Long-term survival after ablation of the atrioventricular node and implantation of a permanent pacemaker in patients with atrial fibrillation. N Engl J Med 344:1043–1051
12. Levy T, Walker S, Mason M, Spurrell P, Rex S, Brant S, Paul V (2001) Importance of rate control or rate regulation for improving exercise capacity and quality of life in patients with permanent atrial fibrillation and normal left ventricular function: a randomised controlled study. Heart 85:171–178
13. Lemke B, Fischer W, Schulten HK (1996) Richtlinien zur Herzschrittmachertherapie. Z Kardiol 85:611–628
14. Irnich W (2002) German pacemaker registry. www.med.uni-giessen.de/technik/index-e.html
15. Schuchert A, Helms S, Meinertz T, on behalf of the LOP Investigators (1999) Effects of the indication for cardiac pacing and the pacing mode on the mortality after pacemaker implantation. Pacing Clin Electrophysiol 22:A18

Device Therapy for Atrial Arrhythmias: Latest Topics from the AT500 Italian Registry

G.L. Botto[1], M. Santini[2], L. Padeletti[3], A. Sagone[1], G. Boriani[4], G. Inama[5], A. Capucci[6], M. Gulizia[7], P. Della Bella[8], F. Solimene[9], M. Vimercati[10], M. Disertori[11], on behalf of the AT500 Italian Registry Investigators

Introduction

Atrial fibrillation (AF) is the most common sustained cardiac arrhythmia in clinical practice, and has been recognized as a cause of morbidity and mortality [1]. Drug treatment is often ineffective, and therefore electrical treatment has been recently suggested.

In many patients with AF a sick sinus syndrome (SSS) or AV conduction disturbances are often present. Atrial pacing in patients with SSS has been associated with a better sinus rhythm maintenance than ventricular pacing [2-4]. Recently, antitachycardia pacing (ATP) has been suggested in the treatment of AF, with some promising results as demonstrated by studies with the dual-chamber defibrillator [5, 6]. To increase the therapeutic options for AF in patients with a dual-chamber pacemaker, a DDDRP device has been developed (Medtronic AT500).

In this paper we report the results in the Italian AT500 Registry, including patients with indication for pacemaker implantation (classes I and II according to the ACC/AHA Guidelines) [7] and/or with AF.

Methods

We studied 330 consecutive patients treated with an AT500 DDDRP pacemaker (Medtronic Inc., Minn., USA) in 21 medical centers (see Appendix) and included in the Italian AT500 Registry. Data collection started on September 1999. The AT500 DDDRP pacemaker used in the present experience is an arrhythmia management device with:

[1]S. Anna Hospital, Como; [2]S. Filippo Neri Hospital, Rome; [3]Careggi Hospital, Florence; [4]S. Orsola Hospital, Bologna; [5]Maggiore Hospital, Crema; [6]Civile Hospital, Piacenza; [7]S. Luigi - Currò Hospital, Catania; [8]Cardiologico Center, Milan; [9]Montevergine Hospital, Mercogliano; [10]Medtronic Italy, Milan; [11]S. Chiara Hospital, Trento, Italy

- An algorithm (PR Logic) to classify the rhythm taking account of the rate and regularity of atrial signals together with AV association
- Three different prevention algorithms that attempt to interact with atrial arrhythmia onset mechanisms
- A programmable set of automatic atrial ATP therapies: "burst±" (constant drive coupled with up to two extrastimuli) and "ramp" (decremental drive) therapies
- An extensive set of diagnostic and monitoring information permitting detailed information - including marker annotation and strips of electrogram (EGM) signal - to be stored.

The primary study outcomes were to measure the number of detected, treated, and successfully terminated episodes, to measure AF burden, and to correlate ATP termination efficacy with AF burden variation between a period with ATP programmed "off" and a period with ATP programmed "on". AF burden was defined as the total amount of time for which the patient was in atrial arrhythmia and was measured in hours per day.

Results

Three-hundred thirty patients (164 male), mean age 71±9 years, were enrolled in the Registry and implanted with the described device with bipolar atrial and ventricular leads. Hypertension was present in 142 (46.1%) patients, valvular disease in 38 (11.5%), 32 (9.6%) patients had a history of myocardial infarction. Left ventricular ejection fraction was 56.2±10.8%. The most common implant indications were SSS in 244 (73.9%) patients and acquired AV block in 41 (12.4%). In 320 (96.9%) patients there was a history of atrial tachyarrhythmias. A bipolar atrial lead was positioned in the right atrial appendage (RAA) in 181 (55%) patients, in the interatrial septum (IAS) in 93 (28%), and in other right atrial (ORA) sites in 56 (17%). Average follow-up duration was 6.3±4.9 months. After pacemaker implantation 123 (37%) patients received no antiarrhythmic therapy, 73 (22%) patients were treated with amiodarone, 72 (22%) with class 1C drugs, 36 (11%) with sotalol, and 26 (8%) with β-blockers.

In order to evaluate the device's ability to detect and terminate atrial arrhythmia, EGMs and marker channels stored in the device memory for 314 episodes in 131 patients were analyzed. Atrial arrhythmia detection was appropriate in 305/314 (97%) episodes. In 9 episodes far-field R wave associated with sinus rhythm led to inappropriate detection. Device-defined termination was appropriate in 256/305 (84%) episodes. In 49 episodes termination classification was inappropriate, mainly because of false far-field R wave (45 episodes) and undersensing of atrial signal (4 episodes).

During the follow-up we did not observe any significant ATP-related complication in the study population.

ATP Efficacy

After discarding inappropriately detected or terminated episodes, we had data on treated episodes stored with EGM information from 52 patients. The device classified 241 (34.8%) of the 693 stored episodes as successfully terminated.

ATP therapy was programmed "off" in the first month after pacemaker implantation to allow lead stabilization, and then switched to "on". The change in AF burden was measured by subtracting AF burden during the ATP "off" period by AF burden during the ATP "on" period. The patients were divided in two groups: group A, in which ATP therapy efficacy defined both as percentage of success and as percentage of treated episodes was higher than one-third and group B, which included all the others.

The mean AF burden reduction for patients in group A was (0.04±2.85) h/day, while the same calculation in group B led to an average value of (2.02±3.17) h/day (p=0.033). A significant correlation was demonstrated between AF burden reduction and ATP therapy efficacy (p<0.05, Spearman nonparametric test).

Analysis of AT/AF Episodes

The device defines the onset of an episode as the moment at which an AT/AF evidence criterion is satisfied. During the episode, the rhythm is continuously classified according to the programmed detection parameters. The device is designed to deliver an ATP therapy whenever the rhythm is classified as AT and the current episode is classified as sustained. Therefore, an episode initially classified as AF may be treated if its characteristics change to AT at any moment of the current episode.

In the subgroup of patients with EGM information available we calculated the number of treated episodes initially classified as AT and AF and measured the difference in therapy efficacy among these two classes. In view of the different atrial lead implant sites, we also evaluated ATP results with the lead location. We also measured the average atrial cycle length at episode onset and the average time from onset to therapy for episodes classified as AT and AF.

AT and AF onset

Among the 693 treated episodes considered, 345 (49.8%) were defined at onset as AT and 348 (50.2%) were defined as AF. One-hundred seventy of the 345 AT-classified episodes (49.3%) and 71 of the 348 AF-classified treated episodes (20.4%) were successfully terminated. The average cycle length at onset of the episodes classified as AT was 271.74±33.78 ms, while the AF episodes had an average median PP interval at onset of 211.18±29.82 ms (p<0.01).

Site of Pacing

With regard to the different possible atrial lead implant sites, we found:

- 46 AT and 94 AF episodes treated in 7 patients with the atrial lead at the RAA
- 22 AT and 47 AF episodes treated in 5 patients with the atrial lead at the IAS
- 27 AT and 20 AF episodes treated in 3 patients with the atrial lead at ORA sites

Because of the small number of patients with leads implanted in ORA sites, we only compared efficacy between implants at the RAA and at the IAS sites. The results are reported in Table 1.

Table 1. ATP therapy efficacy in relation to the different sites of pacing

	Implanation site RAA	IAS	ORA	Total
Patients (n)	7	6	3	16
Episodes (n)	140	69	47	256
Successes (n)	26	41	29	96
Efficacy (%)	18.6%	59.4%		37.5%
	P<0.01			

RAA, right atrial appendage; IAS, interatrial septum; ORA, other right atrium sites

AT and AF Cycle Length

ATP efficacy was evaluated classifying the episodes according to the median PP interval measured before each therapy. We divided the episodes into four groups depending on pretherapy AT/AF cycle length. Efficacies are reported according to median PP interval and to episode classification at onset in Table 2. The respective success rates in the four groups were higher for slower and more organized episodes.

Table 2. ATP therapy efficacy (success/number of episodes) in relation to median PP interval measured before ATP therapy delivery

	PP (ms) <200	200-240	240-290	>290
AF	21/162 (13.0%)	29/129 (22.5%)	21/57 (36.8%)	
AT	3/13 (23.1%)	14/51 (27.5%)	79/153 (51.6%)	74/128 (57.8%)
Total	24/175 (13.7%)	43/180 (23.9%)	100/210 (47.6%)	74/128 (57.8%)

ATP Delay

ATP efficacy was evaluated classifying episodes according to time elapsed from the moment of onset to the moment of the first delivered therapy. We selected a subgroup of 45 patients who had at least one treated episode, thus 374 episodes were analyzed. The efficacy values are reported in Table 3. Our data show that prompt ATP delivery is related to higher efficacy.

Table 3. ATP therapy efficacy (success/number of episodes) in relation to time elapsed from onset of AT/AF episodes and the first therapy

	Time to first therapy			
	<1.5 min	1.5-2.5 min	2.5-4.5 min	>4.5 min
Efficacy	128/248 (51.6%)	17/51 (33.3%)	5/18 (27.8%)	6/57 (10.5%)

Discussion

The present study demonstrates the safety and efficacy of automatic ATP algorithms for detection and termination of AT and/or AF with a sophisticated dual-chamber pacemaker. Atrial ATP terminated a high number of treated AT/AF episodes without any proarrhythmic effects in a population of patients with a history of atrial tachyarrhythmias and indication for pacemaker implantation.

Safety of Atrial ATP

Analysis of the data stored in the device memory showed that the specificity of the AT/AF detection algorithm was 97% and the specificity of device-defined AT/AF termination was 84%. These results are comparable to those of another study using the same AT/AF algorithm [5] and confirm the algorithm's reliability in wide clinical use. However, the use of high bipolar atrial sensitivity may reduce far-field R wave oversensing, particularly in IAS atrial lead implantation, which rarely leads to inappropriate AT detection. The high specificity of the AT/AF detection algorithms explains the absence of any proarrhythmic effect observed during the follow-up period and confirms the results seen in patients with dual-chamber implantable cardioverter/defibrillator systems [5, 6].

Efficacy of Atrial ATP

The analysis of EGM information in a subgroup of patients confirmed the general success rate of ATP, which terminated 241/693 stored AT/AF episodes (34.8%). The effect of ATP on AF burden was, in this subgroup, closely related to the ATP efficacy. The reduction of AF burden was significant only in the patients in whom ATP therapy efficacy was higher in AT/AF termination. This observation firstly suggests the capability of atrial ATP to improve the efficacy of AF prevention by already sophisticated and reliable pacemakers. The experience of the AT500 Italian Registry identifies the subsequent features as mainly related to the success rate of ATP in the termination of AT/AF episodes.

The characteristics of the arrhythmia at onset heavily affect the ATP success rate. The episodes were classified at onset as AT in 49.8% and as AF in 50.2% of the cases. The device is designed to deliver an ATP therapy whenever the rhythm is classified as AT. Therefore, an episode initially classified as AF may be treated if its characteristics (atrial rate or regularity) change to those of AT at any moment of the episode. ATP efficacy was higher in the treatment of episodes classified at onset as AT (49%) than in those classified at onset as AF (20%). In studies with an implantable cardioverter/defibrillator system capable of ATP which used similar criteria for AT detection and definition of ATP success, AT pace-termination was achieved in 45%-71% of episodes [5, 6].

Furthermore, the ATP success rate improved with the increase of pretherapy AT/AF cycle length, from 13.7% for a cycle length below 200 ms to 57.8% when the cycle length was above 290 ms.

The ATP therapy delay also is strictly related to its efficacy. We observed that prolonging the ATP delay impairs the success rate, from 51.6% for ATP therapy within 1.5 min to 10.5% for ATP therapy later than 4.5 min after arrhythmia onset. These results may be explained by the shorter atrial cycle length when the arrhythmia episode starts as AF, and also by short-term metabolic atrial remodeling [8], which could reduce ATP efficacy in an arrhythmia lasting more than a few minutes.

Thus, an arrhythmia episode classified at onset as AT, with a long PP interval, and treated immediately, is more likely to be effectively terminated by ATP than an episode classified at onset as AF and treated late. It has been demonstrated that ATP only achieves local capture in atrial arrhythmias with a very short and irregular atrial cycle length, resulting in failures in terminating AF, as confirmed in some clinical studies [9]. In contrast, ATP efficacy in terminating atrial flutter has been demonstrated [10]. It has also been observed that class I and III class antiarrhythmic agents improve pace-termination of atrial flutter, due to a higher degree of atrial arrhythmia organization and increase of both atrial cycle length and excitable gap [11,12]. It is likely that an association of ATP with antiarrhythmic drugs (hybrid therapy) increases the percentage of patients with satisfactory clinical control of AF.

Finally, the site of atrial pacing affects the efficacy of ATP, showing a significantly higher rate of arrhythmia termination for the IAS than for the RAA pacing site (59.4% versus 18.6%, $p<0.01$). Inhomogeneous electrical activation of the atria has been previously reported during AF [13]. These data suggest the central role of IAS and probably of the Koch triangle, not only in the genesis of AF, but also in its maintenance. However, the mechanisms involved are not completely understood. In our study population the available data did not offer further information.

Conclusions

The present study demonstrates the safety and efficacy of a sophisticated DDDRP pacemaker with automatic ATP therapies for AT/AF termination in patients with AF. The highest ATP efficacy was observed in the treatment of tachyarrhythmia episodes classified at onset as AT with a long PP interval, in patients in whom the IAS site was used for atrial lead implantation. Our results favor the use of the DDDRP pacemaker as a new option in the treatment of AF.

However, besides an history of atrial tachyarrhythmia, most our patients had an indication for pacemaker implantation on the basis of SSS or of AV conduction disturbances. To extend these results to patients with AF alone, not previously selected for pacemaker implantation, we probably need further studies.

Appendix

Participating Centers: Dr. Botto, Dr. Luzi, Dr. Sagone, S. Anna Hospital, Como; Dr. Disertori, Dr. Del Greco, Dr. Gramegna, S. Chiara Hospital, Trento; Dr. Santini, Dr. Ricci, Dr. Pignalberi, S. Filippo Neri Hospital, Rome; Dr. Padeletti, Dr. Pieragnoli, Dr. Colella, Careggi Hospital, Florence; Dr. Dini, Dr. Adinolfi, S. Camillo Hospital, Rome; Dr. Gasparini, Dr. Mantica, Humanitas Hospital, Rozzano; Dr. Proclemer, Dr. Facchin, S. Maria della Misericordia Hospital, Udine; Dr. Capucci, Dr. Marrazzo, Civile Hospital, Piacenza; Dr. Boriani, Dr. Biffi, S. Orsola Hospital, Bologna; Dr. Spampinato, Dr. Martelli, Villa Tiberia Hospital, Rome; Dr. Drago, Dr. Silvetti, Bambino Gesù, Rome; Dr. Inama, Maggiore Hospital, Crema; Dr. Montenero, Multimedica Hospital, Sesto S. Giovanni; Dr. Della Bella, Cardiologico Hospital, Milan; Dr. Adornato, Melacrino Hospital, Reggio Calabria; Dr. Mangiameli, Garibaldi Hospital, Catania; Dr. Gulizia, S. Luigi-S. Currò Hospital, Catania; Dr. Libero, Le Molinette Hospital, Turin; Dr. Senatore, Ciriè Hospital, Ciriè; Dr. Zamparelli, Monaldi Hospital, Naples; Dr. Sassara, Belcolle Hospital, Viterbo; Dr. Puglisi, Fatebenefratelli Hospital, Rome; Dr. Ferri, S. Pietro Hospital, Rome; Dr. Favale, Policlinico di Bari; Dr. Zolezzi, Civile Hospital, Vigevano; Dr F. Solimene Montevergine Hospital, Mercogliano.

References

1. Ryder KM, Benjamin EJ (1999) Epidemiology and significance of atrial fibrillation. Am J Cardiol 84:131R-138R
2. Andersen HR, Nielsen JC, Thomsen PE et al (1997) Long-term follow-up of patients from a randomised trial of atrial versus ventricular pacing for sick-sinus syndrome. Lancet 350:1210-1216
3. Lamas GA, Orav EJ, Stambler BS et al, for the Pace-Maker Selection in the Elderly Investigators (1998) Quality of life and clinical outcomes in elderly patients treated with ventricular pacing as compared with dual-chamber pacing. N Eng J Med 338:1097-1104
4. Padeletti L, Porciani MC, Michelucci A et al (1999) Interatrial septum pacing: a new approach to prevent recurrent atrial fibrillation. J Interv Card Electrophysiol 3:35-43

5. Swerdlow CD, Schols W, Dijkman B et al (2000) Detection of atrial fibrillation and flutter by a dual chamber implantable cardioverter-defibrillator. Circulation 101:878-885
6. Ricci R, Pignalberi C, Disertori M et al (2002) Efficacy of dual chamber defibrillator with atrial antitachycardia function in treating spontaneous atrial tachyarrhythmias in patients with life threatening ventricular tachyarrhythmias. Eur Heart J 23:1471-1479
7. Gregoratos G, Cheltin MD, Conill A et al (1998) ACC/AHA Guidelines for Implantation of Cardiac Pacemakers and Antiarrhythmia Devices: Executive Summary-a report of the American College of Cardiology/American Heart Association Task Force on Practice Guidelines (Committee on Pacemaker Implantation). Circulation 97:1325-1335
8. Allessie MA (1998) Atrial electrophysiologic remodeling: another vicious circle? J Cardiovasc Electrophysiol 9:1378-1393
9. Paldino W, Bahu M, Knight BP et al (1997) Failure of single-and multisite high-frequency atrial pacing to terminate atrial fibrillation. Am J Cardiol 80:226-227
10. Peters RW, Shorofsky SR, Pelini M et al (1999) Overdrive atrial pacing for conversion of atrial flutter: comparison of postoperative with nonpostoperative patients. Am Heart J 137:100-103
11. Tai CT, Chen SA, Feng AN et al (1998) Electrophysiologic effect of class I and class II antiarrhythmic drugs on typical atrial flutter. Insights into the mechanism of termination. Circulation 97:1935-1945
12. Wijffels MCEF, Dorland R, Mast F et al (2000) Widening of the excitable gap during pharmacological cardioversion of atrial fibrillation in the goat. Effects of cibenzoline, hydroquinidine, flecainide, and d-sotalol. Circulation 102:260-267
13. Gaita F, Calo L, Ricciardi R et al (2001) Different patterns of atrial activation in idiopathic atrial fibrillation: simultaneous multisite atrial mapping in patients with paroxysmal and chronic atrial fibrillation. J Am Coll Cardiol 37:534-541

Antiarrhythmic Agents in Atrial Fibrillation: A New Role in the Context of a Hybrid Approach?

G. Boriani[1], M. Biffi[1], C. Martignani[1], C. Camanini[1], C. Valzania[1], I. Diemberger[1], C. Greco[1], G. Calcagnini[2], P. Bartolini[2], A. Branzi[1]

Atrial Fibrillation, Antiarrhythmic Drugs, and Atrial Remodeling

A series of antiarrhythmic agents have been demonstrated to be highly effective in terminating recent-onset atrial fibrillation, with class 1C agents being the most effective [1, 2]. In the conversion of recent-onset atrial fibrillation, flecainide has an efficacy of 65%-96% (intravenous administration) or 78%-95% (oral loading) [1, 2]. In contrast with the high efficacy in recent-onset atrial fibrillation, however, the results obtained in the prevention of atrial fibrillation recurrences are not satisfactory, and this has led to the development both of new nonpharmacological treatments and of combined or hybrid approaches [3-6]. Prevention of atrial fibrillation differs from termination of atrial fibrillation in respect of a series of factors involving the electrophysiological substrate, the pharmacological properties of antiarrhythmic agents, and the influence of the autonomic nervous system (Table 1). Experimental studies have clearly demonstrated that repeated inductions of atrial fibrillation up to the development of stable atrial fibrillation produce important electrophysiological and structural changes in the atria. The most striking electrophysiological alterations are shortening of the atrial effective refractory period and loss of the physiological rate adaptation of refractoriness and were associated with shortening of the atrial fibrillation cycle and development of sustained atrial fibrillation (atrial fibrillation begets atrial fibrillation) [3-5]. The evidence of electrical remodeling has important implications as far as the use of drugs is concerned. First, the development of remodeling (after some hours of atrial fibrillation or brief episodes of paroxysmal atrial fibrillation) may change the electrophysiological substrate for drug action. Second, agents able to counteract development of remodeling and to reduce its severity can be considered in the future as a useful tool to couple with antiarrhythmic drugs or antiarrhythmic interventions used to treat atrial fibrillation.

In experimental studies on chronic atrial fibrillation, electrophysiological remodeling was associated with marked structural changes [6, 7]. The picture of loss of myofibrils, accumulation of glycogen, fragmentation of sarcoplasmic retic-

[1]Institute of Cardiology, University of Bologna; [2]Biomedical Engineering, Istituto Superiore di Sanità, Rome, Italy

Table 1. Main kinds of differences between atrial fibrillation termination (acute conversion) and atrial fibrillation prevention (prophylaxis of recurrences)

Differences in the substrate	Electrophysiological remodeling Structural remodeling
Differences in pharmacological effects	Pharmacokinetics Rate-dependence Reverse rate-dependence Placebo effect
Differences in the effects of the autonomic nervous system	Tonic effects Phasic effects

ulum, dispersion of nuclear chromatin, and increase of myocyte size is very similar to that seen in chronic hibernating myocardium [6] and is associated with reexpression of contractile and cytoskeletal protein suggestive of myocardial atrial dedifferentation [7]. If the same changes occur in humans with chronic persistent atrial fibrillation, it will be quite difficult to speculate on the potential response to antiarrhythmic drugs after conversion to sinus rhythm, and marked alterations in the ionic channels can be expected until reversion of remodeling occurs [3].

Role of Antiarrhythmic Agents in the Context of a Hybrid Therapy for Atrial Fibrillation

According to clinical results and to basic pharmacological investigations it is clear that at the present time we do not have a really "ideal" antiarrhythmic agent to prevent atrial fibrillation recurrences. The same conclusion can be drawn on a purely pharmacological basis (we have neither a tachycardia-specific nor an atrial-specific agent), or taking into account clinical investigations and evidence-based medicine (we do not have an agent with a fully satisfactory risk-benefit profile). Moreover, atrial fibrillation has no single, unique electrophysiological pattern [3] and may show important dynamic changes both in the short and in the long term, and these phenomena may change significantly the response to antiarrhythmic agents.

Although alternative nonpharmacological approaches to prevention of atrial fibrillation have been proposed, they have not been completely validated and their use may be effectively combined with antiarrhythmic drugs. Despite a series of limitations, nonpharmacological techniques may indeed have significant advantages over atrial fibrillation treatment in appropriately selected groups of patients. However, to date no single procedure has been identified that is able to cure drug-refractory atrial fibrillation in a large percentage of patients with the best guarantees for safety and efficacy. The limitations, in terms of efficacy rate, of atrial fibrillation management based on a single treatment has led to the concept of combined or hybrid treatments [8,9].

The rationale of combined or hybrid treatment is to combine different therapeutic modalities in an attempt to achieve a synergistic effect, to improve efficacy over that of single approaches by acting on different targets (the electrophysiological substrate, the anatomical substrate, the triggers, the modulating factors), and also having a rescue treatment in case of failure. In view of the potential effects on different targets (atrial fibrillation termination, atrial conduction and refractoriness, frequency of atrial premature beats, atrial electrophysiological remodeling, atrial size), a series of treatments (antiarrhythmic drugs, internal cardioversion, atrial pacing with/without specific pacing algorithms, focal ablation, linear ablation) may be combined with the aim of achieving a synergistic effect. This approach is therefore justified by two expectations: (1) some nonpharmacological treatments may render atrial fibrillation responsive to previously ineffective drugs, and (2) the combined use of more than one nonpharmacological treatment is expected to be required, alone or in combination to drugs, in some patients, in order to obtain a synergistic effect.

In the contest of hybrid therapy, flecainide may have an important role, and a series of studies has shown very interesting findings for improving our approach to atrial fibrillation therapy. Our group evaluated the effects of flecainide on the threshold of atrial defibrillators and on the electrophysiological patterns of atrial fibrillation as assessed by intra-atrial recordings [10]. The study showed that flecainide significantly reduces the energy requirements for effective defibrillation both in paroxysmal and in chronic atrial fibrillation. This effect was coupled to a significant lengthening of FF cycles, both in the coronary sinus and the right atrial recordings, suggesting that the beneficial effects of flecainide are dependent on a drug-induced change in arrhythmia patterns, with a shift towards a more organized arrhythmia. This paper supports the use of flecainide in combination with devices with pacing-cardioversion capability.

Stabile et al. [11] showed that intravenous flecainide may be a useful test for predicting the long-term efficacy of isthmus ablation, in patients in whom atrial fibrillation was transformed into atrial flutter. This study confirms that the combined use of a class 1C agent plus isthmus ablation may give favorable results in the subgroup of patients with drug-induced transformation of atrial fibrillation into atrial flutter.

In the AT500 Italian Registry [12], involving patients with atrial fibrillation implanted with a DDDRP device, the efficacy of antitachycardia pacing correlated linearly with the cycle of the atrial tachyarrhythmia, and the use of a class 1C agent was associated with longer mean FF cycles compared to patients treated with class 3 agents. These observations stress how class 1C agents may be useful in improving the efficacy of antitachycardia pacing on the burden of atrial tachyarrhytmias detected in atrial fibrillation patients.

Conclusions

Atrial fibrillation is a difficult arrhythmia to treat in view of the multiple factors involved in initiation and maintenance of the arrhythmia and in view of the great variability of the underlying substrate, both from the structural (underlying heart disease) and the electrophysiological point of view. Overall, conventional treatment based on the use of drugs is characterised by a limited efficacy.

Implantable devices for pacing and cardioversion/defibrillation are undergoing very rapid evolution and in selected patients may reduce the incidence of atrial fibrillation and improve quality of life.

In view of the limitations of the conventional approach based on only a single treatment for controlling atrial fibrillation and atrial tachyarrhythmias, a hybrid approach has been proposed [8, 9]. The hybrid approach is based on the use of different therapeutic modalities (pharmacological and nonpharmacological) in an attempt to achieve synergistic effects in order to increase the overall efficacy while decreasing the adverse effects. According to a series of studies, in appropriately selected patients class 1C antiarrhythmic agents may be effectively combined with devices with pacing-defibrillation capabilities.

References

1. Boriani G (2001) New options for pharmacological conversion of atrial fibrillation. Card Electrophysiol Rev 5:195-200
2. Boriani G, Biffi M Capucci A, Botto GL, Broffoni T, Ongari M, Trisolino G, Rubino I, Sanguinetti M, Branzi A, Magnani B (1998) Conversion of recent-onset atrial fibrillation to sinus rhythm: effects of different drug protocols. Pacing Clin Electrophysiol 21:2470-2474
3. Allessie M (1998) Atrial electrophysiologic remodeling: another vicious circle? J Cardiovasc Electrophysiol 12:1378-1393
4. Nattel S (2002) Therapeutic implications of atrial fibrillation mechanisms: can mechanistic insight be used to improve AF management? Cardiovasc Res 54:347-360
5. Wijffels MCEF, Kirchof CJHJ, Dorland R, Allessie MA (1995) Atrial fibrillation begets atrial fibrillation: a study in awake chronically instrumented goats. Circulation 92:1954-1968
6. Ausma J, Wijffels M, Thouè F, Wouters L, Allessie M, Borgers M (1997) Structural changes of atrial myocardium due to sustained atrial fibrillation in the goat. Circulation 96:3117-3163
7. Ausma J, Wijffels M, Van Eys G, Koide M, Ramaekers F, Allessie M, Borgeers M (1997) Dedifferentation of atrial cardiomyocytes as a result of chronic atrial fibrillation. Am J Pathol 151:985-997
8. Lesh MD, Kalman JM, Roithinger FX, Karch MR (1997) Potential role of hybrid therapy for atrial fibrillation. Semin Intervent Cardiol 2:267-271
9. Krol RB, Saksena S, Prakash A (2000) New devices and hybrid therapies for treatment of atrial fibrillation. J Interv Card Electrophysiol 4:163-169
10. Boriani G, Biffi M, Capucci A, Bronzetti G, Ayers GM, Zannoli R, Branzi A, Magnani B (1999) Favorable effects of flecainide in transvenous internal cardioversion of atrial fibrillation. J Am Coll Cardiol 33:333-341
11. Stabile G, De Simone A, Turco P, La Rocca V, Nocerino P, Astarita C, Maresca F, De Mattei C, Di Napoli T, Stabile E, Vitale DF (2001) Response to flecainide in fusion predictes long-term success of hybrid pharmacologic and ablation therapy in patients with atrial fibrillation. J Am Coll Cardiol 37:1639-1644
12. Ricci R, Boriani G, Santini M, Padeletti L, Disertori M, Dini P, Inama G, Gasparini M, Grammatico A (2001) Effect of antiarrhythmic drugs on the atrial arrhythmia cycle length in patients affected by paroxysmal atrial fibrillation: Italian AT 500 Registry. Eur Heart J 22 (abstract suppl):327

10 YEARS OF BIVENTRICULAR PACING IN CONGESTIVE HEART FAILURE

The Electrophysiological Aspect

E. Bertaglia

Introduction

Since the beginning of the 1980s, electrophysiologists have increased their role in the treatment of patients with left ventricular dysfunction: initially, with the introduction of implantable cardioverter-defibrillators (ICDs) to prevent sudden cardiac death [1], more recently, with the wide application of cardiac resynchronization therapy (CRT) to treat patients with heart failure and ventricular conduction delay [2, 3]. Several randomized trials have demonstrated that biventricular (BIV) pacing in conjunction with drug therapy increases cardiac performance, improves quality of life, improves functional capacity, and reduces the hospitalization rate for heart failure (Table 1) [4-8].

It is known that patients with heart failure frequently have dysynchronous contraction of the cardiac chambers. The concept underlying CRT is that the efficiency of the heart as a pump would be increased if the start of the systole could be synchronized by simultaneously pacing the two ventricles [9]. The simplest sign of ventricular conduction delay is a prolongation of QRS duration. It has been calculated that among the heart failure population, 20-40% of subjects have a QRS duration of 120 ms or longer and may be candidates for BIV pacing [10-12]. Yet, the lowest QRS duration that could suggest the presence of dysynchronous ventricular contraction which could be potentially reversed by BIV pacing is still unclear: in the major randomized clinical trials the minimum QRS duration at enrollment ranged between 120 and 150 ms (Table 1). Nevertheless, even among patients with a QRS duration longer than 150 ms there are some nonresponders to CRT. The rate of nonresponse to CRT despite the presence of a ventricular conduction delay ranges between 18% and 30% [13-15]. On the other hand, in the PATH-CHF II study, 40% of patients with a QRS duration shorter than 150 ms demonstrated an increase in peak oxygen consumption greater than 1 ml/kg per minute after CRT [16].

Department of Cardiology, Ospedale Civile, Mirano, Italy

Table 1. Primary and secondary end-points in the major randomized trials on resynchronization therapy

Study	No. of patients	Baseline QRS (ms)	LVEF	LVEDD	Quality of life score	NYHA funct. class	6-min walking test	VO_2	Hospitalizations
MUSTIC[4]	48	> 150	NE	NE					
MIRACLE[5]	453	≥ 130							
PATH-CHF[6]	41	> 120							
CONTAK CD II-III-IV [7]	490	> 120			=	=			=
CONTAK CD III-IV [7]	227	> 120							=
INSYNC ICD III-IV [8]	362	≥ 130	=				=		=

; significantly increased; ; significantly decreased; =; not significantly changed; NE; not evaluated; LVEF; left ventricular ejection fraction; LVEDD; left ventricular end-diastolic diameter; VO_2; peak oxygen consumption

These data suggest that in a nonnegligible percentage of patients with left ventricular dysfunction there is a discrepancy between ventricular conduction delay and ventricular contraction delay. Tissue Doppler imaging seems to better predict patients likely to benefit from CRT [17].

The configuration of the QRS complex that should better identify responders to CRT is unclear too. The great majority of patients enrolled in the observational series and in the randomized trial presented a left bundle branch block (BBB) [4-8]. Left BBB, as a marker of left ventricular contraction delay, was presumed to better predict patients who would benefit by BIV pacing. In contrast with this statement, in the MIRACLE study the magnitude of the effect on the three primary end-points was not influenced by the configuration of the QRS complex (left BBB or right BBB) [5].

Although the value of QRS complex analysis as predictor of responder to BIV pacing is diminished, QRS duration and morphology have been identified as independent predictors of prognosis in patients with heart failure [10,11]. A prolonged QRS duration of 120-149 ms proved to be an independent predictor of increased mortality at 60 months [10]. Patients with a wide QRS complex and complete left BBB presented a 1.62-fold higher risk of death at 1 year than patients with a QRS duration shorter than 120 ms. The same risk was not present in patients with a wide QRS but with a right BBB morphology [11]. In the MADIT II study, a QRS duration of 150 ms or greater (independently of the QRS morphology) was associated with a significant increase in mortality [18].

Conclusions

QRS complex duration and configuration are able to identify the great majority of patients who would benefit from CRT. Doppler Tissue imaging might be more precise in predicting a good response to BIV pacing. Among the heart failure population, analysis of the QRS complex provides useful prognostic information.

References

1. Mirowski M, Reid P, Mower M et al (1980) Termination of malignant ventricular arrhythmias with an implantable automatic defibrillator in human beings. N Engl J Med 303:322-324
2. Cazeau S, Ritter P, Bakdach S et al (1994) Four chamber pacing in dilated cardiomyopathy. Pacing Clin Eelectrophysiol 17:1974-1979
3. Auricchio A, Stellbrink C, Block M et al, for the PATH-CHF Study Group (1999) Effect of pacing chamber and atrioventricular delay on acute systolic function of paced patients with congestive heart failure. Circulation 99:2993-3001
4. Cazeau S, Leclerq C, Lavergne T et al, for the MUSTIC Study (2001) Effects of multisite biventricular pacing in patients with heart failure and intraventricular conduction delay. N Engl J Med 12:873-880

5. Abraham WT, Fisher WG, Smith AL et al (2002) Cardiac resynchronization in chronic heart failure. N Engl J Med 346:1845-1853
6. Stellbrink C, Breithardt O, Franke A et al (2001) Impact of cardiac resynchronization therapy using hemodynamically optimized pacing on left ventricular remodelling in patients with congestive heart failure and ventricular conduction disturbances. J Am Coll Cardiol 38:1957-1965
7. Contak CD Guidant cardiac resynchronization therapy defibrillator system including the CONTAK CD pulse generator and the EASYTRAK left ventricular coronary venous lead. Summary of safety and effectiveness. www.fda.gov
8. Medtronic InSync ICD cardiac resynchronization system. www.fda.gov
9. Haywood G (2001) Biventricular pacing in heart failure: update and results from clinical trials. Curr Control Trials Cardiovasc 2:292-297
10. Shenkman HJ, Pampati V, Khandelwal AK et al (2002) Congestive heart failure and QRS duration: establishing prognosis study. Chest 122:528-534
11. Baldasseroni S, Boffa GM, Camerini A et al, on behalf of IN-CHF Investigators (2002) Left but not bundle branch block is an independent predictor of prognosis in patients with heart failure: report from the IN-CHF registry (abstract). Eur Heart J 23 [Suppl]:645
12. Khan NK, Louis AA, de Silva R et al, on behalf of the Euroheart Failure Investigators (2002) The Euroheart failure survey: the value of the electrocardiogram in the evaluation of heart failure (abstract). Eur Heart J 23 [Suppl]:707
13. Alonso C, Leclerq C, Victor F et al (1999) Electrocardiographic predictive factors of long-term clinical improvement with multisite biventricular pacing in advanced heart failure. Am J Cardiol 84:1417-1421
14. Reuter S, Garrigue S, Barold SS et al (2002) Comparison of characteristics in responders versus nonresponders with biventricular pacing for drug-resistant congestive heart failure. Am J Cardiol 89:346-350
15. Oguz E, Dagdeviren B, Bilsel T et al (2002) Echocardiographic prediction of long-term response to biventricular pacemaker in severe heart failure. Eur J Heart Fail 4:83-90
16. Yu Y, Lamp B, Butter C et al, on behalf of the PATH-CHF II Investigators (2002) Sensitivity and specificity of using QRS duration to predict chronic benefit in heart failure patients with cardiac resynchronization therapy. Eur Heart J 23 [Suppl]:414
17. Soogard P, Egeblad H, Kim Y et al (2002) Tissue Doppler Imaging predicts improved systolic performance and reversed left ventricular remodeling during long-term cardiac resynchronization therapy. J Am Coll Cardiol 40:723-730
18. Moss AJ, Zareba W, Hall J et al, for the MADIT II Investigators (2002) Prophylactic implantation of a defibrillator in patients with myocardial infarction and reduced ejection fraction. N Engl J Med 346:877-883

Pharmacological Trials on Heart Failure: What Can We Translate into Daily Clinical Practice?

G. FABBRI, A.P. MAGGIONI

Adherence to evidence-based medicine is the accepted goal to which doctors should aspire in their clinical practice. In the last 20 years, large-scale controlled trials have been conducted in patients with chronic heart failure. These trials used clinically important outcome measures including death and major morbid events. The assignment of patients to treatments was randomized, the number of patients was adequate, and the follow-up was complete and reasonably long in order to provide the required number of events to generally ensure the necessary statistical power for unequivocal interpretation of the results. Accordingly, there is now evidence on the safety and efficacy of a variety of treatments for heart failure. However, a number of clinical surveys in various countries, both in primary care and in hospital practice, revealed that a significant proportion of eligible patients are not receiving treatments that would increase both the quality and the length of their life. If under-treatment can have an adverse economic effect in terms of increased hospitalizations, incorporating these results into clinical practice would reduce the burden on health care systems [1]. Despite these obvious considerations, however, it appears that translation of the trial results into clinical practice has often been slow and incomplete.

There are several explanations for the delay and the reluctance of doctors to follow guidelines derived from the trials [2, 3]. Patients in clinical trials are generally more selected and homogeneous than those in the community, while large differences exist between the two populations particularly with respect to age, sex distribution, and the presence of comorbid conditions (Table 1). These may be the reasons why clinicians often feel that the typical clinical trial patient is not representative of many patients in their own practice.

Selection bias may considerably limit the generalizability of the data. This is exemplified by results of clinical trials in heart failure that cannot necessarily be transferred to the majority of older patients in the community [4],

Centro Studi ANMCO, Florence, Italy

Table 1. Differences between CHF patients enrolled in clinical trials and in the community

	Clinical trials	Community
Mean age (years)	57-64	70-75
Gender (M:F)	4:1	1:1
EF >40%	Exclusion criterion	Present in >40%
Atrial fibrillation	Present in 20%	Present in 40%
Severe renal dysfunction	Exclusion criterion	Present in 20%-30%
Comorbidities	Exclusion criterion	Frequent
Drug dosage	At target	Low
Compliance	High	Low
Treatment duration	1-3 years	Life-long
1-year mortality	9%-12%	25%-30%

because elderly patients are not usually included in most trials. There are additional subgroups of patients not adequately studied, including patients with heart failure and preserved left ventricular function. Thus, evidence-based recommendations do not cover all the questions that arise in the multifariousness of everyday clinical practice.

The time lag between trial results, the issuing of consensus recommendations, and the appearance of corresponding prescribing behavior [5] has been observed even in the implementation of treatments largely accepted by the medical community, such as ACE inhibitors in heart failure [6,7].

The most important steps in the translation of trial results into clinical practice are: scientific reliability of the studies, proper communication of the results, and methods to facilitate implementation of evidence-based treatments. Many scientific societies have concerned themselves with issuing guidelines or consensus statements, but these strategies have been clearly demonstrated to be insufficient. When the results of a study are valid and considered to be useful in caring for "real world" patients, implementation of the proven treatments should proceed through several phases:

- Observational studies and surveys with the aim of continuously monitoring prescription patterns and use of resources
- Establishment of databases of large cohorts of patients followed in a community setting to collect information on their characteristics and obtain accurate estimates of different outcomes and the factors that affect them
- Feedback programs, including outcomes research studies
- Involvement in research projects of as many cardiology centers as possible in which real patients are managed

All these elements are essential to form a permanent link between research and practice.

This policy has been followed in the past few years by the Italian Association of Hospital Cardiologists (ANMCO). As an example, the Bring-up study [8], conducted by ANMCO with the aim of accelerating the β-blockade use in clinical practice, can be seen as having made possible a rapid impact on the delivery of health care on a national basis [9]. After annual surveys of prescribing patterns through the Italian Network on Congestive Heart Failure [10], a series of regional meetings were organized to discuss (1) the evidence for the use of β-blockers in heart failure, (2) the recommendations on their proper use, and (3) the study design. These meetings involved cardiologists from more than 200 centers. Three thousand patients with heart failure, treated or not treated with β-blockers, were enrolled in 1 month in this prospective study. Both the choice of whether to adopt β-blocker therapy and which drug and dosage to use (carvedilol, metoprolol, or bisoprolol) was left to the clinician responsible. At the beginning of the study 24.9% of patients were already on β-blocker, 32.7% started treatment, and 42.4% were not treated. After 1 year of follow-up 47.9% of the patients were on β-blocker treatment, giving an increase in the proportion of patients treated with β-blocker from a quarter to nearly half.

These results also document the value of the attitude to collaborative work. Operating in real practice, with the recommended combination of total freedom of decision allied with consultation as and when needed, could be seen as a blend of continuity and adaptation of the setting and rules of trials.

Periodical descriptive surveys of practice patterns and analysis of clinical databases developed and maintained with the aim of providing information on the impact of educational campaigns should be regarded as a second choice after active research projects. Their objective is to improve medical practice by understanding physician behaviors and measuring outcome with end-points that are the epidemiological translation of those of controlled trials.

Following the important ad hoc initiatives launched mainly in the United States [11] and the United Kingdom [12] to promote evidence-based practice, scientific societies should develop and test research models in this critical area of medicine. The potential implications of such strategies might be considered either in terms of public health or the cost-benefit profile of medicine, because the investigator networks overlap with the user community.

References

1. Berry C, Murdoch DR, McMurray JJ (2001) Economics of chronic heart failure. Eur J Heart Fail 3:283-289
2. Hobbs FDR, Wilson S, Jones MI et al (2000) European survey on primary care physician perceptions and practice in heart failure diagnosis and management (Euro-HF Study). Eur Heart J 21:1877-1887
3. McMurray JJ, Chen-Solal A, Dietz R et al (2001) Practical recommendations for the use of ACE inhibitors, beta-blockers and spironolactone in heart failure: putting guidelines into practice. Eur J Heart Fail 3:495-502
4. Sharpe N (2002) Clinical trials and the real world: selection bias and generalisability of trials results. Cardiovasc Drugs Ther 16(1) 75-77
5. Felch WC (1997) Bridging the gap between research and practice. The role of continuing medical education. JAMA 277:155-156

6. Houghton A, Cowley A (1997) Why are angiotensin converting enzyme inhibitors under-utilised in the treatment of heart failure by general practitioners? Int J Cardiol 59:7-10
7. Reis SE, Holubkov R, Edmundosicz D et al (1997) Treatment of patients admitted to the hospital with congestive heart failure: specialty related disparities in practice patterns and outcomes. J Am Coll Cardiol 30:733-738
8. Maggioni AP, Tavazzi L (1999) Introducing new treatments in clinical practice: the Italian approach to beta blockers in heart failure. Heart 81:453-454
9. Sleight P (1999) A Napoleonic future for cardiology. Heart 81:455
10. Opasich C, Tavazzi L, Lucci D et al (2000) Comparison of one-year outcome in women versus men with congestive heart failure. Am J Cardiol 86:353-357
11. Woosley RL (2000) Centers for education and research in therapeutics. Clin Pharmacol Ther 68:109-110
12. Rawlins M (1999) In pursuit of quality: the National Institute for Clinical Excellence. Lancet 353:1079-1082

Selection of Patients for Cardiac Resynchronization Therapy

D. GRAS, J.P. CEBRON, P. BRUNEL, B. LEURENT, Y. BANUS

The epidemiologic data recently published with regard to congestive heart failure represent a strong incentive to mobilize all treatment options available. Despite remarkable advances, medical therapy suffers from serious limitations, as does, when all else has failed, cardiac transplantation. In this context, cardiac resynchronization therapy (CRT) has recently been introduced with, as a first objective, the relief of cardiac symptoms refractory to optimal medical therapy [1-4]. Acute hemodynamic studies first demonstrated that CRT could improve left ventricular mechanical function, increase cardiac index, and decrease intrapulmonary pressures [5-8]. These favorable effects were associated with a decrease in myocardial oxygen consumption [9], thus indicating reorganization of the segmental left ventricular contraction sequence and ultimately improved global ventricular function, instead of an increase in contractility at a cellular level.

Recent results of the MUSTIC and MIRACLE trials [10-12] are consistent in showing an improvement of NYHA functional class, quality of life scores, and the distance covered during a 6-min walk. A positive impact on left ventricular function indexes was also reported, as demonstrated by an increase in global ejection fraction, a reverse remodeling effect, and a decrease in mitral regurgitation. In addition, a reduction in hospitalization rate and duration was documented and could further positively impact on health-care-related costs.

These positive results may only be obtained in carefully selected patients, currently those with dilated cardiomyopathy evidenced by a left ventricular end-diastolic diameter greater than 55 mm and global ejection fraction below 35%, of either ischemic or nonischemic origin [12]. As the primary goal of CRT was to improve cardiac symptoms, potential candidates are supposed to be in NYHA functional class III or IV. However, this particular point remains to be further evaluated, as some patients in functional class II could also benefit from the therapy over a longer period of time.

Unité de Soins et de Cardiologie Interventionnelle, Polyclinique Saint Henri, Nantes, France

Individual diagnosis of ventricular dysynchrony is another key parameter before considering CRT, since it is what the treatment intends to remedy. In other words, patients without ventricular dysynchrony are not expected to derive any clinical benefit, and consequently are not considered for this treatment on the basis of present-day knowledge. A first criterion to define ventricular dysynchrony was based on a long QRS duration, with different values considered over 120-150 ms [1-4, 10, 12] depending on authors' definitions. Although it is easy and noninvasive to evaluate on surface ECG, this electrical approach suffers from a lack of clear correlation with the mechanical aspect of dysynchrony, therefore leading to misdiagnosis of potential responders in a subgroup of patients with short or normal QRS duration.

The link between cardiac dysynchrony and ventricular conduction disturbances on the ECG is indeed not straightforward, and the precise value of QRS duration on which we could rely to assess ventricular dysynchrony remains uncertain. This could be explained by the limited information provided by conventional ECG, which does not explore the three-dimensional nature of the electrical disorder. Nevertheless, the longer the QRS, the more likely is ventricular dysynchrony. On the other hand, an extra-long QRS duration may sometimes correlate with very severe disease where the natural process is too advanced to expect any benefit. In the latter case, the indication for CRT could become questionable even though all classical criteria for selecting a potential responder are fulfilled.

Considering the limitations of conventional ECG, echocardiographic parameters were recently proposed to investigate the presence of ventricular dysynchrony [7, 8, 13, 14]. Such parameters are intended to be used to investigate the mechanical consequences of ventricular conduction disorders. In the ongoing CARE-HF study [15], ventricular dysynchrony is evaluated during echocardiography in patients with little increase in QRS duration (120-150 ms) by considering respectively (1) a prolonged aortic pre-ejection delay (> 140 ms), (2) an increased mechanical interventricular delay (> 40 ms), and (3) a left ventricular segmental postsystolic contraction.

The aortic pre-ejection delay is measured between the onset of the QRS complex and the beginning of the aortic flow on pulsed wave Doppler imaging. Prolongation of this delay is explained by delayed left ventricular contraction due to conduction disorders. Together with the prolongation in left ventricular contraction duration, this further translates into a decrease in left ventricular filling duration. This latter is related to delayed early diastolic filling, which ultimately results in a fusion between early and late diastolic filling, as demonstrated by a single transmitral flow on pulsed wave Doppler. A simple rule may be expressed here: the longer the aortic pre-ejection delay, and the shorter the left ventricular filling duration, the more advanced the ventricular dysynchrony.

The mechanical interventricular delay is evaluated during pulsed wave Doppler imaging by the time difference between the onset of the pulmonary flow and the aortic flow. Prolongation of this delay is explained by the loss of coordination of septal activation and contraction. This results in a decrease in regional ejection fraction, thus contributing to a lower left ventricular global ejection fraction.

The left ventricular segmental postsystolic contraction is defined as the maximal local wall inward movement (local peak contraction), using either M-mode or tissue Doppler imaging, occurring later than the start of the transmitral Doppler flow signal. Caution is required to distinguish passive movement correctly from active local contraction. Such a phenomenon is usually documented at the left ventricular posterolateral wall, arguing to consider lateral or posterior coronary sinus tributaries for pacing the left ventricular from this particular region [16, 17]. This particular anomaly may have serious hemodynamic consequences. First, it impairs left ventricular systolic function through lack of coordination in left ventricular segmental contraction. Second, it impairs left ventricular filling because of delayed local relaxation. Third, it may contribute to functional mitral regurgitation, caused by delayed contraction of the papillary muscles, which in turn results in a lack of synchronicity in mitral leaflet closure.

Follow-up visits by recipients of cardiac resynchronization systems in the ambulatory setting are more frequent than by patients with conventional pacemakers, and require additional medical skills. Programming of the CRT system is best performed during echocardiography, with particular attention to the atrioventricular delay, chosen to optimize left ventricular filling as has been previously described in DDD pacing [18, 19]. In individual cases, this optimal interval is based on a longer left ventricular filling period without impingement on the atrial mechanical contribution. Practically, this consists of restoring a more physiologic and longer Doppler echocardiographic transmitral flow (usually by eliminating the fusion pattern), without diminishing the amplitude or area of the A wave. Effectiveness of CRT may also be documented during echocardiography with tissue Doppler imaging techniques, through an improvement in inter- and intraventricular dysynchrony [14, 20].

The recent introduction of systems with programmable interventricular delay makes it possible in some cases to optimize the segmental left ventricular contraction sequence by better correcting the ventricular dysynchrony [21], or by allowing spontaneous nodo-Hisian activation. This new setting may conflict with the atrioventricular delay, which may ultimately need to be reevaluated and reset.

Various types of oversensing may also be observed, which may interfere with proper functioning of the CRT system, including common examples such as inappropriate sensing of an atrial or ventricular electrogram. Sensing by the ventricular channel of a supernumerary signal of right or left ventricular origin, often caused by loss of left ventricular capture in the presence of preserved right ventricular stimulation, is proper to this type of stimulation and may be the source of double counting and erroneous diagnosis of ventricular tachycardia. Furthermore, inhibition of ventricular stimulation may be caused by sensing of a left atrial electrogram at the left ventricular level, which can be prevented by setting a low ventricular sensitivity. The use of modern CRT devices, using independent channels for sensing and pacing right and left ventricles, now allows such oversensing difficulties to be overcome.

References

1. Cazeau S, Ritter P, Lazarus A et al (1996) Multisite pacing for end-stage heart failure: early experience. Pacing Clin Electrophysiol 19:1748-57
2. Gras D, Leclercq C, Tang A, Bucknall C, Luttikhuis HO, Kirstein-Pedersen A (2002) Cardiac resynchronization therapy in advanced heart failure: the multicenter InSync clinical study. Eur J Heart Failure 4:311-320
3. Zardini M, Tritto M, Bargiggia G, and the InSync Italian Registry Investigators (2000) The InSync Italian Registry: analysis of clinical outcome and considerations on the selection of candidates to left ventricular resynchronization. Eur Heart J 2[Suppl J]:J16-J22
4. Auricchio A, Stellbrink C, Sack S, Block M, Vogt J, Bakker P, Huth C, Schöndube F, Wolfhard U, Böcker D, Krahnefeld O, Kirkels H, for the PATH-CHF study group (2002) Long-term clinical effect of hemodynamically optimized cardiac resynchronization therapy in patients with heart failure and ventricular conduction delay. J Am Coll Cardiol 39:1895-1898
5. Leclercq C, Cazeau S, Lebreton H et al (1998) Acute hemodynamic effects of biventricular DDD pacing in patients with end-stage heart failure. J Am Coll Cardiol 32:1825-1831
6. Kass DA, Chen-Huan C, Curry C et al (1999) Improved left ventricular mechanics from acute VDD pacing in patients with dilated cardiomyopathy and ventricular conduction delay. Circulation 99:1567-1573
7. Breithardt OA, Stellbrink C, Franke A, Balta O, Diem BH, Bakker P, Sack S, Auricchio A, for the PATH-CHF Study Group, and Pochet T, Salo R, for the Guidant Congestive Heart Failure Research (2002) Acute effects of cardiac resynchronization therapy on left ventricular Doppler indices in patients with congestive heart failure. Am Heart J 143:34-44
8. Søgaard P, Kim WY, Jensen HK, Mortensen P, Pedersen AK, Kristensen BØ, Egeblad H (2001) Impact of acute biventricular pacing on left ventricular performance and volumes in patients with severe heart failure: a tissue Doppler and three-dimensional echocardiographic study. Cardiology 95:173-182
9. Nelson GS, Berger RD, Fetics BJ et al (2000) Left ventricular or biventricular pacing improves cardiac function at diminished energy cost in patients with dilated cardiomyopathy and left bundle-branch block. Circulation 102:3053-3059
10. Cazeau S, Leclercq M, Lavergne T, Walker S, Varma C, Linde C, Garrigue S, Kappenberger L, Haywood GA, Santini M, Bailleul C, Daubert JC, for the Multisite Stimulation in Cardiomyopathies (MUSTIC) Study Investigators (2001) Effects of multisite biventricular pacing in patients with heart failure and intraventricular conduction delay. N Engl J Med 344:873-880
11. Linde C, Leclercq C, Rex S, Garrigue S, Lavergne T, Cazeau S, McKenna W, Fitzgerald M, Deharo J-C, MD, Alonso C, Walker S, MD, Braunschweig F, Bailleul C, Daubert J-C, on behalf of the MUltisite STimulation In Cardiomyopathies (MUSTIC) Study Group (2002) Long-term benefits of biventricular pacing in congestive heart failure: results from the Multisite STimulation In Cardiomyopathy (MUSTIC) Study. J Am Coll Cardiol 40:111–118

12. Abraham WT, Fisher WG, Smith AL, Delurgio DB, Leon AR, Loh E, Kocovic DZ, Packer M, Clavell AL, Hayes DL, Ellestad M, Messenger J (2002) Cardiac resynchronization in chronic heart failure. N Engl J Med 346:1845-1853
13. Cazeau S, Gras D, Lazarus A, Ritter P, Mugica J (2000) Multisite stimulation for correction of cardiac asynchrony. Heart 84:579-581
14. Yu CM, Chau E, Sanderson JE, Fan K, Tang MO, Fung WH, Lin H, Kong SL, Lam YM, Hill MRS, Lau CP (2002) Tissue Doppler echocardiographic evidence of reverse remodeling and improved synchronicity by simultaneously delaying regional contraction after biventricular pacing therapy in heart failure. Circulation 105:438-445
15. Cleland JGF, Daubert JC, Erdmann E, Freemantle N, Gras D, Kappenberger L, Klein W, Tavazzi L on behalf of the CARE-HF study steering committee and investigators (2001) The CARE-HF study (Cardiac Resynchronisation in Heart Failure study): rationale, design and end-points. Eur J Heart Fail 3:481:489
16. Gras D, Cebron JP, Brunel P, Leurent B, Banus Y (2002) Optimal stimulation of the left ventricle. J Clin Electrophys 13:57-62
17. Butter C, Auricchio A, Stellbrink C, Fleck E, Ding J, Yu Y, Huvelle E, Spinelli J (2001) Effect of resynchronization therapy stimulation site on the systolic function of heart failure patients. Circulation 104:3026-3029
18. Ritter P, Dib JC, Lelievre T et al (1994) Quick determination of the optimal AV delay at rest in patients paced in DDD mode for complete AV block. Eur J CPE 994; 4:39
19. Kindermann M, Frohlig G, Doerr T et al (1997) Optimizing the AV delay in DDD pacemaker patients with high degree AV block: mitral valve doppler versus impedance cardiography. Pacing Clin Electrophysiol 20:2453-2462
20. Ansalone G, Giannantoni P, Ricci R, Trambaiolo P, Fedele F, Santini M (2002) Doppler myocardial imaging to evaluate the effectiveness of pacing sites in patients receiving biventricular pacing. J Am Coll Cardiol 39:489-499
21. O'Cochlain B, Delurgio D, Leon A, Langberg J (2001) The effect of variation in the interval between right and left ventricular activation on paced QRS duration. Pacing Clin Electrophysiol 24:1780–1782

The Perspective of the Emergency Department

L. ZULLI

The physician is the responsible and the real "owner" of the essential actions for the recovery of health. He diagnoses and prescribes therapy.

The doctors are only responsible for the patient's diagnosis and therapy. Thus, they have a particular professional role in taking advantage of resources, using structures, deciding on hospitalizations, defining paths and, finally, determining procedures with their resultant costs. Doctors invoice for services performed and set the revenue of the structure in which they work.

For these reasons, the physician should be considered a "process owner," responsible for the treatment needed by the sick. He should be free to use the qualified resources for the end-point, buying structures, consultants, and drugs and selling services and professional advice.

In a hospital, and in particular in medical enterprises, to manage complicated and defined tasks, physicians are compelled to form teams driven by a director to set up complex operative units. From an economic point of view, too, it is useful to respond to most demands by creating collaborative relationships with other operative units from different branches and specializations. These actions create departments, so that each unit maintains its functional autonomy and is linked to the others in a dynamic, collaborative, and complementary way, something like a "joint venture" [1].

The multifunctional department will be therefore a strategic alliance based on complementary resources provided by the different ICUs, dedicated to complex services such as rescuing the health of the sick/customer. The integrated departments should be distributed among the great operative areas of Medicine, Surgery, Emergency, and Specialist fields as ICCU or Pneumology ward [2] (Fig. 1).

The scientific development, the CQI (continuous quality improvement) in the management of the patient, the progresses of the clinical methodology and of the surgical and electrical treatments show that in emergency conditions,

Dipartimento di Emergenza e Accettazione, UOC Medicina d'Urgenza e di Pronto Soccorso, ACO S. Filippo Neri, Rome, Italy

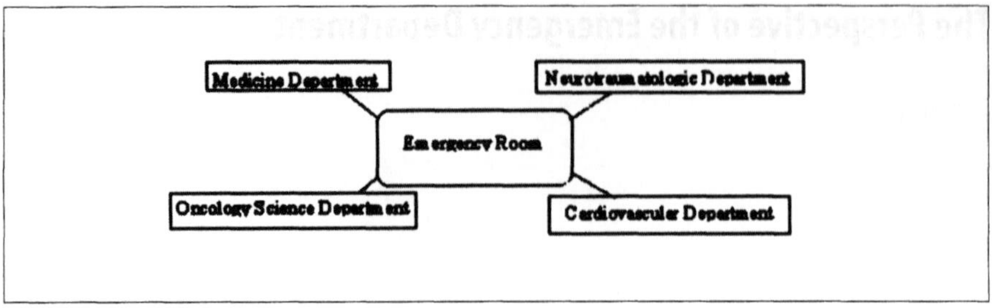

Fig. 1. ED-crossroad intra-H

the *golden hour* is very important. However, in absolute terms the *most* important thing is primary and secondary prevention. The greatest emphasis of health policy should therefore be applied to the population in general, without neglecting individual risk in an appropriate primary prevention project.

The first aid station and the emergency department (ED) are crucial points for a project of prevention: the crossroads at the entrance for disease, the filter for patient stabilization, and the fulcrum of all-inclusive emergency intervention, which from extra-hospital stage includes first aid in the intra-hospital period and afterward in the ICU [3, 4].

The principal activity of emergency medicine is the diagnosis and treatment of acute pathologies, but it should also recognize and predict all events that cause acute illnesses. Really the ED for its particular position is a bridge between extra-hospital and intra-hospital domains, in constant contact with both extra-hospital generalist and the intra-hospital specialist, from today on it should dedicate major time and resources to prevention [5].

Thus, the ED is the prototype of the multifunctional and integrated department that occurs today in emergency care, studying and taking account of the prevention and origin of disease.

For this reason we have focused our studies on syncope and heart failure projects [6], the principal objectives of which are to reduce unexpected deaths and to select men and women for intracardiac cardioverter-defibrillator implantation and cardiac resynchronization [7]. Our first purpose, however, is acute failure. Therefore, in ED we select patients with chest pain and acute myocardial infarction, with critical conditions of life and with red codex of *triage*. In these conditions, the first hour of treatment is essential for life, survival, and prognosis. The first hour is called *golden hour*; in our hospital this means percutaneous coronary angioplasty (PTCA). From November or December we shall be taking part in the Finesse study on PTCA facilities. The new ED, then, is a new reality and always has new perspectives for its multiple targets: AMI/ictus/trauma/respiratory disease/abdominal pain. In the case of traumatic pathologies we focus attention on patients in the *golden hour*, but we follow them for a *golden day* and a *golden week*. The purpose of this behavior is to avoid deaths.

In the end, the perspective of the ED for the treatment of Acute Myocardial Infarction is the creation of a *fast track* to shorten door-to-needle and door-to-balloon times, and the perspective for the treatment of trauma is the institution of trauma centers.

References

1. Gaia E (1997) Il dipartimento integrato come risposta polufunzionale. In: Organizzazione e finanziamento del dipartimento ospedaliero. Edizioni Minerva Medica, Turin, pp 15-24
2. Lomastro M, Vichi MC (1999) Il percorso del paziente ospedaliero. Mecosan 32:75-90
3. Karimi A (1999) Excerpt from recommendations on problems in emergency and intensive care medicine in D I V I, Karimi A, Dick W (eds). Cologne, pp 6-55
4. Oakley PA, Coleman NA (2001) Intensive care of trauma patients. Resuscitation 48:37-46
5. Gai V (1999) Rapporti tra medicina interna e medicina d'urgenza. G Ital Med Urg Pronto Secorso 4:125-129
6. Hershberger RE, Ni H, Nauman DJ et al (2001) Prospective evaluation of an outpatient heart failure management program. J Card Fail 7:64-74
7. Cassin M, Macor F et al (2002) Management of patients with low risk chest pain at the time of admission: a prospective study on a non-selected population from the Emergency Department. Ital Heart J 7:399-405

Ventricular Pacing in Congestive Heart Failure: The Role of the Internist

M. Pagani[1], F. Lo Presti[2]

Congestive heart failure (CHF) is a complex clinical syndrome caused by multiple structural and functional alterations which together induce left ventricular dysfunction. Throughout the world CHF affects more than 22 million individuals and 4%-6% of the population over 65 years of age. With 2 million new cases every year, it has become a social and health program problem of immense proportions. At 5 years after diagnosis the survival rate is only 50%. The two main causes of death are pump dysfunction and arrhythmias.

The role of electrostimulation therapy in CHF has progressively gained momentum over recent years to become one of the topics of major interest in the pathophysiology of CHF, and the approach itself has become more widely used in clinical application. Initially patients with CHF could be fitted with a pacemaker to correct low frequency and to improve the atrioventricular (AV) interval. In patients with severe cardiac dysfunction the AV interval can be a critical parameter, as the hemodynamic profile can vary in relation to the length of this interval.

Recently, a new pathophysiological concept has been defined relative to the electromechanical coupling of the heart and the profound mechanical alterations which can result from an improper contraction sequence during cardiac activity. In dilated cardiomyopathy, regional ischemic alterations of electromechanical activation negatively influence ventricular efficiency. In patients with intraventricular conduction disturbances, such as left bundle branch block (LBBB), asynchronous myocardial activation renders ventricular contractions asynchronous as well, associated with delayed depolarization and contraction of the free wall of the left ventricle in respect of the intraventricular septum and the right ventricle. According to the available literature, the prevalence of ventricular dysfunction associated with excessive length of QRS from the surface ECG (>120 ms) varies between 23% and 53%. It is known that the widening of QRS due to delayed intraventricular conduction (in particular LBBB) is an independent prognostic factor of or contributor to a negative prognosis.

[1]Centro Terapia Neurovegetativa, University of Milan; [2]Departments of Medicine and Cardiology, L. Sacco Hospital, Milan, Italy

In cases of ventricular asynchrony, biventricular pacemaker therapy has been proposed to improve the mechanical performance of the heart by simultaneous stimulation of the right and left ventricles, minimizing the mechanical intraventricular delay and improving the dynamics of the pulmonary and aortic valves. Biventricular electric stimulation can be guided by the sinoatrial (SA) node (DDD stimulation method) or, in the case of atrial fibrillation, by VVI. Biventricular pacing, besides improving left ventricular mechanical performance, reduces both mitral regurgitation and left ventricular volume, leading to inverse remodeling of the left ventricle.

Another electric stimulation therapy that can improve the survival of patients with CHF is implantation of an automatic intracardiac cardioverter defibrillator (ICD). Sudden death, principally secondary to lethal arrhythmias, is the main cause of death in patients with NYHA class II and III disease. Several multicenter studies have shown ICD implantation to be a highly efficient preventive treatment for sudden death caused by sustained ventricular tachycardia or ventricular fibrillation. Other studies, however, have shown the persistence of sudden death in patients with CHF notwithstanding ICD implantation. This is probably due to irreversible electromechanical disassociation.

The possibility of combining biventricular stimulation and ICD properties in a single device opens new possibilities for treating the two major causes of death in CHF patients. A series of ongoing studies (MIRACLE ICD, CONTAK CD, InSync ICD, BELIEVE, Ventak CHF) aim to evaluate, in patients with refractory CHF, the efficacy in terms of morbidity and mortality of this type of combined electrostimulation therapy. In this context, the role of the internist is best seen as one component in a multidisciplinary continuous chain of care in which the specialized hospital cardiology units are linked with everyday management by the GP. As is by now well recognized, ancillary therapies and care, including the use of simple telematic (e.g. INCAS) approaches can dramatically improve treatment adherence, and, consequently, in the well being of patients, with a drastic reduction of unnecessary emergency admissions to hospital, with improved use of resources and, ultimately, greater quality of life.

Suggested Reading

Abrahm WT (2002) Cardiac resynchronization therapy for heart failure: biventricular pacing and beyond. Curr Opin Cardiol 17:346-352

Santini M, Ricci R (2002) Biventricular pacing in patients with heart failure and intraventricular conduction delay: state of the art and perspectives. Eur Heart J 23:682-686

Legge D, Leper B (2002) Management of heart failure: use of biventricular pacing. J Cardiovasc Pacing 16:72-81

Pavia SV, Wilkoff BL (2001) Biventricuar pacing for heart failure. Cardiol Clin 19:637-651

Barold SS (2001) What is cardiac resynchronization therapy? Am J Med 111:224-232

Role of Electrical Therapy in Patients with Left Ventricular Dysfunction: The Clinical Cardiologist's Experience

F. Nacci[1], F. Fino[1], V.F. Napoli[2]. S. Favale[1]

Introduction

The prevalence of intraventricular conduction delays in patients with left ventricular (LV) systolic dysfunction and chronic heart failure (CHF) has been estimated at 30%-50%. These abnormalities negatively affect both systolic and diastolic ventricular function causing uncoordinated contractions between the left and the right ventricles and between the various segments of the LV wall [1-9], and have been associated with an unfavorable prognosis [10-15]. The most common expression of the presence of intraventricular conduction delays is left bundle branch block (LBBB). Cardiac resynchronization by LV or biventricular pacing has recently been introduced to treat patients with chronic heart failure (CHF) who respond poorly to optimal medical therapy, LV systolic dysfunction, and intraventricular conduction delays, based on the hypothesis that LV pacing, possibly associated with right ventricular pacing, can restore the physiological coordination of ventricular contraction.

Randomized Trials

Acute studies have demonstrated that biventricular pacing improves both systolic and diastolic function of the LV in patients with CHF secondary to LV systolic dysfunction and LBBB [16-22]. More recent nonrandomized clinical studies showed an improvement in symptoms, functional capacity, and quality of life after cardiac resynchronization therapy (CRT) [23-35].

Three randomized clinical trials which enrolled more than 400 patients have been carried out. The PAcing THerapies for Congestive Heart Failure (PATH-CHF) trial [36], which was a single-blind, randomized, uncontrolled study of

[1]Istituto di Cardiochirurgia, Università di Bari; [2]Fondazione S. Maugeri IRCCS, Divisione di Cardiologia, Cassano Murge, Bari, Italy

biventricular pacing versus LV pacing over periods of 4 weeks and using a crossover design, enrolled patients in NYHA class III-IV despite optimal medical therapy, a LV ejection fraction (LVEF) of 35% or less, QRS duration above 120 ms, and PR duration above 160 ms. The LV pacing system was implanted via thoracotomy. At follow-up the 42 patients enrolled (mean age 60 years) showed a significant reduction in NYHA class and a significant increase in maximal oxygen uptake at stress testing during the period in which CRT was active, with no significant differences between biventricular and LV pacing.

The recently published MUSTIC study [37] (MUltisite STimulation in Cardiomyopathies), a single-blind, randomized, controlled trial using a crossover design of biventricular pacing versus placebo over periods of 3 months, is the first comparative study in which the LV pacing system was transvenously implanted in all patients. The inclusion criteria were: NYHA class III despite optimal medical therapy, LVEF 35% or less, LV end-diastolic diameter (LVEDD) greater than 60 mm, QRS duration less than 150 ms, and a 6-min walking distance of less than 450 m. The study separately evaluated patients with chronic atrial fibrillation, for whom enrollment criteria were the same as for patients with sinus rhythm except that QRS duration had to be greater than 200 ms during right ventricular stimulation. The trial enrolled 48 patients (mean age 63 years) in sinus rhythm, with a mean LVEF of 22% and mean QRS duration of 176 ms, and 41 patients (mean age 65 years) in chronic atrial fibrillation, with a mean LVEF of 19% and mean QRS duration of 206 ms. At follow-up patients in sinus rhythm showed a significant reduction in NYHA class (-0.7), a significant improvement in the 6-min walking distance (+23%), maximal oxygen uptake at stress testing (+8%), and quality of life score (+32%), and a significant reduction in number of hospitalizations (3 in the period of pacing on versus 9 in the period of pacing off.)

The MIRACLE trial [38] (Multicenter InSync Randomized Clinical Evaluation) is the first double-blind, randomized, controlled study with a parallel arm design to evaluate the efficacy of CRT in the treatment of CHF with a large number of patients enrolled. Enrollment criteria were: NYHA class III-IV despite optimal medical therapy, LVEF 35% or less, LVEDD greater than 55 mm, and QRS duration greater than 130 ms. Two hundred and sixty-six patients (mean age 64 years) were enrolled, with a mean LVEF of 22% and mean QRS duration of 165 ms. Six-month follow-up data were similar to those presented in other studies: there was a significant reduction in NYHA class (almost 1 class in 69% of patients), and a significant improvement in quality of life score (+13%), 6-min walking distance (+13%), number of hospitalizations, number of days spent in hospital, and in LVEF and LVEDD.

Unresolved Issues

Although the results of the clinical trials are very encouraging, some caution is required. Some aspects still have to be clarified: patient selection, effect on mortality, and combination with the implantable cardioverter defibrillator (ICD) are the most relevant.

At present the most important criteria for the selection of patients for CRT are: NYHA class III-IV while on optimal medical therapy, LVEF of 35% or less, and LBBB with QRS duration greater than 130 ms. However, approximately 25% of patients who fulfill these criteria do not respond to biventricular pacing therapy. While it was suggested that NYHA class, basal QRS duration and reduction of QRS duration during biventricular pacing may be predictive markers of the efficacy of CRT [39], in the InSync Italian Registry [27] patients responding to biventricular pacing could not be predicted by exercise tolerance, LVEF, QRS duration, LV pacing site, or the presence of sinus rhythm or chronic atrial fibrillation. In the latter study only cardiac dyssynchrony, as evaluated by echocardiogram (interventricular mechanical delay greater than 40 ms, aortic pre-ejection delay greater than 140 ms, and activation of the posterolateral wall after aortic valve closure) effectively identified responder patients.

An unresolved issue is whether CRT may be beneficial to patients with chronic atrial fibrillation. Some studies [40] have suggested its usefulness, but the results of MUSTIC-AF are not conclusive. On the other hand, in some patients enrolled in the latter study constant pacing was not obtained, even though all had previously undergone atrioventricular ablation. Moreover, VVIR stimulation may have led to an increase in mean paced frequency. These may have been the reasons for the attenuated benefits of CRT in these patients compared to the group of patients in sinus rhythm.

Another unresolved issue is whether CRT may benefit patients with CHF, LV systolic dysfunction with indications for ventricular pacing but without signs of ventricular dyssynchrony. In fact, as demonstrated in some small studies, stimulation at the right ventricular apex may not be the ideal approach in this subset of patients [41, 42].

It is not yet clear whether CRT has at a long-term follow-up positive effects on mortality, which is an extremely important endpoint considering that the majority of other therapeutic options in CHF not only improve symptoms but also reduce mortality. Few data are available concerning patients enrolled in the InSync study, in which the 1-year mortality rate was 22% (48% sudden) and in the InSync Italian Registry, in which the 10-month mortality rate was 7% (38% sudden). The 2- and 3-year mortality rates of patients enrolled in the PATH-CHF study were 14% and 25%, respectively. In the MUSTIC study the 6-month mortality was 6.2% (75% sudden).

There are two ongoing trials dealing with the effect of biventricular stimulation on mortality. The first is Cardiac Resynchronization in Heart Failure (Care-HF), an open, randomized trial of biventricular stimulation versus control, which will enroll 800 patients who are in NYHA class III-IV while on optimal medical therapy and have a LVEF of 35% or less, LVEDD of 30 mm/m (height) or more, and QRS duration of more than 150 ms or more than 120 ms if echo criteria for ventricular dyssynchrony are present. Primary endpoints are total mortality and nonprogrammed cardiovascular hospitalizations.

The second is COmparison of Medical therapy, Pacing, ANd defibrillation In cONgestive heart failure (COMPANION), an open, randomized trial of biventricular stimulation versus biventricular stimulation plus ICD versus control, which will enrol 2500 patients who are in NYHA class III-IV while on optimal medical therapy, who have a LVEF of 35% or less, LVEDD of 60 mm or greater, QRS duration greater than 150 ms, and PR greater than 120 ms. Primary endpoints are total mortality and hospitalization for any cause.

It has been suggested that biventricular stimulation can reduce ventricular arrhythmias compared with sinus rhythm and right ventricular stimulation [43]. Moreover, in VENTAK-CHF, a trial which enrolled patients with symptoms of heart failure, a LVEF of 35% or less, QRS duration greater than 120 ms, and indications for ICD implantation, appropriate ICD interventions were significantly lower during the period of biventricular stimulation than during the period of nonstimulation [44]. Several trials are specifically evaluating the efficacy of CRT associated with ICD. The MIRACLE-ICD, a randomized trial with a crossover design over periods of 3 months, will enroll patients in NYHA class II-IV while on optimal medical therapy, who have a LVEF of 35% or less, QRS duration greater than 130 ms, and indications for ICD implantation, and randomize them to ICD without biventricular stimulation or ICD with stimulation. Primary endpoints are the 6-min walking distance and quality of life.

The INSYNC-ICD, a nonrandomized trial, will enroll patients in NYHA class III-IV while on optimal medical therapy, with a LVEF of 35% or less, QRS duration greater than 130 ms, and indications for ICD implantation in order to evaluate the safety and efficacy of a new biventricular ICD at 6-month follow-up. Primary endpoints are the 6-min walking distance and quality of life.

The BELIEVE study, a randomized trial with a crossover design over periods of 3 months, will enroll patients in NYHA class II-IV while on optimal medical therapy, with a LVEF of 35% or less, QRS duration greater than 130 ms, and indications for ICD implantation, randomizing them to ICD plus left ventricular stimulation or ICD plus biventricular stimulation. Primary endpoints are echocardiographic parameters.

Conclusions

CRT by biventricular pacing restores the coordination of contractions between the right and left ventricles and between the segments of the LV wall in patients with moderate to severe CHF secondary to severe LV systolic dysfunction and LV conduction delays. The effects are short-term improvement in cardiac performance and long-term improvement in clinical status (symptoms, functional capacity, and quality of life). CHR, therefore, may be considered a promising new option in the treatment of this group of patients.

While these results are encouraging, experience of this new technique is limited to a restricted number of patients. It is hoped that the several ongoing randomized trials will provide more data on the benefits of CRT on morbidity and mortality in the long term and more specific criteria for the selection of patients for whom CRT could be a therapeutic option.

References

1. Wilensky RL, Yudelman P, Cohen Al et al (1988) Serial electrocardiographic changes in idiopathic dilated cardiomyopathy confirmed at necropsy. Am J Cardiol 62:276-283
2. Xiao HB, Roy C, Fujimoto S et al (1996) Natural history of abnormal conduction and its relation to prognosis in patients with dilated cardiomyopathy. Int J Cardiol 53:163-170
3. Xiao HB, Roy C, Gibson DG (1994) Nature of ventricular actìvation in patients with dilated cardiomyopathy: evidence for bilateral bundle branch block. Br Heart J 72:167-174
4. Askenazi J, Alexander JH, Koenigsberg DI et al (1984) Alteration of left ventricular performance by left bundle branch block simulated with atrioventricular sequential pacing. Am J Cardiol 53:99-104
5. Rosenqvist M, Isaaz K, Botvinick EH et al (1991) Relative importance of activation sequence compared to atrioventricular synchrony in left ventricular function. Am J Cardiol 67:148-156
6. Murkofsky RL, Dangas G, Diamond JA et al (1998) A prolonged QRS duration on surface electrocardiogram is a specific indicator of left ventricular dysfunction. J Am Coll Cardiol 32:476-482
7. Hamby RI, Weissman RH, Prakash MN et al (1983) Left bundle branch block: a predictor of poor left ventricular function in coronary artery disease. Am Heart J 106:471-477
8. Auricchio A, Salo RW (1997) Acute hemodynamic improvements by pacing in patients with severe congestive heart failure. Pacing Clin Electrophysiol 20:313-324
9. Grines CL, Bashore TM, Boudoulas H et al (1989) Functional abnormalities in isolated left bundle branch block: the effect of interventricular asynchrony. Circulation 79:845-853
10. Wilensky RL, Yudelman P, Cohen AI et al (1988) Serial electrocardiographic changes in idiopathic dilated cardiomyopathy confirmed at necropsy. Am J Cardiol 1988;62:276-283
11. Aaronson KD, Schwartz JS, Chen TM et al (1997) Development and prospectíve evaluatíon of a clinical index to predict survival in ambulatory patients referred for cardiac transplant evaluation. Circulation 95:2660-2667
12. Shamim W, Francis DP, Yousufùddin M. et al (1999) Intraventricular conduction delay: a prognostic marker in chronic heart failure. Int J Cardiol 70:171-178
13. Likoff MJ, Chandler SL, Kay HR (1987) Clinical determinants of mortality in chroníc congestive heart fàilure secondary to idiopathic dilated or to ischemic cardiomyopathy. Am J Cardiol 59:634-638
14. Venkateshar K, Gottipaty SLF et al, for the VEST investigators (2000) The resting electrocardiograrn provides a sensitive and inexpensive marker of prognosis in patients with chronic congestive heart failure (abstract). J Am Coll Cardiol 33:145A
15. Silvet H, Padmanabham S, Pai R (1999) Increased QRS duration reduces survival in patients with left ventricular dysfunction: results from a cohort of 2263 patients (abstract). J Am Coll Cardiol 33:145A

16. Auricchio A, Stellbrink C, Block M et al (1999) Effect of pacing chamber and atrioventricular delay on acute systolic function of paced patients with congestive heart failure. Circulation 99:2993-3001
17. Etienne Y, Mansourati J, Gilard M et al (1999) Evaluation of left ventricular based pacing in patients with congestive heart failure and atrial fibrillation. Am J Cardiol 83:1138-1140
18. Leclercq C, Cazeau S, Le Breton H et al (1998) Acute hemodynamic effects of biventricular DDD pacing in patients with end-stage heart failure. J Am Coll Cardiol 32:1825-1831
19. Blanc JJ, Etienne Y, Gilard M et al (1997) Evaluation of different ventricular pacing sites in patients with severe heart failure. Results of an acute hemodynamic study. Circulation 96:3273-3277
20. Foster AH, Gold MR, McLauglin JS (1995) Acute hemodynamic effects of atrio-biventricular pacing in humans. Ann Thorac Surg 59:294-300
21. Kass D, Chen-Huan C, Curry C et al (1999) Improved left ventricular mechanics from acute VDD pacing in patients with dilated cardiomyopathy and ventricular conduction delay. Circulation 99:1567-1573
22. Saxon LA, Kerwin WF, Cahalan MK et al (1998) Acute effects of intraoperative multisite ventricular pacing on left ventricular function and activation/contraction sequence in patients with depressed ventricular function. J Cardiovasc Electrophysiol 9:13-21
23. Gras D, Mabo P, Tang T et al (1998) Multisite pacing as a supplemental treatment of congestive heart failure: preliminary results of the Medtronic Inc In Sync Study. Pacing Clin Electrophysiol 21:2249-2255
24. Gras D, Ritter P, Lazarus A et al (2000) Long-term outcome of advanced heart failure patients with cardiac resynchronization therapy (abstract). Pacing Clin Electrophysiol 23:658
25. Bakker P, Chin K, Sen A et al (1995) Biventricular pacing improves functional capacity in patients with end-stage congestive heart failure. Early experience. Pacing Clin Electrophysiol 19:1748-1757
26. Braunschweig F, Linde C, Gadler F, Rydén L (2000) Reduction of hospital days by biventricular pacing. J Heart Fail 2:399-406
27. Zardiní M, Tritto M, Bargiggia G et al (2000) The InSync Italian Registry: analysis of clinical outcome and considerations on the selection of candidates to left ventricular resynchronization. Eur Heart J Supplements 2 [Suppl J]: J16-J22
28. Porciani MC, Puglisi A, Colella A et al (2000) Echocardiographic evaluation of the effect of biventricular pacing: the InSync Italian Registry. Eur Heart J Supplements 2 [Suppl J]: J23-J30
29. Leclercq C, Cazeau S, Ritter P et al (2000) A pilot experience with permanent biventricular pacing to treat advanced heart failure. Am Heart J 140:862-870
30. Bakker PF, Meijburg H, de Vries JW et al (2000) Biventricular pacing in end-stage heart failure improves functional capacity and left ventricular function. J Interv Card Electrophysiol 4:395-404
31. Cazeau S, Ritter P, Bakdach S et al (1994) Four chamber pacing in dilated cardiomyopathy. Pacing Clin Electrophysiol 17:1974-1979
32. Cazeau S, Ritter P, Lazarus A et al (1996) Multisite pacing for end-stage heart failure: early experience. Pacing Clin Electrophysiol 19:1748-1757
33. Auricchio A, Stellbrink C, Block M, Mortensen P (1998) Clinical and objective improvements in severe congestive heart failure patients using univentricular or biventricular pacing: preliminary results of a randomized prospective study (abstract). J Am

Coll Cardiol 31[Suppl A]:31A
34. Auricchio A, Stellbrink C, Sack S et al (1999) The Pacing Therapies for Congestive Heart Failure (PATH-CHF) study: rationale, design, and endpoints of a prospective randomized multicenter study. Am J Cardiol 83[Suppl 5B]:130D-135D
35. Saxon LA, Boehmer JP, Hummel J et al (1999) VIGOR CHF and VENTAK CHF Investigators. Biventricular pacing in patients with congestive heart failure: two prospective randomized trials. Am J Cardiol 83[Suppl 513]:120D-123D
36. Auricchio A, Stellbrink C, Sack S et al (2000) Chronic benefit as a result of pacing in congestive heart failure: results of the PATH-CHF trials (abstract). Circulation 102:3352A
37. Cazeau S, Leclercq C, Lavergne T et al (2001) Effects of multisite biventricular pacing in patients with heart failure and intraventricular conduction delay. N Engl J Med 344:873-880
38. Abraham WT, Fisher W, Smith A et al (2002) Cardiac resynchronization in chronic heart failure. N Engl J Med 24:1845-1853
39. Alonso C, Leclercq C, Victor F et al (1999) Electrocardiographic predictive factors of long-term clinical improvement with multisite biventricular pacing in advanced heart failure. Am J Cardiol 84:1417-1721
40. Leclercq C, Victor F, Alonso C et al (2000) Comparative effects of permanent biventricular pacing for refractory heart failure in patients with stable sinus rhythm or chronic atrial fibrillation. Am J Cardiol 85:1154-1156
41. Gold MR, Feliciano Z, Gottlieb SS, Fisher ML (1995) Dual-chamber pacing with a short atrioventricular delay in congestive heart failure: a randomized study. J Am Coll Cardiol 26:967-973
42. Linde C, Gadler F, Edner M et al (1995) Results of atrioventricular synchronous pacing with optimized delay in patients with severe congestive heart failure. Am J Cardiol 75:919-923
43. Walker S, Levy TM, Rex S et al (2000) Usefulness of suppression of ventricular arrhythmia by biventricular pacing in severe congestive cardiac failure. Am J Cardiol 86:231-233.
44. Higgins SL, Yong P, Scheck D et al (2000) Biventricular pacing diminishes the need for implantable cardioverter defibrillator therapy. J Am Coll Cardiol 36:824-827

Echocardiography in the Identification of Responders: The Novel Role of Tissue Doppler Imaging and Strain Imaging

S. Carerj, C. Zito

Biventricular pacing (BivP) has been proposed as an adjunctive nonpharmacological therapy for patients with chronic heart failure (HF) who have electromechanical delay. It is already known that BivP improves symptoms, exercise capacity, quality of life and systolic function in these patients. The French pilot study, the Insync PATH-CHF I study, and the recent MUSTIC and MIRACLE trials have shown the improvement of outcome in HF patients calculated in different ways: myocardial oxygen consumption, distance covered during a 6-min walking test, estimation of NYHA functional class, and assessment of quality of life [1]. Recently, it has been demonstrated that BivP is effective in regressing left ventricular (LV) remodeling.

Up to 50% of patients with chronic HF have interventricular conduction delay such as left bundle branch block (LBBB), resulting in abnormal electrical depolarization of the heart. Prolonged QRS duration results in abnormal interventricular septal wall motion, decreased contractility, shortening of LV diastolic filling time, and prolonged mitral regurgitation, which places the failing heart at a significant mechanical disadvantage, with prolonged LV ejection time and asynchrony between right ventricular (RV) and LV contraction. Prolonged QRS duration has been associated with poor outcome in HF patients [2].

Another key factor in these patients is the optimization of the atrial-ventricular (AV) delay, since the atrial contraction is very important for cardiac performance. In patients with HF, a prolonged AV delay impairs LV performance. Moreover, optimization of the AV interval abolishes the diastolic mitral regurgitation that arises when LV diastolic pressure is higher than atrial pressure, so that atrial contraction leads to incomplete and untimely closure of the mitral valve. Optimization of the AV delay thus prevents the increase of LV end-diastolic pressure and decreases left atrial (LA) pressure.

Dipartimento Clinico-Sperimentale di Medicina e Farmacologia, Policlinico G. Martino, Università di Messina, Italy

Doppler echocardiography is a useful tool by which to predict responders to BivP and to objectively demonstrate the benefits from this procedure on LV function. In fact, this technique in its standard different applications [B-mode pulsed-wave (PW) and continuous-wave (CW) Doppler] now has an established role in:

- The selection of patients who may benefit from permanent pacing
- Showing the improvement in some parameters studied before pacemaker implantation, such as ejection fraction, RV and LV diameters and volumes, cardiac output, LV electromechanical delay (LVED), RV electromechanical delay (RVED), interventricular delay (IVD), LV filling time (LVFT), RV filling time (RVFT), LV ejection time (LVET), RV ejection time (RVET), etc [3].

PW and CW Doppler analysis can be helpful to identify patients who are potential responders to BivP; e.g., a duration of mitral regurgitation of 450 ms or more and a LV diastolic filling time of 200 ms or less are two markers predicting the efficacy of cardiac resynchronization therapy (CRT) [4]. Echocardiographic analysis may also show the possible deleterious effects of a nonoptimal delay between LA and LV contraction. It is a useful guide for seeking the best AV delay that will lead to the best hemodynamic results. This is possible by means of PW Doppler analysis of LV diastolic filling before and during BivP. Optimization of the AV delay leads to a significant increase in the LV filling time, calculated between the beginning of the E wave and the end of the A wave.

To date, the proposed criteria to be included for BivP are: functional class NYHA III-IV; QRS duration >120-150 ms, LV ejection fraction <35%; LV end-diastolic diameter >60 mm; pharmacological therapy optimized with ACE inhibitors and β-blockers; and relative stabilization of clinical status.

How can new Doppler-derived techniques help us in the identification of responders to CRT? Recently introduced tissue Doppler imaging (TDI) permits accurate quantification of regional and global LV function and volumes. Moreover, from digitally recorded TDI loops of one or more heart beats, two new TDI modalities can be derived: tissue tracking and strain rate. Tissue tracking visualizes the longitudinal motion amplitude in each myocardial segment during systole, and strain rate analysis can be used to determine whether this motion represents contraction or is merely passive. By using TDI it is possible to perform serial and quantitative assessment of regional cardiac function and synchronicity before pacing. It is also possible to quantify the degree of LV mechanical asynchrony by the extent of myocardium at the LV base displaying delayed longitudinal contraction (DLC). The number of segments with DLC is the only covariate to predict short-term response to CRT. Recently, Søgaard et al. have shown that CRT improved LV function and a parallel reduction in LV volumes (reversed LV remodeling) during long-term follow-up [5]. Patients likely to benefit from CRT can be identified by TDI before implantation of a biventricular pacemaker. In other words, the extent of the LV base DLC, as detected by TDI before pacemaker implantation, predicted the long-term efficacy of CRT. In this study, QRS duration, which in the MUSTIC trial is considered the major determinant for selection of the responders to CRT, failed to predict resynchronization efficacy. It appears that the detection of mechanical asynchrony as reflected by DLC is a better predictor of CRT efficacy. Moreover, patients who died during this study had QRS widths comparable to those of survivors. Thus, preimplantation TDI screening could improve the selection of candidates likely to benefit from CRT - a hypothesis that is currently being tested in a substudy of the Cardiac Resynchronization in Heart Failures (CARE-HF) study.

Strain rate analysis is a valuable tool to document when DLC represents contraction and thus a potential contractile "reserve" that could be resynchronized into systole [5].

In a recent study, it has also been shown that using TDI it is possible to demonstrate the presence of LV systolic dyssynchrony in patients before pacing therapy by the significant regional difference in time to peak sustained systolic contraction (t_s) (being earliest in the basal anteroseptal segment and latest in the basal lateral segment) and the marked increase in the standard deviation of t_s (t_s-SD) among the different LV segments. The improvement in intraventricular synchronicity after BivP was reflected by the loss of regional difference in t_s as well as the significant reduction in t_s-SD. BivP improves LV synchronicity by homogeneously delaying those sites with early peak systolic contraction, causing all segments to contract late with respect to the QRS onset but simultaneously with respect to each other. Furthermore, some patients actually have paradoxical septal motion so that sustained systolic contraction is earlier in the lateral wall. In this situation, BivP helps by abolishing the abnormal septal motion together with delaying the t_s in the lateral wall, so that synchronicity is successfully achieved.

Thus, the proposed mechanisms of BivP benefits suitable to be studied with TDI are the following:

- By delaying the t_s in the LV segments so that intraventricular synchronicity is improved, systole becomes more effective, ejection fraction and cardiac output are improved, and LV end-systolic volume is reduced.
- By synchronizing the contraction, thus reducing mechanical mitral regurgitation due to distortion of mitral apparatus and left atrial pressure. As a result, LV end-diastolic pressure and volume are decreased.
- By shortening the isovolumic contraction time after optimization of AV delay with increased diastolic filling time and stroke volume.
- By improving the interventricular synchrony between the left and the right ventricle. This benefit may be mediated through ventricular interdependence. This results in a gain in RV cardiac output so that LV filling is augmented [6].

Finally, since the rationale of BivP is to stimulate the most delayed LV wall, the left pacing site could provide additional benefit when it is concordant with the most delayed site. In accordance with this hypothesis, Ansalone et al. used TDI to define the most delayed wall and to verify whether LV performance showed a greater improvement in patients paced at the most delayed site than in patients paced at any other site [7]. The activation delay was in this study calculated as the time interval between the end of the A wave (named "C point") and the beginning of the E wave (named "O point") from the basal level of each wall. Patients paced at the most delayed site showed a greater improvement than did patients paced at any other site in respect of LV end-systolic volume, LV ejection fraction, bicycle stress testing work, time between closure and reopening of mitral valve (cardiac output) and LV isovolumetric contraction time.

Regional quantitative TDI analysis is an effective noninvasive technique that can also be useful to assess the severity of the regional delay in activation at each LV wall in patients with LBBB and HF who are candidates for BivP treatment [7].

Mele et al. used quantitative TDI to achieve direct measurement of intraventricular synchronicity, providing new indexes that also localize the level of dyssynchrony [septum-lateral wall synchronicity index (ms); intraseptal synchronicity index (ms), and intralateral synchronicity index (ms). They also concluded that TDI can be helpful to guide CRT in heart failure [8].

Based on similar assumptions, a new ultrasonographic method of quantifying regional deformation has been introduced to study both patients who are potential candidates for CRT and patients with a biventricular pacemaker already implanted, in order to define the benefits provided by this new mode of pacing. This technique is based on measurements of the strain and strain rate. Strain is defined as the deformation af an object, normalized to its original shape; strain rate is the speed at which deformation (i.e., strain) occurs [9].

Because myocardial velocities are dependent on overall heart motion, strain rate and strain calculation (based on regional velocity gradients) are able to reveal true regional deformation properties independent of global heart motion and might thus be sensitive for detection of contractile asynchrony. Breithardt et al. have shown that by means of strain rate imaging it is possible to study the regional inhomogeneity between midseptal and lateral wall segments before CRT and the relative improvement that occurs after BivP. Strain rate imaging offers new insight into the pathophysiology of LBBB and CRT [10].

References

1. Gras D, Leclercq C, Tang AS et al (2002) Cardiac resynchronization therapy in advanced heart failure: the multicenter InSync clinical study. Eur J Heart Fail 4:311-320
2. Abraham WT (2000) Rationale and design of a randomized clinical trial to assess the safety and efficacy of cardiac resynchronization therapy in patients with advanced heart failure: the Multicenter InSync Randomized Clinical Evaluation (MIRACLE). J Card Fail 6:369-380
3. Porciani MC, Puglisi A, Colella A et al, on behalf of the InSync Italian Registry Investigators (2000) Echocardiographic evaluation of the effect of biventricular pacing: the InSync Italian Registry. Eur Heart J [Suppl J]:J23-J30

4. Brecker SJ, Gibson DG (1996) What is the role of pacing in dilated cardiomyopathy? Eur Heart J 17:819-824
5. Søgaard P, Egeblad H, Yong Kim W et al (2002) Tissue doppler imaging predicts improved systolic performance and reversed left ventricular remodeling during long-term cardiac resynchronization therapy. J Am Coll Cardiol 40:723-730
6. Yu CM, Chau E, Sanderson JE et al (2002) Tissue Doppler echocardiographic evidence of reverse remodeling and improved synchronicity by simultaneously delaying regional contraction after biventricular pacing therapy in heart failure. Circulation 105:438-445
7. Ansalone G, Giannantoni P, Ricci R et al (2002) Doppler myocardial imaging to evaluate the effectiveness of pacing sites in patients receiving biventricular pacing. J Am Coll Cardiol 39:489-499
8. Mele D, Aggio S, Pasanisi G et al (2002) Quantitative tissue doppler can measure and localize improvement of ventricular dyssynchrony in dilated cardiomyopathy after biventricular pacing. Eur Heart J 4[Abstr. Suppl]:651
9. D'Hooge J, Heimdal A, Jamal F et al (2000) Regional strain and strain rate measurements by cardiac ultrasound: principles, implementation and limitations. Eur J Echocardiogr 1:154-170
10. Breithardt OA, Stelbrinck C, Herbots L et al (2002) Effects of cardiac resynchronization therapy on regional myocardial deformation as measured by echocardiographic strain rate imaging. Eur Heart J 4[Abstr. Suppl]:3

How to Follow Resynchronized Paced Patients

G. De Martino, T. Chiriaco, G. Pelargonio, A. Dello Russo, T. Sanna, C. Ierardi, D. Gabrielli, L. Messano, P. Zecchi, F. Bellocci

Biventricular stimulation is a new promising therapy for the treatment of moderate-to-severe heart failure in patients refractory to drug treatment and with contractile dyssynchrony due to conduction delay. The principle on which the resynchronization therapy is based is the reactivation of homogeneous and synchronized contraction by means of atrial-biventricular stimulation. The restoration of greater contraction synchrony seems to produce beneficial effects in the short (e.g., improvement in cardiac output, reduction of mitral regurgitation, increase of dP/dt, reduction of pulmonary wedge pressure) and the medium term (e.g., reduction of left ventricular diameters, increase of ejection fraction, reduction of mitral regurgitation, and reduction of sympathetic activity).

Two large clinical randomized and controlled studies (MUSTIC[1] and MIRACLE[4]) have demonstrated that in the medium term (six months follow-up) biventricular stimulation improves exercise capacity and quality of life. It has been recently reported that these beneficial effects are still present after 1 year of follow-up [5].

The current indications for implantation of a biventricular device are restricted to patients with heart failure in NYHA functional class III-IV despite optimal medical treatment (ACE-inhibitors, diuretics, digoxin, β-blockers), ejection fraction below 35%, left bundle branch block and QRS duration ≥ 130 ms. Both the follow-up and the pacemaker/implantable cardioverter-defibrillator (PM/ICD) implantation have only few aspects in common with those of a normal PM/ICD. Unlike most patients with a singular/dual-chamber pacemaker, who generally only need an instrumental follow-up and an ordinary clinical evaluation, patients with biventricular devices need a more complex clinical evaluation because of their severe symptoms. In fact, even the instrumental evaluation is more difficult in those patients, because the device is more complex. The two kinds of evaluation (instrumental and clinical) must be done together and need greater organizational effort than those for the common devices.

Department of Cardiology, Catholic University, Rome, Italy

Instrumental Follow-Up of Biventricular PM/ICD

Instrumental follow-up must be set on course at the moment of implantation, when the capture threshold, sensitivity, and impedance of the implanted leads must be measured with the utmost precision. Obviously maximum attention must be paid to the lead placed in the coronary sinus; its position must be photographed with three acquisitions anteroposterior, left anterior oblique (45°), and right anterior oblique (45°) projections. This information can turn out to be valuable during follow-up because they provide a basis for comparison if displacement is suspected. During the implantation it is worth looking for a diaphragmatic contraction activating the left lead at 10 V and on forced in and out breathing. The supine position can hide a diaphragmatic stimulation which might occur only in the upright standing position.

The state of the pacing/sensing and impedance values of the left lead seem to overlap with those of the right one. Actually, even if the left acute thresholds are higher than the right ones, their time trends are similar. In the Insync Registry [6] and in the Alonso et al. study [7], the average left ventricular lead capture threshold was 1.1±0.7 V/0.5 ms at the moment of implantation, reached its peak value within 3 months, and then remained at the value of 1.9±0.9 V/0.5 ms after 18 months of follow-up. Therefore the first instrumental follow-up can be carried out when the chronic threshold has been reached, i.e., after 3 months and then at regular 6-month intervals. The type of the lead (over the wire or preshaped leads) and the technique used (transvenous or by thoracothomy) do not seem to influence the acute or chronic threshold [8].

Before discharge, a radiographic follow-up which includes oblique projections and an ECG may be useful to look for early displacement of the left lead. For the same reason it can be useful to repeat the same studies after 1 month. The displacements can occur both early or at a later date, but generally if it happens it is within 3 months. The incidence of displacement is 5%-11% [7, 8].

The electrode threshold evaluation involves quite peculiar problems. Although it is relatively simple to check the devices with a separate channel for the left lead, it is more complex for the majority of devices, because in these the two ventricular channels are joined in parallel in the internal circuit of the device. In these cases the left and right threshold evaluation can be done by analyzing the paced QRS morphology changes.

Another important aspect is the optimization of the AV interval to permit optimal left ventricular filling. The best way to regulate it is using the echo-guided technique, which uses the transmitral pulsed Doppler pattern [9, 10]. This programming must be done before discharge and possibly at all follow-up ECGs.

The remainder of the instrumental follow-up is similar to the common one used for single/dual-chamber devices and must include checking the state of the battery, the sensing and impedance values, the ICD detection of malignant ventricular arrhythmias, and diagnostic data stored on the devices improved with Holter functions.

Clinical Evaluation of the Patient

As previously reported, the clinical evaluation of the patient must be conducted thoroughly and in parallel to the instrumental one of the device. All patients are suffering from a severe heart failure and their poor hemodynamic status necessitates assiduous clinical monitoring and frequent changes of medical treatment. Before implantation, in addition to a standard clinical evaluation useful to assess the general state of health, it's important to define exactly the echocardiographic and functional status of the patient in order to provide a point of comparison useful for later follow-up. The later evaluations will allow an assessment of the response to the resynchronization therapy.

The ECG evaluation has a key role because it allows us to obtain information about dimensions, kinetics, left ventricular systolic and diastolic function, and valvular function. Obviously the exam must be done before and after implantation, and preferably at every follow-up device check. The ECG must be done together with the instrumental checking-up of the devices to allow optimization of the AV interval.

The functional capacity can be more easily evaluated with the 6-min walking test or when available, with the cardiopulmonary treadmill test, which allow more precise determination of O_2 consumption, anaerobic threshold, etc. This test must also be done after implantation and regularly at every follow-up exam.

It is obvious that the organization for the follow-up of these patients needs an organizational effort, which cannot and must not fall exclusively on the electrophysiologist. Ideally, the follow-up of the patient with biventricular PM/ICD would be conducted with the collaboration of the heart failure outpatient's department, to whom must be more properly entrusted the clinical and ECG evaluation and the medical treatment, and the electrophysiologist, to whom should be entrusted the instrumental evaluation of the device.

References

1. Cazeau S, Leclerq C, Lavergne T et al for Multisite Stimulation in Cardiomyopathy (2001) Effects of multisite heart failure and intraventricular conduction delay. N Engl J Med 12: 873-880
2. Leclerq C, Walker S, Linde C et al on behalf of the MUSTIC Study Group (2000) Comparative effects of permanent biventricular and right univentricular pacing in heart failure patients with chronic atrial fibrillation. Am J Cardiol 85:1154-1156
3. Abraham WT (2000) Rationale and design of randomized clinical trial to assess the safety and efficacy of cardiac resynchronization therapy in patients with advanced heart failure: the Multicenter InSync Randomized Clinical Evaluation (MIRACLE). J Card Fail 6:369-380
4. Abraham WT, Fisher WG, Smith AL et al (2002) Cardiac resynchronization in chronic heart failure. N Engl J Med 346:1845-1853

5. Linde C, Leclercq C, Rex S et al (2002) Long-term benefits of biventricular pacing in congestive heart failure: results from the MUltisite STimulation in cardiomyopathy (MUSTIC). J Am Coll Cardiol 40:111-118
6. Gras D, Mabo P, Pang T et al (1999) Multisite pacing as supplemental treatment of congestive heart failure: preliminary results of the Medtronic InSync Study. Pacing Clin Electrophysiol 21:2249-2255
7. Alonso C, Leclercq C, d'Allonnes FR et al (2001) Six year experience of transvenous left ventricular lead implantation for permanent biventricular pacing in patients with advanced heart failure: technical aspects. Heart 86(4):405-410
8. Daoud EG, Kalbfleisch SJ, Hummel JD et al (2002) Implantation techniques and chronic lead parameters of biventricular pacing dual-chamber defibrillators. J Cardiovasc Electrophysiol 13(10):964-970
9. Naito M, Dreifus LS, Mardelli TJ et al (1980) Echocardiographic features of atrioventricular and ventriculoatrial conduction. Am J Cardiol 46(4):625-633
10. Pearson AC, Janosik DL, Redd RR et al (1988) Doppler echocardiographic assessment of the effect of varying atrioventricular delay and pacemaker mode on left ventricular filling. Am Heart J 115(3):611-621

Which Congestive Heart Failure Patient Needs to Be Studied in Haemodynamic Laboratory and When?

C. Vassanelli[1], G. Menegatti[2]

Introduction

Heart failure has emerged as a major challenge of increasing prevalence as age-adjusted rates of myocardial infarction and stroke decline [1]. In Italy, it has been estimated that congestive heart failure accounts for 800 000 days of hospitalization per year in cardiological units [2]. Invasive investigation is generally not required to establish the presence of chronic heart failure, but it may be important in elucidating the cause or to obtain prognostic information. Three diagnostic tools may be helpful in different situations: coronary angiography, hemodynamic monitoring, and endomyocardial biopsy. None of these is indicated as a routine procedure.

Coronary Angiography

Systolic Dysfunction

Although it was previously believed that myocardial ischemia either was short-lived and resulted in little or no muscle dysfunction or led to infarction with permanent damage, it is now clear that a middle state may exist in which chronic ischemic dysfunctional myocardium is present, to which function may return after myocardial revascularization [3, 4]. This intermediate state has been termed "myocardial hibernation."

Although most cases of myocardial dysfunction secondary to coronary artery disease are probably irreversible when due to infarction and subsequent ventricular remodeling (so-called ischemic cardiomyopathy) [5], some

[1]Divisione Clinicizzata di Cardiologia, Università del Piemonte Orientale, Azienda Ospedaliera "Maggiore della Carità", Novara; [2]Servizio di Cardiologia, Policlinico "G.B. Rossi", Verona, Italy

patients with hibernating myocardium have been shown to experience a marked improvement of resting ejection fraction and resolution of congestive heart failure after coronary revascularization [6, 7]. In most cases of hibernation, however, a marginal increase of ejection fraction of about 5% occurs after revascularization [8]. In view of this phenomenon, the possibility of reversible myocardial systolic dysfunction should always be considered, especially before a cardiac transplantation is contemplated. Usually, segmental wall motion abnormalities in ischemic cardiomyopathy coupled with perfusion defects during myocardial scintigraphy allow the diagnosis of ischemia as a probable cause of myocardial dysfunction before angiography. Likewise, the presence of thin-walled dilated cardiomyopathy with homogeneously poor wall motion and normal myocardial scintigraphy strongly suggests that nonischemic cardiomyopathy is present [9]. However, the two conditions may overlap such that some patients with idiopathic dilated cardiomyopathy may have regional wall motion abnormalities, whereas some patients with ischemic cardiomyopathy may have global left ventricular dysfunction. If noninvasive techniques suggest the presence of an area of viable myocardium, coronary angiography should be performed to identify potential revascularization targets.

It is worth noting that most centers do perform coronary angiography in the workup for cardiac transplantation.

Diastolic Dysfunction

Isolated diastolic dysfunction is the cause of heart failure in up to 30% of patients. This disorder is more common in elderly people with hypertension and often is suspected because of concentric left ventricular hypertrophy, normal systolic function, and abnormal transmitral flow velocity patterns on echocardiography [10]. However, in some patients with normal systolic function, the abrupt onset of pulmonary edema raises the suspicion that transient ischemia may be the mechanism of acute decompensation, because often elderly hypertensive patients have, by definition, at least two risk factors for coronary disease. In these patients, who are often unable to perform stress testing, coronary angiography may be necessary to establish or rule out the diagnosis of ischemia-related diastolic dysfunction and heart failure.

Coronary Artery Disease with Angina

Coronary artery bypass grafting has been shown to improve symptoms and survival in patients with heart failure and angina, although patients with severe symptoms of heart failure or markedly reduced ejection fraction were not included in these studies [11]. Because revascularization is recommended in individuals with ischemic chest pain regardless of the degree of ischemia or viability, there would appear to be little role for noninvasive cardiac testing in such patients. Clinicians should proceed directly to coronary angiography in patients who have angina and impaired ventricular function [12].

Up to one-third of patients with nonischemic cardiomyopathy complain of chest pain, which may resemble angina or may be atypical in nature. Because coronary revascularization would play a role in the management of these patients if their chest pain were related to the presence of coronary artery disease, coronary angiography is generally recommended in these circumstances to define the presence or absence of large-vessel coronary obstructions. Although many physicians perform noninvasive testing before coronary angiography in these patients, inhomogeneous nuclear images and abnormal wall-motion patterns are common in patients with a nonischemic cardiomyopathy. Hence, in most situations, clinicians should proceed directly to coronary angiography in patients who have heart failure and chest pain.

How should physicians evaluate patients with heart failure due to left ventricular dysfunction who do not have chest pain and who do not have a history of coronary artery disease? The use of coronary angiography appears reasonable in young patients to exclude the presence of congenital coronary anomalies. In older patients, however, efforts to detect the presence of coronary artery disease may not be worthwhile, because revascularization has not been shown to improve clinical outcomes in patients without angina [12].

Coronary Artery Disease Without Angina

The clinician has often to deal with cases of incident heart failure where the patients survive the initial presentation, do not have cardiac catheter data, lack clear noninvasive evidence of coronary artery disease, or whose suspected etiology is hypertension, alcohol, arrhythmia, or undetermined. The diagnosis of coronary artery disease as etiological factor in a patient's heart failure requires not only the presence of coronary artery disease, but evidence that the coronary artery disease is responsible for the development of heart failure. Coronary angiography remains the definitive method of identifying coronary anatomy, but the functional importance of the coronary artery disease needs to be determined. Increasing evidence suggests that revascularization is a treatment option in patients with significant hibernating myocardium [13, 14]. Controlled trials have not addressed the issue of whether coronary revascularization can improve clinical outcomes in patients with heart failure without anginal symptoms. Nevertheless, the 1999 ACC/AHA Guidelines for Coronary Artery Bypass Graft Surgery [12] recommend revascularization in patients with extensive myocardium at risk (significant left main stenosis and large areas of noninfarcted but hypoperfused and hypocontractile myocardium on noninvasive testing). Observational studies have shown that revascularization can favorably affect left ventricular function in some patients with impaired yet viable myocardium, but it is not clear how such patients should be identified because the sensitivity and specificity of an abnormal imaging test have not been validated in patients with heart failure. Additional studies are needed to determine whether the presence of myocardial ischemia or viability should be routinely evaluated to assess the contribution of coronary artery disease in patients with heart failure due to left ventricular systolic dysfunction who do not have angina.

Until now there have been no data on the prevalence of hibernating myocardium amongst incident heart failure cases in a population setting. The only data have come from highly selected cohorts of patients awaiting revascularization. One study suggested improvement in left ventricular function in 18/84 (33%) of such patients, implying the presence of hibernating myocardium prior to revascularization [15]. This figure may have little relevance to incident heart failure cases in the general population, and in particular amongst cases of heart failure who would not normally be considered for revascularization on the basis of their angina status.

Epidemiological studies of heart failure have allocated etiology without using invasive investigations such as angiography. The Framingham study [16] described hypertension as present in 70% and coronary artery disease in 59% of men and 48% of women. In a report from a cohort from Hillingdon, in west London, UK, coronary artery disease was present in 60% of those with an identifiable etiology. Fox et al. [17] sought to identify all incident cases of heart failure in a population of 292 000 in south London, UK, by monitoring patients admitted to hospital and through a rapid-access heart failure clinic. On the basis of angiographic data, 71 of the 136 patients (52%) under the age of 75 years had coronary artery disease causing heart failure. Probably, some of the 23 patients with noninvasively assigned etiologies other than coronary artery disease who did not undergo angiography had significant coronary artery disease, and hence the proportion of all cases due to coronary artery disease could be higher than 52%. Assuming the proportion of significant coronary artery disease in these patients was the same as in those who did undergo angiography would raise the overall proportion with coronary artery disease as etiology in the 136 cases of heart failure under 75 years to 59%. Ischemia was reported as the cause of heart failure in 33% in the SEOSI registry performed in 1995-1996 [2] and increased to 41% in the more recent IN-CHF (Italian Network of Chronic Heart Failure [18]). The finding of coronary artery disease has additional treatment implications beyond revascularization. Secondary prevention interventions such as aspirin treatment and, particularly, lipid-lowering therapy, are aimed at reducing the incidence of coronary events but might also prevent deterioration in left ventricular function [19].

Coronary angiography is indicated in patients with depressed left ventricular function and automatic defibrillator implanted in case of recurrent uncontrolled arrhythmias (the syndrome known as "arrhythmic warm-up"). In patients with diffuse coronary artery disease, the incidence of false-negative noninvasive tests is high: the coronary angiography might show changes in anatomy and lead to mechanical revascularization which, in some cases, is effective in controlling the arrhythmic warm-up [20].

Guidelines

According to the guidelines of the European Society of Cardiology [21], coronary angiography should be considered in patients with acute or acutely decompensated chronic heart failure and in the presence of severe heart failure (shock or acute pulmonary edema) not responding to initial treatment. Coronary angiography should also be considered in patients with angina pectoris or any other evidence of myocardial ischemia if not responding to appropriate anti-ischemic treatment. Angiography is required to exclude coronary artery disease when a diagnosis of idiopathic dilated cardiomyopathy is considered. Coronary angiography is also indicated in patients with refractory heart failure of unknown etiology and in patients with evidence of severe mitral regurgitation or aortic valve disease. Conversely, cardiac catheterization is not recommended in end-stage patients, in patients not considered as candidates for myocardial revascularization or valvular surgery, or in patients with known coronary anatomy in the absence of new episodes of myocardial infarction.

Hemodynamic Monitoring

In most patients the hemodynamic profile can be easily and quickly assessed at the bedside on the basis of signs and symptoms. This evaluation is frequently enough to guide initial treatment, although bedside skill in estimating hemodynamics has been challenged [22]. Invasive hemodynamic monitoring is often used when more precise measurement of filling pressures, perfusion, and systemic vascular resistances are desired. Urgent assessment is needed to guide initial intervention in critical situations when therapies must be provided rapidly to avoid circulatory collapse.

Invasive hemodynamic monitoring is useful if:

- Comorbidities (e.g., pulmonary disease) make management difficult
- The profile is not clear from clinical assessment and response
- Multiple therapies need to be adjusted simultaneously
- Initial treatments fail or intravenous inotropic agents cannot be withheld

Despite widespread use of the pulmonary artery catheter (PAC) in the last 30 years, recently the safety of its use has been challenged [23]. A recent multi-institutional, case-matched study assessing PAC safety in nine disease categories raised perhaps the greatest concern on potential harm associated with PAC use [24]. Some large observational studies have even suggested that the use of the PAC is associated with excess morbidity and mortality. An actual cause-and-effect relationship has not been established because there are no sufficiently powered randomized trials evaluating the safety or clinical efficacy of the PAC, and clinical trials are needed [25]. Multiple potential factors such as operational problems, errors in data interpretation, and exaggerated or inappropriate therapeutic responses to data obtained through use of the PAC have been implicated, singly or in combination, to explain these observations. However, a number of factors including reluctance of physicians to manage critically ill patients without a PAC, patient crossovers in randomized trials, and legal and ethical considerations have been implicated as barriers to a prospective randomized controlled trial in critically ill and other high-risk patients.

The results of the ESCAPE trial, in which conventional clinical management is compared with that using a PAC, will provide information about the utility of invasive monitoring in patients with advanced heart failure [26].

Guidelines

The guidelines of the European Society of Cardiology state that monitoring of hemodynamic parameters by means of a PAC is useful to assess the diagnosis and exclude correctable causes of heart failure [21]. It is also useful in directing treatment of patients with chronic congestive heart failure in the following circumstances: acutely decompensated heart failure not responding promptly to initial and appropriate treatment, dynamic mitral regurgitation in conjunction with volume overload or exercise, when chronic lung disease is a differential diagnosis, and in patients with refractory heart failure not responding to appropriate treatment. Routine right heart catheterization should not be used to tailor chronic therapy.

Endomyocardial Biopsy

One-third of patients with heart failure due to left ventricular dysfunction have normal coronary arteries on coronary angiography, and in such individuals myocardial disorders are responsible for the development of cardiomyopathy. Most patients with a cardiomyopathy have no identifiable causative factor (i.e., idiopathic dilated cardiomyopathy), but in some patients the cardiomyopathy is related to a systemic disorder (e.g., hyperthyroidism, hemochromatosis, or hypocalcemia), to exposure to a cardiotoxic agent (alcohol, cocaine, anthracycline, or trastuzumab), or to the presence of myocardial inflammation or infiltration, which can be diagnosed by endomyocardial biopsy. However, the overall usefulness of endomyocardial biopsy in the evaluation of patients with a cardiomyopathy of unknown cause is not clear [27]. The biopsy has been advocated as a means of making the diagnosis of myocardial disorders that might not be suspected otherwise, but most patients with a nonischemic cardiomyopathy show nonspecific changes on biopsy (including hypertrophy, cell loss, and fibrosis), and biopsy findings (even when positive) frequently do not have a material effect on patient management [28]. For example, the biopsy can detect inflammatory cell infiltrates attributed to viral myocarditis in some patients with acute or chronic heart failure, but many patients with acute myocarditis improve with supportive care without specific antiviral or anti-inflammatory treatment, and the prognosis of chronic cardiomyopathy does not appear to be influenced by immunosuppression, whether or not histological criteria for myocarditis are fulfilled [29]. Similarly, the biopsy can be used to make a diagnosis of sarcoidosis and amyloidosis, but changes characteristic of these disorders are often missed on histological evaluation, and there is no evidence that treatment can favorably affect the course of these diseases. Hence, the weight of available evidence suggests a limited role for endomyocardial biopsy in the evaluation of patients with heart failure. Tissue obtained by biopsy can be used to make the diagnosis of hemochromatosis, endocardial fibroelastosis, and Loeffler's syndrome in patients in whom these disorders are suspected on clinical grounds. Biopsy tissue may also be used to assess the risk of continued anthracycline therapy in patients with cancer, especially when combined with imaging of ventricular function [30, 31]. Biopsies can confirm the presence of cardiac disorders that might disqualify patients for heart transplantation (e.g., amyloidosis).

Biopsy can be used to identify patients with giant-cell myocarditis, who generally progress rapidly to death and are unresponsive to treatment and who thus may be considered for immediate heart transplantation [32]. Thus, endomyocardial biopsy is not indicated in the routine evaluation of cardiomyopathy. Although the risk of a serious complication is less than 1%, biopsies should be performed only when there is a strong reason to believe that the results will have a meaningful effect on subsequent therapeutic decisions.

Guidelines

The use of endomyocardial biopsy is limited to selected patients with unexplained (myocardial ischemia excluded) heart failure and may help to differentiate between constrictive and restrictive etiologies [21].

Special Situations

Coronary sinus venography is performed, usually in the electophysiology laboratory, to guide the correct positioning of electrodes to pace the left ventricle for electrical resynchronization treatment.

References

1. American Heart Association (2001) Heart and Stroke 2000 Statistical Update. American Heart Association, Washington, DC
2. The SEOSI Investigators (1997) Survey on heart failure in Italian hospital cardiology

units. Eur Heart J 18:1457-1464
3. Dilsizian V, Bonow RO (1993) Current diagnostic techniques of assessing myocardial viability in patients with hibernating and stunned myocardium. Circulation 87:1-20
4. Braunwald E, Rutherford JD (1986) Reversible ischemic left ventricular dysfunction: evidence for the "hibernating myocardium." J Am Coll Cardiol 8:1467-1470
5. Greenberg B, Quinones MA, Koilpillai C et a (1995) Effects of long-term enalapril therapy on cardiac structure and function in patients with left ventricular dysfunction: results of the SOLVD echocardiography substudy. Circulation 91:1573-1581
6. Akins CW, Pohost GM, Desanctis RW, Block PC (1980) Selection of angina-free patients with severe left ventricular dysfunction for myocardial revascularization. Am J Cardiol 46:695-700
7. Rankin JS, Newman GE, Muhbaier LH, Behar VS, Fedor JM, Sabiston DCJ (1985) The effects of coronary revascularization on left ventricular function in ischemic heart disease. J Thorac Cardiovasc Surg 90:818-832
8. Dilsizian V, Bonow RO, Cannon ROI et al (1988) The effect of coronary artery bypass grafting on left ventricular systolic function at rest: evidence for preoperative subclinical myocardial ischemia. Am J Cardiol 61:1248-1254
9. Tauberg SG, Orie JE, Bartlett BE, Cottington EM, Flores AR (1993) Usefulness of thallium-201 for distinction of ischemic from idiopathic dilated cardiomyopathy. Am J Cardiol 71:674-680
10. Bonow RO, Udelson JE (1992) Left ventricular diastolic dysfunction as a cause of congestive heart failure: mechanisms and management. Ann Intern Med 117:502-510
11. Alderman EL, Fisher LD, Litwin P et al (1983) Results of coronary artery surgery in patients with poor left ventricular function (CASS). Circulation 68:785-795
12. Eagle KA, Guyton RA, Davidoff R et al (1999) ACC/AHA guidelines for coronary artery bypass graft surgery: a report of the American College of Cardiology/American Heart Association Task Force on Practice Guidelines (Committee to Revise the 1991 Guidelines for Coronary Artery Bypass Graft Surgery). J Am Coll Cardiol 34:1262-1347
13. Perrone-Filardi P, Pace L, Prastaro M et al (1995) Dobutamine echocardiography predicts improvement of hypoperfused dysfunctional myocardium after revascularisation in patients with coronary artery disease. Circulation 91:2556-2565
14. Bax JJ, Cornel J, Visser FC et al (1997) F18-Fluorodeoxyglucose single-photon emission computed tomography predicts functional outcome of dyssynergic myocardium after surgical revascularization. J Nucl Cardiol 4:302-308
15. Christian TF, Miller TD, Hodge DO, Orszulak TA, Gibbons RJ (1997) An estimate of the prevalence of reversible left ventricular dysfunction in patients referred for coronary artery bypass surgery. J Nucl Cardiol 4:140-146
16. McKee PA, Castelli WP, McNamara PM, Kannel WB (1971) The natural history of congestive heart failure: the Framingham study. N Engl J Med 285:1441-1446
17. Fox KF, Cowie MR, Wood DA et al (2001) Coronary artery disease as the cause of incident heart failure in the population. Eur Heart J 22:221-236
18. Maggioni AP, Luci D, Gorini M et al (1996) The epidemiological profile of an Italian population of outpatients with congestive heart failure. Eur Heart J 17:437
19. Kjekshus J, Pederson T, Olsson AG, Faergeman O, Pyorala K (1997) The effects of simvastatin on the incidence of heart failure in patients with coronary heart disease. J Card Fail 3:249-254
20. Paffoni P, Bortnik M, Pedrigi C, Perucca A, Occhetta E, Vassanelli C (2000) La rivascolarizzazione miocardica come risoluzione del riscaldamento aritmico in pazienti con cardiovertitore-defibrillatore impiantabile: due casi clinici. Ital Heart J 1:1591-1596

21. Task Force for the Diagnosis and Treatment of Chronic Heart Failure of the European Society of Cardiology (2001) Guidelines for the diagnosis and treatment of chronic heart failure. Eur Heart J 22:1527-1560
22. Badget RG, Lucey CR, Mulrow CD (1997) Can the clinical examination diagnose left-sided heart failure in adults? JAMA 277:1712-1719
23. Zion MM, Balkin J, Rosenmann D et al, for the SPRINT Study Group (1990) Use of pulmonary artery catheters in patients with acute myocardial infarction. Chest 98:1331-1335
24. Connors AFJ, Speroff T, Dawson NV et al, for the SUPPORT Investigators (1996) The effectiveness of right heart catheterization in the initial care of critically ill patients. JAMA 276:889-897
25. Bernard GR, Sopko G, Cerra F et al (2000) Pulmonary artery catheterization and clinical outcomes. National Heart, Lung, and Blood Institute and Food and Drug Administration Workshop Report. JAMA 283:2568-2572
26. Shah MR, O'Connor CM, Sopko G et al (2001) Evaluation study of congestive heart failure and pulmonary artery catheterization effectiveness (ESCAPE): design and rationale. Am Heart J 141:528-545
27. Lie JT (1988) Myocarditis and endomyocardial biopsy in unexplained heart failure: a diagnosis in search of a disease. Ann Intern Med 109:525-528
28. Chow LC, Dittrich HC, Shabetai R (1988) Endomyocardial biopsy in patients with unexplained congestive heart failure. Ann Intern Med 109:535-539
29. Mason JW, O'Connell JB, Herskowitz A et al (1995) A clinical trial of immunosuppressive therapy for myocarditis. The Myocarditis Treatment Trial Investigators. N Engl J Med 1995:269-275
30. Mason JW, Bristow MR, Billingham ME, Daniels JR (1978) Invasive and noninvasive methods of assessing adriamycin cardiotoxic effects in man: superiority of histopathologic assessment using endomyocardial biopsy. Cancer Treat Rep 62:857-864
31. Alexander J, Dainiak N, Berger HJ et al (1979) Serial assessment of doxorubicin cardiotoxicity with quantitative radionuclide angiocardiography. N Engl J Med 300:278-283
32. Cooper LTJ, Berry GJ, Shabetai R (1997) Idiopathic giant-cell myocarditis natural history and treatment. Multicenter Giant Cell Myocarditis Study Group Investigators. N Engl J Med 336:1860-1866

Biventricular Pacing with ICD Backup: A Luxury or a Necessity?

S. Nisam, C. Duby

Introduction

The prevalence of heart failure (HF) in Europe has recently been estimated to be on the order of 6.5 million individuals [1]. HF is the only major cardiovascular disease that is increasing in incidence [2] with approximately 580 000 new cases diagnosed each year. The treatment of HF includes oral administration of β-blockers, ACE inhibitors/AT II receptor antagonists, diuretics, spironolactone, and digitalis. Nitrates and intravenously administered inotropes can be added for acute periods of hemodynamic decompensation. Nonetheless, many patients remain severely symptomatic despite optimal medical therapy. Cardiac resynchronisation therapy (CRT), also called biventricular pacing, can profit somewhere between 10% and 30% of patients with HF [3, 4]. The indications for CRT are the coexistence of symptomatic HF, including left ventricular dysfunction, and a wide QRS complex, such as is demonstrated by left bundle branch block (LBBB). There is a fast growing body of evidence suggesting that CRT may be a beneficial adjunct in the treatment array for chronic HF. In respect of short- and medium-term hemodynamic and efficacy parameters, patients in the PATH-CHF [5] and the MIRACLE [4] randomized controlled trials have demonstrated significant improvement in both maximal and submaximal exercise as well as in quality of life. The short-term beneficial effect of CRT is also maintained in the long term for patients in NYHA classes II, III, and IV [6, 7].

Need for ICD Backup

There is growing evidence supporting the need for backup of CRT by the capacity of an implantable cardioverter-defibrillator (ICD) to protect against

Guidant Europe, Diegem, Brussels, Belgium

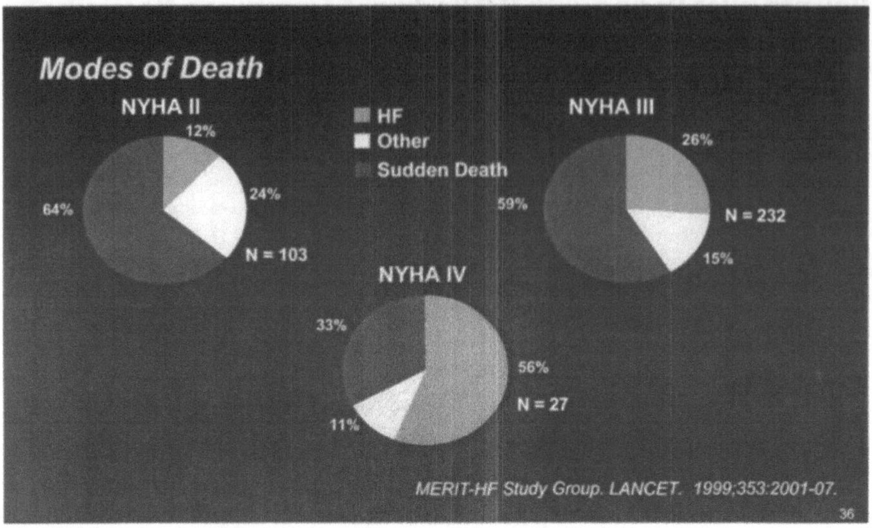

Fig. 1. Proportions of different modes of death in the different NYHA classes. (From [11], reproduced with permission)

sudden cardiac death (SCD) [8, 9]. The large multicenter MERIT-HF trial [10] was a double-blind, controlled, randomized study investigating the effect of metoprolol on survival. In that trial, the NYHA class III patients - considered to be those best suited for CRT - had a nearly 60% incidence of SCD (Fig. 1). In more recently published studies relating to CRT without ICD backup such as MUSTIC [11] and MIRACLE [4], half of all cardiac deaths were sudden. Moreover, interventricular conduction delay and LBBB, which result in a wide QRS complex, have both been demonstrated to be independent predictors of mortality [12, 13], thereby signifying the increased risk to patients indicated to receive CRT. The fact that more than 95% of patients suffering a SCD episode die before reaching a hospital [14] shows the vital necessity of protecting these patients in the event they suffer such episodes. They certainly do not have the "luxury" of out-of-hospital resuscitation. Not surprisingly, the vast majority of these deaths are due to ventricular tachyarrhythmias [15], making the case for ICD backup yet more evident.

Protecting Against SCD

With the notable exception of β-blockers, which have been clearly shown to reduce mortality from SCD, none of the other standard HF medications (ACE inhibitors, AT II receptor antagonists, diuretics, digoxin) have demonstrated this effect. The COMPANION trial [16] is an ongoing randomized three-arm study of patients with NYHA class III or IV heart failure, a left ventricular ejection fraction (LVEF) of 35% or less, and a QRS duration greater than 120

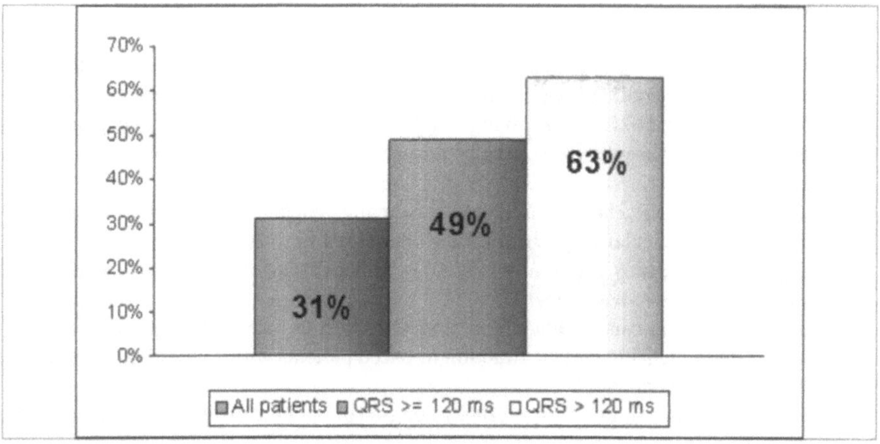

Fig. 2. Reduction in mortality among patients randomized to receive ICDs in the MADIT II study, according to different QRS widths on ECG

ms. The enrolment has to date reached 1600 of the 2200 patients needed, and the main objective is to determine whether optimal pharmacological therapy used with CRT alone or in combination with ICD backup is superior to optimal pharmacological therapy alone in reducing mortality. While awaiting the results, we can draw inspiration ourselves from the results of MADIT II [17], which involves essentially a HF patient population (two-thirds in NYHA class II/III), who have suffered a myocardial infarction and have a LVEF of 30% or less. In addition, 50% of these patients had a wide QRS of 120 ms or more. Patients in both limbs of the study received optimal pharmacological therapy. Those randomized to receive ICDs had a 31% reduction in mortality ($p = 0.02$) compared to the control limb. The benefit of the ICD was even greater for patients with increasing QRS width (Fig. 2). As regards the main issue in this article, by 2 years approximately 40% of the MADIT II patients had received appropriate therapy from the ICD. As these were patients with HF without a previous history of sustained ventricular tachycardia or ventricular fibrillation, it is clear that they were nonetheless highly vulnerable to ventricular tachyarrhythmias, and that these episodes were treatable by the ICD.

Conclusions

Approximately 60% of patients in HF NYHA class II/III die of SCD. The ICD has been shown conclusively to be the therapy of choice to protect patients against SCD. Therefore, for the cohort of patients with HF who qualify for CRT, it appears to be a necessity, not a luxury, to provide them with ICD backup. However, definitive confirmation of this will have to await the outcome of the COMPANION trial results.

References

1. New Medicine Inc (1977) Congestive heart failure: worldwide markets, clinical status and product development opportunities. Medicine Inc, pp 1-40 (www.newmedinc.com)
2. Massie BM, Shah NB (1997) Evolving trends in the epidemiologic factors in heart failure; rationale for preventive strategies and comprehensive disease management. Am Heart J 133:703-712
3. Farwell D, Patel NR, Hall A et al (2000) How many people with heart failure are appropriate for biventricular resynchronization? Eur Heart J 21:1246-1250
4. Abraham W, Fisher W, Smith A et al (2002) Cardiac resynchronization in chronic heart failure. N Eng J Med 346:1845-1853
5. Auricchio A, Stellbrink C, Block M et al (1999) Effect of pacing chamber and atrioventricular delay on acute systolic function of paced patients with congestive heart failure. Circulation 99:2993-3001
6. Linde C, Leclercq C, Rex S et al (2002) Long-term benefits of biventricular pacing in congestive heart failure: results from the multisite stimulation in cardiomyopathy (MUSTIC) study. J Am Coll Cardiol 40:111-118
7. Molhoek S, Bax J, Van Erven L et al (2002) Efficacy of resynchronization therapy in patients with end-stage heart failure. Am J Cardiol 90:379-383
8. Uretsky B, Sheahan R et al (1997) Primary prevention of sudden cardiac death in heart failure: will the solution be shocking? J Am Call Cardiol 30:1589-1597
9. Gaita F, Bocchiardo M, Porciani M et al (2000) Should stimulation therapy for congestive heart failure be combined with defibrillaiton backup? Am J Cardiol 86 (9A):165-168
10. Merit-HF study group (1999) Effect of metoprolol CR/XL in chronic heart failure: metoprolol CR/XL randomized intervention trial in congestive heart failure (MERIT-HF). Lancet 353:2001-2007
11. Linde C, Leclercq C, Rex S et al (2002) Long-term benefits of biventricular pacing in congestive heart failure: results from the multisite stimulation in cardiomyopathy (MUSTIC) study. J Am Coll Cardiol 40:111-118
12. Shamin W, Francis DP, Yousufuddin M et al (1999) Intraventricular conduction delay: a prognostic marker in chronic heart failure. Int J Cardiol 70:171-178
13. Baldasseroni S, Opasich C, Gorini M et al (2002) Left bundle-branch block is associated with increased 1-year sudden and total mortality rate in 5517 outpatients with congestive heart failure: a report from the Italian Network on Congestive Heart Failure. Am Heart J 143:398-405
14. American Heart Association (2001) Heart and Stroke Statistical Update
15. Tedesco C, Reigle J, Bergin J et al (2000) Sudden cardiac death in heart failure. J Cardiovasc Nurs 14:38-56
16. Bristow MR, Feldman AM, Saxon LA et al (2000) Heart failure management using implantable devices for ventricular resynchronization: comparison of medical therapy, pacing, and defibrillation in chronic heart failure (COMPANION) trial. COMPANION steering committee and COMPANION clinical investigators. J Card Fail 6:276-285
17. Moss A, Zareba W, Hall J et al (2002) Prophylactic implantation of a defibrillator in patients with myocardial infarction and reduced ejection fraction. N Engl J Med 346:877-883

Biventricular Cardiac Resynchronization in Moderate-to-Severe Heart Failure: Analysis of Hospital Costs and Clinical Effectiveness (Brescia Study)

A. Curnis[1], F. Caprari[2], G. Mascioli[1], L. Bontempi[1], A. Scivales[2], F. Bianchetti[1], S. Nodari[1], L. Dei Cas[1]

Introduction

Heart failure is a chronic condition of complex physiopathologic origin which involves escalating clinical costs [1-3]. Cardiac resynchronization therapy is a novel treatment for the one in every six heart failure patients whose condition is refractory to optimized drug treatment, with evidence of ventricular dysynchrony which leads to a deterioration of hemodynamics and a higher risk of death [4-7]. In such hearts the regions which activate in advance will experience or receive a lower afterload, and the rapid presystolic contraction does not convert into a rise in pressure, because the other parts of the myocardium are still inactive. As a consequence, most myocardial activity is wasted in transferring the ejection from one part of the heart to another. This results in a lengthening of the ventricular pre-ejection period, a reduction of the contraction and the relaxation period, a reduction of the ejection fraction, and a rise in mitral regurgitation.

In biventricular pacing, simultaneous delivery of an electric stimulus to both ventricular chambers almost completely cancels the interventricular delay. Furthermore, if the left ventricular lead (electrode) is positioned in a tributary vein to the left ventricular tract with delayed contraction, it is possible to significantly shorten the intraventricular delay. Biventricular stimulation has been shown to deliver considerable economic advantages [8, 9].

Aim of The Study

The aim was to evaluate the impact biventricular pacing can have on this clinical condition and on the hospital costs in a group of patients with severe heart failure that is refractory to drug treatment. The study compared specific clinical and economic parameters 1 year before and 1 year after the implantation of a biventricular stimulation system.

[1]Department of Cardiology, University and Spedali Civili of Brescia; [2]Fondazione Medtronic Italia, Milan, Italy

Patients

Between October 1998 and December 1999, 30 patients were enrolled in the study and were implanted with a biventricular stimulator. See Table 1 for patients' characteristics.

Table 1. Clinical characteristics of the study group (n=30). Values represent percentage of patients except where otherwise indicated

Age at implant (years)	67.2 ±7.71 (range 52-80)
Male gender	80
Idiopathic dilated cardiomyopathy	37
Postinfarction cardiomyopathy	63
Coronary artery bypass graft	20
Chronic obstructive broncopneumopathy	17
Atrial fibrillation	17
Mean ejection fraction (%) measured by angiocardiography	23±8 (range 9-40)
QRS > 150 ms	100
NYHA class III	94
NYHA class IV	6

Methods

The study was carried out according to an observational method using a single group of patients, retrospectively for a 1-year period preceding the implantation and prospectively for a 1-year period following the implantation. The variables taken into account for the clinical and economic assessment of the pathology were: ejection fraction, New York Heart Association (NYHA) class, number of hospitalizations in the cardiology ward or ICU (intensive care unit), days of hospitalization in the cardiology ward or ICU, number of clinic visits (outpatients), number of day hospital visits, number of days free from acute events requiring hospitalization or clinic visits, and the cost of the healthcare delivered. All data collected in the year following the device implantation were compared to those collected during the year preceding the implant.

Economic Evaluation

In order to evaluate the economic impact (from a hospital point of view) of biventricular stimulation in patients with heart failure, the activity-based costing was used where possible. When budget information did not allow an assessment of real costs, the cost of diagnostic tests and outpatient visits were calculated according to the current outpatient rates, except for coronary angiography, for which an accurate cost analysis was already available from the Hemodynamic Cost Center Accounting Report (1999). See Table 2 for cost sources.

Table 2. Sources of cost information

Type cost	Source
Drugs	Italian National Formulary 1999
Instrumental tests	Current outpatient rates
Coronary angiography	Hemodynamic cost center accounting report (1999)
Day hospital visits	DRG ex DGR n. VI/37597 (1998)
Outpatient clinic visits	Current outpatient rates
Pacemaker	Cardiology cost center accounting report (1999)
Electrophysiology performance	Electrophysiology cost center accounting report (1999)
In-hospital stay	Cardiology & ICU cost center accounting report (1999)
Doctor and nurse assistance	Evaluation according to the NLC

DRG, Disease Related Group; DGR, Delibera Giunta Regionale; NLC, National Labour Contract

Statistical Methods

Results given are mean ± 1 SD. The differences pre- and post-implant regarding ejection fraction, heart failure episodes, number of hospital days and hospitalizations, and number of days free from hospitalizations and/or day hospital visits, were analyzed using Student's t-test (paired comparison). A two-tailed p-value below 0.05 was considered statistically significant.

Results

In the 12 months following implantation, the patients' symptoms improved considerably, as quantitatively demonstrated by a significant reduction in functional NYHA class (3.0±0.3 vs. 2.1±0.3, $p< 0.05$). Although not a statistically significant change, ejection fraction increased from 23%±8% to 27%±10%.

Six of the 30 patients had arrhythmias that required implantation of a device for biventricular stimulation, as well as high-energy therapies for ventricular fibrillation. The clinical and economic evaluation of these patients was restricted to the part of their therapy related to their heart failure, i.e., the part related to biventricular pacing. Therefore, during the economic evaluation, the devices implanted were considered as biventricular stimulators and subsequent care considered was restricted to that required to treat heart failure.

At 6 months two patients died and one dropped out of the study for a heart transplantation. Their results were multiplied by two to account for the whole year.

Clinical improvement was shown by a significant reduction in all the assessed morbidity indexes (Table 3).

There were no significant changes in drug therapy, except for the dosages of β-blockers and ACE inhibitors. The previous years' costs include the full cost of hospitalization except for the procedure cost, which has been added to the second-year cost.

Table 4 shows the total management cost for the 30 patients during the year

Table 3. Mean results per patient

	Baseline	12 months follow up	Change (%)	*p*-value
Number of hospitalizations:				
- Cardiology ward	1.83 ± 1.21	0.30 ± 0.70	- 84	< 0.001
- intensive care unit	0.97 ± 1.27	0.13 ± 0.51	- 86	< 0.01
- other	0.70 ± 2.73	0.03 ± 0.18	- 95	< 0.05
Total	3.50 ± 2.89	0.47 ± 0.82	- 87	< 0.001
Days of hospitalization:				
- Cardiology	37.57 ± 34.15	2.63 ± 6.26	- 93	< 0.001
- intensive care unit	2.57 ± 3.29	0.13 ± 0.37	- 95	< 0.001
- others	1.90 ± 4.59	0.07 ± 0.51	- 96	< 0.05
Total	42.03 ± 37.51	2.83 ± 6.36	- 93	< 0.001
Day hospital visits	2.6 ± 1.8	4.2 ± 2.7	± 64	< 0.05
Outpatient visits	3.5 ± 2	4.4 ± 2.3	± 28	NS
Total hospital care (days of hospitalization ± day hospital ± outpatient visits)	48.07 ± 37.84	11.47 ± 9.08	- 76	< 0.001
Days free from acute events	104 ± 123	266 ± 137	± 156	< 0.001
Worsening heart failure episodes	2.8 ± 0.6	0.5 ± 0.5	- 82	< 0.001
NYHA class	3 ± 0.3	2.1 ± 0.3	- 30	< 0.001
Ejection fraction (%)	23 ± 8	27 ± 10	± 17	< 0.05

Table 4. Total management costs for 30 patients for the one year before and one after implanation

	1 year before implant (€)	1 year after implant (€)
Stay in cardiology ward	27 8781	19 294
Stay in ICU	67 007	3 481
Drug therapy	2 688	298
Procedures	16 780	6 207
Pacemaker implant cost	0	231 341
Day hospital visits	16 543	27 071
Outpatient visits	1 719	2 198
Total	383 518	289 890
Total cost excluding implant cost	383 518	58 549
Cost per patient	12 784	9 663
Cost per patient excluding implant cost	12 784	1 952

before and the year after device implantation, calculated according to the above-mentioned criteria. These costs decreased from € 383519 to € 289890 including the implant costs (device plus electrophysiology procedure cost) and to € 58549 excluding the latter. The cost per patient decreased from €12784 to €9663 including implant cost and to €1952 excluding it (Fig. 1).

If we examine each single variable, excluding implant costs, it is clear that it is the implant that determines a change in care, because the patient is monitored more and more as an outpatient (see Fig. 2 for the distribution of total hospital care).

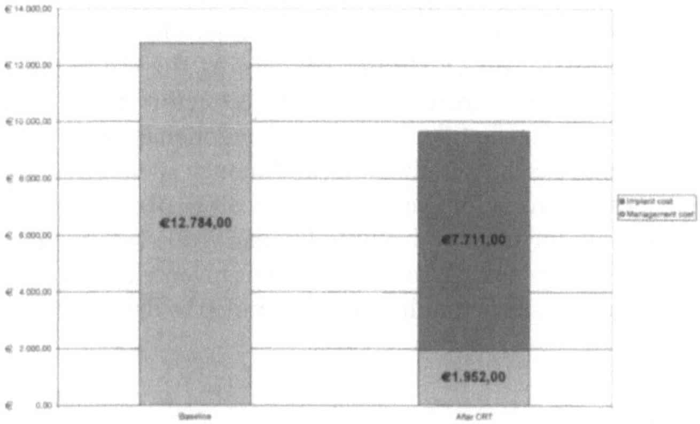

Fig. 1. Cost per patient/year before and after CRT

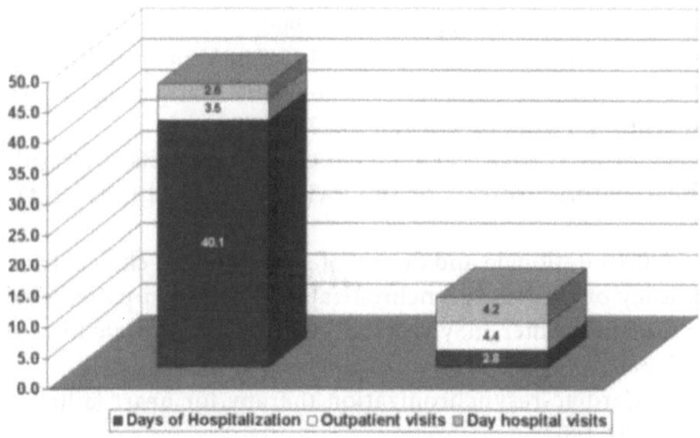

Fig. 2. Breakdown of total hospital care into types before and after CRT

Discussion

The results of this analysis are consistent with the literature [5, 10, 11]. They provide useful indications for those responsible for adopting new techniques with regard to budgets at every level of the system: the department of cardiology, the general management of the hospital, and regional health care services.

This trial demonstrates how:

1. Biventricular stimulation reduces the need for hospitalizations, delivering advantages for national health care system through:
   - A reduced need for hospital care
   - A reduction in the number of DRG cases to be reimbursed to hospitals
2. This technology reduces the portion of the hospital ward's budget allocated to treatment of heart failure, thus increasing productivity and reducing the risk of budget overruns.

If the randomized trials currently being undertaken, confirm the data highlighted in these preliminary studies concerning the efficacy of biventricular pacing in the long-term treatment of drug-refractory heart failure, this technology will contribute significantly to reducing management costs. The reduction in the number of hospitalizations and money spent on heart failure could free important resources for the treatment of other patients.

While waiting for hard end-points [7] (survival) results, the US Food and Drug Administration has approved the use of biventricular pacing for moderate-to-severe heart failure that has not responded to drug therapy [12].

References

1. Schweiger C, Maggioni AP (2001) Scompenso cardiaco ancora in attesa di strategie. Sole 24ore Sanità. 20-26 november
2. Ministero della Salute (2001) Clinical Evidence Edizione Italiana
3. Ministero della Salutre (2000) Rapporto SDO 2000
4. Kervin WF, Botvinick EH, O'Connel JW et al (2000) Ventricular contraction abnormalities in dilated cardiomiopathy: effect of biventricular pacing to correct interventricular dyssynchrony. J Am Coll Cardiol 35:121-127
5. Auricchio A, Stellbrink C, Sack S et al (2000) Chronic benefits as a result of pacing in congestive heart failure: results of the PATH-CHF Trial (abstract). Circulation 102:3352A
6. Abraham WT (2000) Rationale and design of a randomized clinical trial to assess the safety and efficacy of cardiac resynchronization therapy in patients with advanced heart failure: the Multicenter InSync Randomized Clinical Evaluation (MIRACLE). J Card Fail 6:369–380
7. Hare JM (2002) Cardiac-resynchronization therapy for heart failure (editorial). N Engl J Med 346:1902-1904
8. Braunschweig F, Linde C, Gadler F, Rydén L (2000) Reduction of hospital days by biventricular pacing. Eur J Heart Failure 2:399-406
9. Dixon LJ, Thompson G, Harbinson M et al (2002) Cardiac resynchronisation therapy - a cost effective treatment for cardiac failure. Eur Heart J 4 (Abstr Suppl):3
10. Ryden-Bergsten T, Andersson F (1999) The health care costs of heart failure in Sweden. J Intern Med 246:275-284
11. Cazeau S, Leclercq C, Lavergne T et al (2001) Effects of multisite biventricular pacing in patients with heart failure and intraventricular conduction delay. N Engl J Med 344:873-880
12. Leclerq C, Kass DA (12) Retiming the failing heart: principles and current clinical status of cardiac resynchronization. J Am Coll Cardiol 39:194-201

ATRIAL ARRHYTHMIAS: DRUGS, DEVICES OR ABLATION FOR THE PREVENTION AND TREATMENT OF THE RECURRENCES?

Atrial Fibrillation and Flutter: Sympathetic Nervous System and Arrhythmogenesis

F. Lombardi, D. Tarricone, F. Tundo, F. Colombo, S. Belletti

In the last few years, several studies have investigated the role of autonomic dysfunction in atrial fibrillation (AF) onset. In most instances, particularly in subjects with paroxysmal AF, a distinct proarrhythmic effect of sympathetic or vagal activation was found.

A simple method [1] that allows an appropriate evaluation of autonomous nervous system modulation and its relationship with AF is the analysis of heart rate variability (HRV) carried out on Holter recordings during sinus rhythm preceding the onset of the arrhythmia. In a recent report, Herweg et al. [2] analyzed HRV in a group of 29 patients during sinus rhythm just before the onset of episodes of paroxysmal AF, and observed an increase in the high frequency (HF) component, suggesting a proarrhythmic role of vagal mechanisms. This pattern was particularly evident before nocturnal episodes, especially in younger patients with structurally normal hearts ("lone fibrillators"). Another study [3] carried out in 26 patients undergoing coronary artery bypass surgery described the changes in sympathovagal balance in the hour preceding AF episodes. It was observed that the low frequency/high frequency (LF/HF) ratio was lower 30 min before AF onset and higher immediately before initiation of the arrhythmia. These findings led the authors to conclude that a shift in the autonomic balance with a loss of vagal tone and a moderate increase in sympathetic tone characterized the time before AF onset.

Similar findings were reported by Wen et al. [4], who studied 12 patients with paroxysmal atrial flutter: the analysis of the HRV in the frequency domain demonstrated an increase in the normalized value of the LF component and in the LF/HF ratio and a decrease in the normalized value of the HF component. These changes started 6 min before the onset of episodes of paroxysmal atrial flutter, suggesting a shift in the sympathovagal balance toward sympathetic predominance.

Cardiology, Department of Medicine, Surgery and Dentistry, Ospedale San Paolo, University of Milan, Italy

Other authors [5] evaluated the LF/HF ratio at different times before the onset of 17 episodes of AF. There were no significant differences in the HF values before the onset of arrhythmia, but the LF/HF ratio increased progressively from about 30 min to just before its onset.

More recently, Bettoni and Zimmermann [6] reported the results of a study carried out in a larger group of patients, in which 147 episodes of paroxysmal AF (>30 min) were analyzed using time and frequency domain methodologies. A significant increase in the HF component and a progressive decrease in the LF component were observed immediately before the arrhythmic event. The LF/HF ratio increased linearly until 10 min before AF, followed by a sharp decrease confined to the minutes before AF onset. These changes were consistent with a complex pattern of autonomic dysfunction, with a primary increase in adrenergic modulation followed by a late parasympathetic activation buffering the adrenergic predominance. In this study, no difference was observed between patients with "lone" AF and patients with structural heart disease.

All the above studies seem therefore to support the hypothesis that the autonomous nervous system plays an important role in the genesis and maintenance of AF, particularly in subjects with no evidence of organic heart disease.

We have recently moved our attention to new areas of interest: the relationship between the type of initiation of AF and autonomic balance, and the effect of restoration of sinus rhythm on autonomic control mechanisms [7]. Analysing Holter recordings containing episodes of paroxysmal AF lasting more than 30 s, we examined the role of the autonomous nervous system in relation to the onset, maintenance, and spontaneous termination of AF. One hundred ten episodes of paroxysmal AF lasting at least 30 s were studied. The mean age of patients was 67±10 years (range 47-87 years). The pharmacological therapy included digoxin in 4 patients, class I antiarrhythmic drugs in 17 patient, beta-blockers in 8 patients, class III anti-arrhythmic drugs in 13 patients, and calcium antagonists in 7 patients; 29 patients had no drug therapy. Clinical characteristics of individual patients were as follows: systemic hypertension, 35%; coronary artery disease, 19%; sick sinus syndrome, 8%; valvular disease, 8%; lone AF, 30%.

Two-channel 24-h electrocardiographic recordings were analyzed using a commercially available digital scanner (Synetec, V 1.20, Ela Medical, Paris, France). The electrocardiogram was digitally sampled at 128 samples per second and data were then transferred from the scanner to an IBM PC-compatible computer for HRV analysis. Data relative to 75 patients and 110 episodes of paroxysmal AF were used as a basis to estimate short-term variability during the control period, the 5 min of sinus rhythm immediately preceding the onset of AF, and the 5 min after its spontaneous termination. Details of the performance of spectral computations and discussion of the physiological interpretation of spectral components have been reported elsewhere [8-11]. Arrhythmic episodes were divided into two groups on the basis of the prevalence of LF over HF, using a lowermost cut-off value of the LF/HF ratio of 2, a value known to reflect a shift of sympathovagal balance toward sympathetic activation [8-11].

The mean duration of AF was 154±20 min (range 0.5-1020 min). Sixty-five episodes (59%) happened during the day time, 45 episodes (41%) at night time. On the basis of the presence or absence of a "short-long-short" sequence before AF onset, arrhythmic episodes were classified as type 1 (T1, n= 37) and type 2 (T2, n= 73). Taking all AF episodes as a whole, we observed that the LF/HF ratio before AF onset was significantly greater than that measured upon restoration of sinus rhythm (6.2±1.1 vs 3.3±0.6). The analysis of HRV in relation to the type of onset revealed a greater increase in LF component in T1 than in T2 onsets (61.8±4.1 vs 53±3.2). Furthermore, the duration of AF episodes with T1 onset was significantly shorter than that of episodes with T2 onset (68±16 vs 197±27 min, p<0.001). On the other hand, no significant difference between day-time and night-time episodes was discovered in respect of duration (165±16 vs 146±24 min) or mean values of RR interval, variance, LF, HF, and LF/HF ratio.

Using a cut-off value for the LF/HF ratio of 2, signs of sympathetic predominance were observed in 73 cases, whereas a parasympathetic predominance was detectable in the remaining 37 events. Moreover, when we analyzed HRV in the minutes immediately following the spontaneous recovery of sinus rhythm, patients with an initial LF/HF ratio of 2 (or greater) presented a significant increase in the HF components and a reduction of the LF components and of the LF/HF ratio, whereas patients with an initial LF/HF ratio lower than 2 showed an increase in the LF component and the LF/HF ratio toward values consistent with a more physiological sympathovagal balance.

Finally, we analyzed the standard deviation and the coefficient of variation of RR interval at the beginning, central, and final part of AF. No differences in any of these parameters were observed, indicating that no pseudoregularization of the ventricular response appears to occur before spontaneous termination of paroxysmal AF episodes.

Conclusions

Our results are well in agreement with previous studies suggesting that alteration of autonomic control mechanisms is frequently detectable in the minutes preceding the onset of paroxysmal AF. In most instances, signs of sympathetic activation and of reduced vagal modulation are clearly evident, but in about one-third of the episodes parasympathetic control mechanisms appear to prevail. Immediately after spontaneous recovery of sinus rhythm, signs of sympathetic activation are no longer evident but are replaced by an HRV pattern consistent with a more physiological modulation of sinus node. Also in patients with signs of vagal activation before AF episodes, a more physiological sympathovagal balance is present at the end of the arrhythmic episodes. Whether the observed changes in autonomic control mechanisms might contribute to the termination of the arrhythmic events or simply reflect the hemodynamic consequences of AF remains to be assessed. Nevertheless, the minutes preceding and following AF episodes appear to be characterized by fluctuations in sympathovagal balance, with variable shifting toward distinct patterns of autonomic imbalance.

References

1. Task Force of the European Society of Cardiology and the North American Society of Pacing and Electrophysiology (1996) Heart rate variability. Standards of measurement, physiological interpretation, and clinical use. Circulation 93:1043-1065
2. Herweg B, Dalal P, Nagy B, Schweitzer P (1998) Power spectral analysis of heart period variability of preceding sinus rhythm before initiation of paroxysmal atrial fibrillation. Am J Cardiol 82:869-874
3. Dimmer C, Tavernier R, Gjorgov N et al (1998) Variations of autonomic tone preceding onset of atrial fibrillation after coronary artery bypass grafting. Am J Cardiol 82:22-25
4. Wen ZC, Chen SA, Tai CT, Huang JL, Chang MS (1998) Role of autonomic tone in facilitating spontaneous onset of typical atrial flutter. J Am Coll Cardiol 31:602-607
5. Tomoda Y, Uemura S, Fujimoto S, Yamamoto H, Matsukura Y, Hashimoto T, Dohi K (1998) Assessment of autonomic nervous activity before the onset of paroxysmal atrial fibrillation. Am J Cardiol 31:11-71
6. Bettoni M, Zimmermann M (2002) Autonomic tone variations before the onset of paroxysmal atrial fibrillation. Circulation 105: 2753-2759
7. Lombardi F, Tundo F (2002) Autonomic nervous system and atrial fibrillation. G Ital Aritmol Cardiostimol 5:23-27
8. Pagani M, Lombardi F, Guzzetti S et al (1986) Power spectral analysis of heart rate and arterial pressure variabilities as a marker of sympathovagal interaction in man and conscious dog. Circ Res 59:178-197
9. Malliani A, Pagani M, Lombardi F, Cerutti S (1991) Cardiovascular neural regulation explored in the frequency domain. Circulation 84: 482-492
10. Lombardi F, Malliani A, Pagani M, Cerutti S (1996) Heart rate variability and its sympathovagal modulation. Cardiovasc Res 32:208-216
11. Lombardi F (2000) Chaos theory, heart rate variability, arrhythmic mortality. Circulation 101:8-10

Current Approach and Treatment in Acute Atrial Fibrillation

G. Chiarandà[1], A. Busà[1], A. Lazzaro[2], T. Regolo[3]

In the clinical setting, the most frequently observed arrhythmia is atrial fibrillation (AF). Its prevalence is rising [1], and at present it involves 0.3%-0.4% of the general population. There are 2.3 million cases in the USA, and the projection for the year 2050 is about 5.6 millions [2]. Several clinical surveys, including the Framingham Heart Study [3], indicate a steady increase in the incidence and prevalence of AF in the elderly, starting with 0.1% in subjects below 55 years of age, and reaching 9% in those over 80 years old. This is in agreement with the Cardiovascular Heart Study, which found a 5% prevalence of AF in subjects older than 65 years [4].

AF is associated with an increase in overall and cardiovascular morbidity and mortality [5], though the prognosis depends on the underlying heart disease, as can be deduced from the survival curves of the main published case series [6]. The high prevalence of AF causes a large number of hospitalizations [7]; hence, the therapy of acute AF, and the prevention of relapses, may have a strong socioeconomic impact.

From the therapeutic viewpoint, the most useful classification for AF is presently derived from the ESC guidelines [8] and includes: single AF episode or recurrent AF (if two or more episodes); acute AF (shorter than 24-48 h); or chronic AF. The latter includes paroxysmal recurrent AF, persistent AF, and permanent AF. Paroxysmal recurrent AF is characterized by spontaneous termination of episodes; persistent AF lasts longer than 7 days and requires electrical or pharmacological cardioversion; permanent AF is resistant to cardioversion procedures.

[1]U.O. di Cardiologia con UTIC Ospedale Muscatello, Augusta (SR); [2]Cardiologia, Ospedale Gravina, Caltagirone (CT); [3]U.O. di Cardiologia, Ospedale Ferrarotto, Catanzaro, Italy

Therapy of Acute AF

When evaluating a patient with AF, it is important to determine the clinical importance of the arrhythmia, and to identify all the possible accompanying pathologies. In particular, a complete clinical approach should include the following:

- Evaluation of the indication, the time, and the method of cardioversion to sinus rhythm
- Evaluation of the indication for anticoagulant therapy, to prevent thromboembolic accidents
- Control of ventricular rate while in AF

Prompt conversion to sinus rhythm may improve hemodynamic conditions (restoring functional atrial contraction and normalizing RR intervals), reduce thromboembolic risk, and prevent electrophysiological remodeling of the atrium. Intuitively, it can be inferred that early cardioversion may reduce hospitalization time and costs.

Cardioversion is indicated in patients who fulfill the following conditions:

- No frequent relapses (i.e., more than one episode every 2-3 months), despite prophylaxis with optimal doses of antiarrhythmic medications (i.e., refractoriness to at least three different drugs, or drug intolerance)
- No documented atrial thrombosis in the presence of contraindications to anticoagulant therapy
- No uncontrolled thyrotoxicosis
- No myocarditis or pericarditis
- No arrhythmic atrial disease uncured with a pacing device
- No left atrial enlargement (> 60 mm)
- Duration of AF less than 1 year

The choice of the right moment for cardioversion is directly related to the time of onset of AF and to the clinical presentation. It is necessary to evaluate all possible triggers (electrolytic alterations, thyrotoxicosis, acute pericarditis, myocarditis, myocardial infarction, pheochromocytoma, pulmonary embolism, etc.), which have to be corrected before trying cardioversion.

Hemodynamically Unstable AF

In situations of hemodynamic instability, such as in patients with low throughput or those with Wolff-Parkinson-White (WPW) syndrome, or discrepancy angina secondary to tachycardia (which could cause severe complications [5, 9]), the first-line therapy is emergency transthoracic cardioversion. Hemodynamically unstable conditions are usually associated with heart disease or acute systemic disease. Cardioversion has a greater success rate (>95%) when class III antiarrhythmic medications are preventively administered [5].

If enough time is available, sedation should be performed with diazepam, escalating doses of morphine, or a short-lasting barbiturate, possibly with anesthesiological assistance; in addition, anticoagulation with unfractioned heparin should be started after transthoracic cardioversion [10].

Hemodynamically Stable AF, >48 h

The risk of a thromboembolic accident discourages cardioversion in asymptomatic patients when the duration of AF is uncertain or greater than 48 h. In such cases, there are currently two possible strategies: (1) anticoagulation therapy for the 3 weeks preceding and the 4 weeks following cardioversion [11, 12], combined with pharmacological control of heart rate when necessary (with β-blockers, verapamil, diltiazem, digitalis); or (2) transesophageal echocardiography, then, if atrial thrombosis is excluded, infusion of unfractionated or low-molecular-weight heparin, embricated with a dicumarol, then DC shock, and anticoagulation for 4 weeks.

Hemodynamically Stable AF, < 48 h

Cardioversion may be attempted in recent-onset AF (< 48 h) in asymptomatic patients without the trigger factors and contraindications listed above. When cardioversion is indicated, anticoagulant medications must be started in patients with high thromboembolic risk, since intra-atrial thrombosis has been observed even in AF of less than 3 days' duration [13]. A high risk of thromboembolism is present in patients with rheumatic disease, mitral valve substitution, past embolism or myocardial infarction, heart failure, hypertension, or sick sinus syndrome.

In some patients with well-tolerated AF, especially if they are young and free of organic heart disease, a watchful waiting strategy may be feasible, based on ventricular rate control. In fact, 50%-70% of AF episodes lasting less than 24 h spontaneously revert to sinus rhythm [15]. Recently, additional elements which may predict an easier return to sinus rhythm during placebo treatment have been recognized, such as the absence of structural heart disease and age below 60 years.

Methods of Cardioversion

Cardioversion may be accomplished by means of electrical currents (external, by DC shock with biphasic or monophasic waves; or internal, with low-energy or transesophageal catheterization), or pharmacologically. Pharmacological cardioversion, which has a greater success rate in AF of less than 7 days' duration, is the first-choice, standard procedure. Although its efficacy is lower than that of electrical cardioversion, it has the important advantage that it does not require anesthesia [8].

External Electrical Cardioversion

External electrical cardioversion has a satisfactory success rate, reaching 95% in cases of recent-onset AF [16]. It is indicated in the following conditions:

- In emergency, when AF induces hemodynamic instability
- In recent-onset AF (< 48 h), usually after an unsuccessful trial of pharmacological cardioversion

Typically, a series of synchronized shocks of increasing energy are delivered. There is no consensus about the initial energy to use: 100 J is effective in 50% of cases, while 200 J has a 65%-85% success rate. Although on the one hand it is useful to deliver low energies, to avoid the negative effects of cardioversion on myocardial inotropism, on the other hand it may then be necessary to repeat the procedure, since low-energy shocks have a low success rate, resulting in secondary damage to the heart. It is possible to enhance the success rate by acute pretreatment with antiarrhythmic drugs (e.g., intravenous verapamil [17], sotalol [18], amiodarone [19] or ibutilide [20]) to reduce the defibrillation threshold and the risk of early recurrence.

Very high success rates (94%) have been recently obtained by delivering a biphasic wave shock [21]. Some authors used additional energy (up to 720 J) given through two defibrillators, with an 84% success rate and no major complications such as transient hemodynamic imbalance and stroke [22]. Electrical cardioversion with additional energy may represent a valuable alternative to intracavitary cardioversion, having similar efficacy and safety, but with the advantage of being performed in the same setting, without discontinuing ongoing anticoagulation therapy. The success rate increases if the plaques are in an anteroposterior arrangement, using plaque surfaces proportional to the total body area, interposing a saline gel between skin and electrodes, mildly increasing the pressure on the electrodes at the time of shock, and delivering the shock at the end of expiration [8]. The advantages of external electrical cardioversion include:

- High success rate
- No need for reducing anticoagulation
- Low cost
- Short hospitalization period

It also have some disadvantages:

- High energies must be delivered, due to the high impedance of the thorax
- General anesthesia is necessary, and an anesthesist is required
- There is a risk of causing thoracic burns
- The success rate is low (< 50%) in obese or emphysematous subjects
- Atrial pacing cannot be performed in sick sinus disease, ventricular pacing is impossible if there is a risk of postshock asystolia.

Renewed anesthesia is necessary in cases of early recurrence of AF after cardioversion.

Intracavitary Electrical Cardioversion

Low-energy intracavitary electrical cardioversion, a recently developed technique, is performed by inserting three catheters: two, for shock delivery, into the distal portion of the coronary sinus (anode) and into the lateral wall of the right atrium (cathode), and the third into the apex of the right ventricle, to synchronize shocks on the QRS wave and for a backup if a bradyarrhythmia appears. A single electrocatheter may also be used, positioned in the pulmonary artery branches, preferably the left one. The best configuration for a low stimulatory threshold involves the coronary sinus and lateral wall of the right atrium [23]; low-energy (2-8 J) biphasic shocks are delivered, synchronized with the QRS complex. The success rate in paroxysmal AF is 92%-100%. Pretreatment with antiarrhythmics from class IC (flecainide) or class III (ibutilide or sotalol) allows reduction of the defibrillation threshold and of the incidence of early arrhythmic recurrences [24]. The advantages are a high success rate, absence of anesthesia, the possibility of stimulating both atrium and ventricle, low energy delivered, and the possibility of repeating the procedure if there is early recurrence of AF. The disadvantages are: invasiveness, the need for fluoroscopy and electrophysiological equipment, need for lower anticoagulation, longer hospitalization, higher cost, and lack of effect on atrial stunning. At present, indications are still limited to patients who:

- Have AF resistant to transthoracic cardioversion
- Have AF induced during an electrophysiological study
- Have contraindications to general anesthesia
- Are obese, or have a pulmonary disease, where it is known that external cardioversion has a low success rate

Transesophageal Electrical Cardioversion

More recently, intracavitary cardioversion has been simplified, with the first decapolar catheter placed into the esophagus (near the left atrium) and the second into the right atrium. In this way, it is not necessary to be trained to place an electrocatheter into the coronary sinus or into the left branch of pulmonary artery. A 94% success rate has been reported [25].

Drugs Used in the Cardioversion of AF

Several papers show the efficacy of antiarrhythmic drugs with different electrophysiological properties in restoring sinus rhythm. Data from the literature show success rates ranging from 6% to 81%. The choice of the best antiarrhythmic medication should be driven by careful evaluation of the clinical context of each patient. Class IC drugs (propafenone and flecainide) are the most effective in recent-onset AF (< 48 h), in patients with normal left ventricular function, without significant disturbances of intraventricular conduction.

In a hospital setting, this intervention has been shown to be safe. Amiodarone should be used preferably in patients with heart failure, myocardial infarction, after aortocoronary bypass, or bundle branch block. In patients with WPW syndrome, if emergency electrical cardioversion is not required, the first-choice therapy includes intravenous procainamide, propafenone, or flecainide.

It is now widely accepted that drugs like digitalis and β-blockers are not particularly useful in converting AF to sinus rhythm, except for the use of β-blockers in patients with postsurgical AF.

Class IA Drugs

Quinidine

Quinidine is one of the most used drugs for restoring sinus rhythm. Success rates have been reported at 30%-90% [26]. It is given as 200 mg every 2 h for 5-6 times, up to 1200 mg, or 300-400 mg every 6 h. In recent-onset AF, quinidine should be combined with conduction-blocking drugs (digitalis, β-blockers), due to its vagolytic effect. Compared to class IC drugs, quinidine shows a delayed onset of action and lower therapeutic efficacy [27, 28], although greater than that of sotalol [29]. Quinidine therapy is combined, after the restoration of sinus rhythm, with lengthening of the QT interval and ventricular tachiarrhythmias, including torsades de pointes. Hence, quinidine should be started cautiously, and when risk factors of ventricular arrhythmia are present, hospitalization for 24-72 h is required [30]. A meta-analysis by Coplen and coworkers [31] on the use of quinidine in AF shows that the treated group has a mortality rate at 1 year about three times that of the control group.

Procainamide

Procainamide is used only intravenously for the treatment of AF in patients with a healthy heart or postsurgical AF [32]. Various trials have compared procainamide with class IC (propafenone) and class III drugs (amiodarone), showing comparable effects [33, 34].

Class IC Drugs

Propafenone and Flecainide

Propafenone and flecainide are frequently used, with success rates of 70%-85% within 8 h [35]. More recently, oral loading treatment has been adopted, also because of its ease of use. Propafenone is given intravenously in a bolus (2 mg/kg in 10 min), followed by an infusion of 0.0078 mg/kg per min for 2 h, or orally (600 mg single dose, or 450 mg if body weight <50 kg). Its efficacy is similar to that of intravenous amiodarone but with a shorter onset of action [36]. The oral and intravenous routes of administration are equipotent [37, 38], and have no significant proarrhythmic effects (i.e., 1:1 atrial flutter) [39].

A recent meta-analysis by Khan [40] evaluates the efficacy and safety of cardioversion with a single oral loading dose of propafenone; such treatment performed better than placebo at 8 h, but not at 24 h. Oral administration had a lower success rate at 2 h than intravenous administration, but equal performance thereafter. In comparison studies, oral loading with propafenone had the same efficacy as flecainide, and better efficacy than the same regimen with quinidine or amiodarone. No severe adverse events were encountered, and in particular no threatening arrhythmias. The efficacy and safety of propafenone are also confirmed by two recent Italian studies. Propafenone and flecainide have a negative inotropic effect, and are virtually proarrhythmic; hence their utilization, both intravenously and orally, must be preceded by careful selection of patients on the basis of specific exclusion criteria. In fact, these drugs are contraindicated in the following cases: age above 80 years; heart failure (NYHA class > II); left ventricular dysfunction (EF < 40%); ischemic heart disease with transient myocardial ischemia; mean ventricular rate below 70/min; QRS > 0.11 s; prior findings of second- or third-degree AV block; sick sinus syndrome; liver or kidney failure; hypopotassemia; simultaneous treatment with other antiarrhythmic drugs.

Flecainide has a quick onset of action, and its effect is proportional to plasma levels; it may be administered intravenously (2 mg/kg bolus in 10 min), or orally (300 mg single dose, or 200 mg if body weight < 50 kg). The main adverse effect of these drugs (3.5%-5%) is the transformation of AF into atrial flutter with 1:1 conduction, resulting in hemodynamic disturbances.

The efficacy of oral propafenone and flecainide suggests their utilization in recent-onset AF (< 48 h) in a hospital setting, as listed in Table 2, but also in a possible outpatient approach [41] in selected patients with infrequent tachiarrhythmic recurrences (<1 episode per week), good compliance, no contraindications, and who have been treated at least 2-3 consecutive times as inpatients. Patients with conduction disturbances, low ejection fraction, recent acute myocardial infarction or angina, or AF duration >48 h in the absence of anticoagulant therapy must be excluded from such therapeutic approach.

Class III Drugs

Amiodarone

Intravenous amiodarone has long been used for recent-onset AF, with extremely variable success rates (43%-92%) [15, 42, 43]. Most trials agree that intravenous amiodarone (5 mg/kg bolus, followed by the infusion of 1.5-1.8 g in 24 h) has a limited role, with late onset, in the restoration of sinus rhythm. Hou et al. [44], to maximize its efficacy, propose a protocol that reaches peak plasma levels within 1 h, showing high success rates, though at the price of prominent adverse effects. Cotter et al. [45], using higher doses of amiodarone (3 g in 24 h), reported a 92% success rate. Indeed, in a recent meta-analysis by Hilleman and Spinler [46], amiodarone does not differ significantly from other antiarrhythmic drugs in terms of efficacy (72.1% vs 71.9%), or adverse effects (12.2%

vs 14%), but it is better than placebo (82.4% vs 59.7%), though with more frequent adverse effects (26.8% vs 10.8%), especially phlebitis at the infusion site, bradycardia, and hypotension.

Intravenous amiodarone is the first-choice medication in AF complicating acute myocardial infarction or aortocoronary bypass surgery. The treatment of AF in patients with ventricular pre-excitation is controversial, given the risk of onset of ventricular fibrillation.

Ibutilide

Ibutilide is a pure class III antiarrhythmic; its main effect is prolongation of the action potential, due to the inactivation of a potassium outward current. Ibutilide is administered intravenous (0.01-0.025 mg/kg in 10 min), and has low efficacy (27%-40%) in restoration of sinus rhythm from recent-onset AF [40], with a better performance in atrial flutter (30%-71%). As an advantage, ibutilide is devoid of negative inotropism. Instead, the main adverse effect is dose-related enlargement of the QT interval, associated with polymorphic ventricular tachiarrhythmias including torsades de pointes (3%-4% of cases). Ibutilide may be given also in combination with calcium channel inhibitors, on account of the documented lack of interference of these drugs on the success rate of cardioversion.

Dofetilide

When administered intravenously, dofetilide is less effective than class IC drugs in AF conversion (12.5%-31%, related to dose) [48]. A recent randomized controlled trial shows that in WPW syndrome, one or two intravenous doses of dofetilide (the second given if the first was ineffective) performed better than placebo (71% vs 20%), without significant adverse effects. The incidence of torsades de pointes is about 3%.

Control of Ventricular Rate

Control of the ventricular rate has a key role in the treatment of AF, since an excessive rate may be unacceptable, especially in the elderly, resulting in dyspnea, angina, and syncope. Rate control must be performed in symptomatic, hemodynamically stable patients when immediate cardioversion is not feasible (AF >48 h or uncertain or long duration, very old subjects, presence of severe mitral pathology and enlarged left atrium, presence of high thromboembolic predisposition and lack of transesophageal echography, continuously recurring AF with inadvisability of further cardioversion, or presence of transient pathologies that discourage cardioversion at the moment).

There is no clear definition of controlled ventricular rate in the literature, partly because there are no data available to demonstrate that rate reduction may improve performance. An arbitrary definition of controlled ventricular rate in AF is 60-90 bpm at rest, and 90-115 bpm during mild exercise. The AFFIRM study takes for controlled an 80-bpm ventricular rate at rest. To reduce ventricular response, usually digitalis, β-blockers and non-dihydropiridine calcium channel blockers are used.

Digitalis

Digitalis has some drawbacks: long latency, need for stepwise loading, dependence on renal functionality, and insufficient activity during sympathetic activation. The effect of digitalis on the atrioventricular node is indirect and mediated by vagal activation. Hence, digitalis reduces the heart rate at rest, but this effect is blunted during physical exercise. Intravenous digitalis performs better than placebo at 2 h and thereafter, but the reduction in ventricular rate is modest, by only about 10 bpm. It can be used in elderly patients with heart failure.

Non-Dihydropyridine Calcium Channel Blockers

Intravenous verapamil is effective in acutely reducing ventricular rate during AF. The peak effect is reached at 2-3 min, and dosing can be repeated as 5 mg boli, up to 20 mg in total. Its effect is independent of adrenergic activation, but is quite short. Diltiazem is equally effective in controlling heart rate; its effect starts shortly after 4 min. A 10-15 mg/h diltiazem infusion is enough to modulate ventricular response. Verapamil and diltiazem cause hypotension and negative inotropism, which could precipitate an acute heart failure; thus, it may be useful to add a digitals-based drug, especially in the course of ischemic heart disease and hypertension.

β-Blockers

β-adrenergic blockers are strongly effective in controlling ventricular rate in AF. There are reports concerning esmolol (which, because of its short half-life, has the advantage of easy control of adverse effects and the disadvantage of needing continuous infusion), atenolol, metoprolol, and carvedilol. Their efficacy is comparable to that of calcium channel blockers. A recent paper from Farshi et al. [49], comparing digitalis plus atenolol to digitalis plus diltiazem, showed that the combination of atenolol and digitalis is more effective, both at rest and during exercise.

Antiarrhythmic Drugs

Neither class I nor class III antiarrhythmic drugs are indicated for rate control in AF. Amiodarone, however, may be used with good results in cases of acute myocardial infarction, dilated cardiomyopathy, or hyperkinetic ventricular arrhythmias. In WPW syndrome, intravenous digitalis or calcium channel blockers are contraindicated, while it is possible to use class III medications and β-blockers.

References

1. Braunwald E (1997) Shattuck lecture. Cardiovascular medicine at the turn of the millennium: triumphs, concerns and opportunities. N Engl J Med 337:1360–1369
2. Go AS, Hylek EM, Phillips KA et al (2001) Prevalence of diagnosed atrial fibrillation in adults. JAMA 285:2370–2375
3. Wolf PA, Benjamin EJ, Belanger AJ et al (1996) Secular trends in the prevalence of atrial fibrillation. The Framingham Study. Am Heart J 131:790–795
4. Furberg CD, Psaty BM, Manolio TA (1994) Prevalence of atrial fibrillation in elderly subjects (the Cardiovascular Health Study). Am J Cardiol 74:236–241
5. Narayan SM, Cain ME, Smith GP (1997) Atrial fibrillation. Lancet 350:943–950
6. Benjamin EJ, Wolf PA, D'Agostino RB (1998) Impact of atrial fibrillation on the risk of death. The Framingham Heart Study. Circulation 98:946–952
7. Bialy D, Lehman MH, Schumaker DN et al (1992) Hospitalization for arrhythmias in the United States: importance of atrial fibrillation. J Am Coll Cardiol 19:41 (abstract)
8. Fuster V, Ryden LE, Asinger RW et al (2001) Guidelines for the management of patients with atrial fibrillation. A report of the American College of Cardiology/American Heart Association Task Force on Practice Guidelines and the European Society of Cardiology Committee for Practice Guidelines and Policy Conferences (Committee to develop guidelines for the management of patients with atrial fibrillation) developed in collaboration with the North American Society of Pacing and Electrophysiology. Eur Heart J 22:1852–1923
9. Falk RH (2001) Atrial fibrillation. N Engl J Med 344:1067–1078
10. Albers JW, Dale JE, Laupacis A, Manning WJ, Petersen P, Singer DE (2001) Antithrombotic therapy in atrial fibrillation. Chest 11:194S–206S
11. Laupacis A, Albers G, Dunn M, Feinberg W (1992) Antithrombotic therapy in atrial fibrillation. Chest 102[Suppl 4]:426S–433S
12. Prystowsky EN, Benson DW, Fuster V et al (1996) Management of patients with atrial fibrillation. A statement for healthcare professionals from the subcommittee on electrocardiography and electrophysiology, American Heart Association. Circulation 93:1262–1277
13 Stoddard MF, Dawkins PR, Prince CR, Ammash NM (1995) Left atrial thrombus is not uncommon in patients with acute atrial fibrillation and a recent embolic event: a transesophageal echocardiographic study. J Am Coll Cardiol 25:452–459
14. Danias PG, Caufield TA, Weigner MJ et al (1998) Likelihood of spontaneous conversion of atrial fibrillation to sinus rhythm. J Am Coll Cardiol 31:588–592
15. Donovan KD, Power BM, Hockings BEF, Dobb GJ, Lee KY (1995) Intravenous flecainide versus amiodarone for recent-onset atrial fibrillation. Am J Cardiol 75:693–697
16. Boriani G, Biffi M, Capucci A, Pergolini F, Botto GL, Branzi A, Magnani B (1999) La cardioversione farmacologica della fibrillazione atriale. G Ital Aritmol Cardiostim 2:7–13
17. Daoul EG, Hummel JD, Augostini R, Williams S, Kalbfleisch SJ (2000) Effect of verapamil on immediate recurrence of atrial fibrillation. J Cardiovasc Electrophysiol 11:1231–1237

18. Lai LP, Lin JL, Lien WP, Tseng JZ, Huang SK (2000) Intravenous sotalol decreases transthoracic cardioversion energy requirement for chronic atrial fibrillation in humans: assessment of the electrophysiological effects by biatrial basket electrodes. J Am Coll Cardiol 35:1434–1441
19. Van Noord T, Van Gelder IC, Schoonderwerd BA, Crijns HJ (2000) Immediate reinitiation of atrial fibrillation after electrical cardioversion predicts subsequent pharmacologic and electrical conversion to sinus rhythm with amiodarone. Am J Cardiol 86:1384–1385
20. Oral H, Souza JJ, Michaud JF (1999) Facilitating transthoracic cardioversion of atrial fibrillation with ibutilide pretreatment. N Engl J Med 340:1849–1854
21. Mittal S, Ayati S, Stein KM et al (2000) Transthoracic cardioversion of atrial fibrillation. Comparison of rectilinear biphasis versus damped sine wave monophasic shock. Circulation 101:1282
22. Saliba W, Juratli N, Chung MK et al (1999) Higher energy synchronized external direct current cardioversion for refractory atrial fibrillation. J Am Coll Cardiol 34:2031–2034
23. Cooper RA, Alferness CA, Smith WM, Ideker RE (1993) Internal cardioversion of atrial fibrillation in sheep. Circulation 87:1673–1686
24. Boriani B, Biggi M, Capucci A et al (1999) Favorable effects of flecainide in transvenous internal cardioversion of AF. J Am Coll Cardiol 33:333–341
25. Santini M, Pandozi C, Colivicchi F, Ammirati F, Carmela Scianaro M, Castro A, Lamberti F, Gentilucci G (2000) Transoesophageal low-energy cardioversion of atrial fibrillation. Results with the oesophageal-right atrial lead configuration. Eur Heart J 21:848–855
26. Hurst JW, Paulk EA, Proctor HD et al (1964) Management of patients with atrial fibrillation. Am J Med 37:728
27. Borgeat A, Goy JJ, Maendly R et al (1985) Flecainide versus quinidine for conversion of recent onset atrial fibrillation to sinus rhythm. Am J Cardiol 58:496–498
28. Capucci A, Boriani G, Rubino I et al (1993) A controlled study on oral propafenone versus digoxin plus quinidine in converting recent onset atrial fibrillation to sinus rhythm. Int J Cardiol 43:305–313
29. Halinen MO, Huttunen M, Paakkinen S et al (1995) Comparison of sotalol with digoxin-quinidine for conversion of acute atrial fibrillation to sinus rhythm (The Sotalol-Digoxin-Quinidine Trial). Am J Cardiol 76:495–498
30. Grace AA, Camm, AJ (1998) Quinidine. N Engl J Med 33:35–45
31. Coplen SE, Antmann EM, Berlin JA et al (1990) Efficacy and safety of quinidine therapy for maintenance of sinus rhythm after cardioversion: a meta-analysis of randomized control trials. Circulation 82:1106–1116
32. De Haas DD, Tagliaferro EH, Amin MN et al (1988) Intravenous procainamide for the conversion of new onset atrial fibrillation in emergency department setting. J Emerg Med 6:185–187
33. Volgman AS, Carberry PA, Stamgler B et al (1998) Conversion efficacy and safety of intravenous ibutilide compared with intravenus procainamide in patients with atrial flutter or fibrillation. J Am Coll Cardiol 31:1414–1419
34. Mattioli AV, Lucchi VR, Vivoli D et al (1998) Propafenone versus procainamide for conversion of atrial fibrillation to sinus rhythm. Clin Cardiol 21:763–766
35. Capucci A, Villani GQ, Piepoli MS et al (1999) The role of IC antiarrhythmic drugs in terminating atrial fibrillation. Curr Opin Cardiol 14:48
36. Blanc JJ, Voinov C, Marek M et al (1999) Comparison of oral loading dose of propafenone and amiodarone for converting recent onset atrial fibrillation. PARSIFAL Study

Group. Am J Cardiol 84:1029–1032
37. Capucci A, Villani GQ, Aschieri D et al (1999) Safety of oral propafenone in the conversion of recent onset atrial fibrillation to sinus rhythm: a prospective parallel placebo-controlled trial. Int J Cardiol 68:187–196
38. Botto GL, Bonini W, Broffoni T et al (1998) Randomized, cross over controlled comparison of oral loading versus intravenous infusion of propafenone in recent onset atrial fibrillation. Pacing Clin Electrophysiol 21(11Part2):2480–2484
39. Boriani G, Capucci A, Botto GL et al (1998) Conversion of recent-onset atrial fibrillation to sinus rhythm: effects of different drug protocols. Pacing Clin Electrophysiol 21(11Part2):2470–2474
40. Khan IA (2001) Single oral loading dose of propafenone for pharmacological cardioversion of recent-onset atrial fibrillation. J Am Coll Cardiol 37:542–547
41. Botto JL, Bonini W, Broffoni T et al (1996) Conversion of recent-onset atrial fibrillation with single oral dose of propafenone: is in-hospital admission absolutely necessary? Pacing Clin Electrophysiol 19(Part2): 1939–1943
42. Galve E, Rius T, Ballester R et al (1996) Intravenous amiodarone in treatment of recent-onset atrial fibrillation: results of randomized controlled study. J Am Coll Cardiol 27:1079–1082
43. Negrini N, Gibelli G, De Ponti C (1991) Propafenone compared with amiodarone for conversion of paroxysmal atrial fibrillation to sinus rhythm (abstract). J Am Coll Cardiol 17:131A
44. Hou ZY, Chang MS, Chen CY et al (1995) Acute treatment of recent-onset atrial fibrillation and flutter with a tailored dosing regimen of intravenous amiodarone. A randomized digoxin-controlled study. Eur Heart J 16:521–528
45. Cotter J, Blatt A, Kaluski E et al (1999) Conversion of recent-onset paroxysmal atrial fibrillation to normal sinus rhythm: the effects of no treatment and high-dose amiodarone. A randomized placebo-controlled study. Eur Heart J 20:1833–1842
46. Hilleman DE, Spinler SA (2002) Conversion of recent-onset atrial fibrillation with intravenous amiodarone: a meta-analysis of randomized controlled trial. Pharmacotherapy 22:66–74
47. Falk RH (1992) Proarrhythmia in patients treated for atrial fibrillation or flutter. Ann Intern Med 117:141–150
48. Noogard BL, Watchell K, Christensen PD et al (1997) Efficacy and safety of intravenously administered dofetilide in the acute termination of atrial fibrillation and flutter. A multicenter, randomized, double-blind, and placebo-controlled trial. J Am Coll Cardiol 29[Suppl A]:442A
49. Farshi R, Kistner D, Sarma JS, Longmate JA, Singh BN (1999) Ventricular rate control in chronic atrial fibrillation during daily activity and programmed exercise: a crossover open-label study of five drug regimens. Am Coll Cardiol 33:304–310

Role of the Implantable Loop Recorder in the Management of Patients with Atrial Fibrillation

A.S. Montenero[1], A. Quayyum[1], P. Franciosa[1], D. Mangiameli[1], A. Antonelli[1], M. Dell'Orto[1], M. Vimercati[2], N. Bruno[1], F. Zumbo[1]

Introduction

Target sites for successful arrhythmia ablation can be characterized as being either discrete anatomic elements critical to maintaining the arrhythmia, or electrophysiologic markers which bode well for the procedure. Accessory atrioventricular connections are examples of relatively well defined discrete anatomical targets as the accessory pathways potential appear to be relatively specific electrophysiologic markers.

At the present time, techniques being studied for ablation of atrial fibrillation (AF) address neither known critical anatomic elements nor well-defined electrophysiologic markers, although they are conceptually based on the "multiple wavelets" or "focal origin" hypotheses [1, 2]. There are few data on AF ablation based on catheter-mediated linear lesions; those that exist show success rates ranging between 25% and 67% [3-6]. Moreover, paroxysmal atrial fibrillation (PAF) is an arrhythmia with a high recurrence rate, and although patients usually enrolled in studies are very symptomatic, the success rate of any treatment cannot be defined only on the basis of symptoms because of the high rate of asymptomatic recurrences. Therefore, in this subset of patients with an unpredictable follow-up, the accuracy of recurrence detection becomes very important. The present study investigates whether the linear ablation approach still may have a role in treating PAF, and whether the loop recorder system would be a helpful aid in refining ablation targets in the future.

Materials and Methods

Patient Selection

Nine patients (seven men, two women, mean age 63.8±5.9 years) who had been

[1]Department of Cardiology and Arrhythmia Center, Policlinico MultiMedica, Sesto S. Giovanni (MI); [2]Medtronic Italy, Milan, Italy

suffering from AF PAF for many years were referred to our institution to undergo AF ablation.

The primary inclusion criterion was a history of at least two symptomatic episodes of AF per week for at least 1 year, the episodes defined as AF that did not require pharmacologic or electrical cardioversion for termination. Although all patients had had most episodes documented by ECG for many years and were aware of the symptoms related to AF, they had a Reveal Plus implantable loop recorder (ILR) (Medtronic, Minn., USA) implanted 1 month before the ablation. Even though the ILR was programmed to detect any arrhythmic event automatically, patients were asked to record at least one episode of spontaneous AF to prove the relationship between symptoms and AF. The duration and intensity of symptoms were also reported by the patients in a daily diary. Patients were asked to discontinue any antiarrhythmic treatment during this month; for those receiving amiodarone, the treatment was stopped 4 months before inclusion in the study.

Additional inclusion criteria were normal left ventricular function and atrial size (cardiac two-dimensional color Doppler echocardiogram), absence of valvular or coronary artery disease, and absence of hypertension or thyroid dysfunction.

All patients gave written informed consent in accordance with the protocol approved by the institutional ethics committee.

ILR System: Implantation and Programming

The ILR was implanted subcutaneously in the right parasternal location and positioned on the basis of P wave amplitude during sinus rhythm according to the following criteria:

- The R wave to T wave amplitude ratio was required to be 3:1 or greater, in order to avoid improper activation due to T wave oversensing.
- The R wave to P wave amplitude was required to be about 5:1, in order to have a visible P wave stored in the device memory for all patients.

The devices were programmed to:

- Store up to 42 min of ECG data, distributed among patient-activated episodes (PAE) and automatically activated episodes (AAE).
- Store 10 min ECG data for up to three symptomatic AF episodes for each follow-up period (PAE). To achieve this, the patients were asked to use an external activator.
- Detect and save 2 min of spontaneous ECG tachyarrhythmic episodes (up to six episodes per follow-up period) (automatic episodes). In fact, the ILR is able to self-activate whenever the ventricular rate exceeds the programmable rate (130 bpm was chosen for this study).
- So far as possible, avoid false activations due to undersensing. For this reason, bradycardia options were programmed as follows: the lower rate limit for bradycardia-induced self-activation was 30 bpm and the time for pause-induced self-activation was set at 4 s.

Electrophysiologic Study: Diagnostic and Ablation Catheters

To map the right atrium (RA), a 7F, 24-pole catheter (Orbiter large, USCI-Bard, USA) with alternating 2- and 10-mm interelectrode distance (2-mm interpolar distance) was placed via the right femoral vein in the trabeculated RA to simultaneously record the right atrial free wall, the atrial roof, and the anterior septum. A 10-pole catheter (USCI-Bard, USA) was placed in the coronary sinus (CS) via the left subclavian vein to record the left atrium (LA) and part of the inferoposterior atrial septum. A four-pole catheter was inserted via the right femoral vein and positioned along the atrial septum in the region of the His bundle.

A braided, 64-electrode array 8.5F catheter (MEA Endocardial Solutions Inc., Minn., USA) was inserted via the right femoral vein and deployed via a 7.5-ml balloon filled with a mixture of saline and contrast medium in the right atrium to build a three-dimensional reconstruction of the right atrium using the EnSite3000 system (Endocardial Solutions). This technique allows the proper construction of reliable models of atria, definition of the site and extent of ablation lines, and thus enable gaps in the lines to be avoided [7].

The catheter used for making radiofrequency (RF) linear lesions was a specially designed, deflectable 7F catheter which included six successive coiled 6-mm electrodes (Amazr, Medtronic) with an interelectrode distance of 1.5 mm. To make linear lesions, this catheter was advanced through the right femoral vein to the RA. Ablation of the subeustachian isthmus was performed with a 7F four-pole catheter with an 8-mm tip electrode (RF Conductr MC, Medtronic).

ILR Recording Analysis

The analysis of ILR recordings was performed weekly during the first month before ablation. Two groups of recordings were analyzed: group 1 (PAEs) and group 2 (AAEs). For both groups a further analysis of appropriateness and inappropriateness of recordings was done in order to discriminate between symptomatic and asymptomatic arrhythmic episodes and validate automatic detection.

A detection was defined as appropriate whenever it was consistent with an episode of atrial tachyarrhythmia, irrespective of the type of the arrhythmia.

Electrogram Recording

Bipolar intracardiac electrograms filtered between 30 and 250 Hz were digitally recorded and stored on a Lab System 3.57 (Bard), simultaneously with a two-lead surface ECG. Over 3300 virtual electrograms recording beat by beat were acquired and stored on the EnSite 3000 (Endocardial Solutions) workstation from the MEA balloon catheter. These signals were processed in real time to allow visualization of both isopotential and isochronal activation maps of the RA and 3D navigation of the ablation catheter.

Baseline Electrophysiologic Study and Ablation Procedure

In all patients a basal electrophysiologic study was performed in SR to exclude any other electrical disease that might be responsible for the AF episodes. A bipolar electrode of the Orbiter catheter close to the right atrial auricula was chosen as pacing site. Stimuli were twice the diastolic threshold and 2 ms long.

All patients underwent ablation in SR. A temperature-controlled power generator (AtakrII, Medtronic) was used to make linear lesions. After insertion of the Amazr ablation catheter, care was taken to obtain a stable catheter position with a good electrode-endocardium contact, as judged by fluoroscopy and by recording of stable electrograms. The applications of RF energy (50 W, 55 °C for 60 s) were delivered in unipolar fashion between the selected electrodes and the external back paddle, beginning at the first electrode (distal) and then sequentially through the more proximal ones.

After ablation, a more than 30% decrease in the amplitude of the electrograms recorded in SR by the ablation catheter was considered to indicate lesion effectiveness at each site. Noncontact mapping techniques allowed by the EnSite3000 system were used to build an activation map before and after the procedure, to verify the presence of a line of block along the ablation line and to close any gaps left between or along the lines.

The ablation catheter was initially placed under fluoroscopic guidance in a vertical position on the posterior right atrial wall behind the crista terminalis, from the orifice of the SVC to the orifice of the IVC. When this lesion was complete, the ablation catheter was placed on a nearly horizontal plane, from the posteroseptal mid-right atrium to the crista terminalis close to the mouth of the CS, and was then withdrawn posteriorly behind the crista to the smooth atrium.

A third lesion was made at the subeustachian isthmus to create a bidirectional block between the isthmus and the CS (lesion C). RF energy at the isthmus was delivered in unipolar fashion between the tip of the Conductr catheter and an external back paddle with the same temperature-controlled power generator (target temperature 65 °C).

Heparin (1000 IU/h) was injected continuously during the procedure with a permanent ACT value of 250.

Follow-up

ILR recordings were analyzed weekly throughout the 6 months after ablation. Each patient kept a daily diary of the number and duration of events during the follow-up period. Event rates before and after ablation were compared.

Statistical Analysis

Statistical comparisons were performed using nonparametric tests, Student's *t*-test, paired or unpaired, and the χ^2 test when considered appropriate. The choice of test to use was made according to the measured statistical distribution for the analyzed variable. A value of $p<0.05$ was considered statistically significant. Values were expressed as mean ± SD.

Results

Electrophysiologic Study

Seven out of nine patients (six men and one woman) underwent baseline EFH and were assigned to receive an ILR. In all seven patients electrophysiologic study showed the absence of other electrical diseases, including AVNRT, WPW, and ectopic atrial tachycardia. Specific attempts to identify a focal atrial source of AF were not performed and AF was never induced in any patient. At the end of EFH an ILR was implanted in all of them.

Spontaneous Episodes of AF Before Ablation

Seven patients completed the 1-month pre-ablation monitoring (mean 35.2±11.2 days). Of the 178 ILR events detected in these patients, 54 were PAEs (30%) and 124 AAEs (70%), as depicted in Table 1.

Of the 54 PAEs, 37 (69%) were appropriate detections and 17 (31%) were inappropriate, while for AAEs the number was 89 (67%) and 41 (33%), respectively (Table 2). Note that patient 1 did not have PAEs.

Reasons for inappropriate detections are indicated in Table 3. From this table it can be seen that premature atrial or ventricular contractions represent the majority of symptom-related activations, while undersensing very frequently led to automatic activation of the device.

The onset of the arrhythmia was properly identified in four patients (44%). Of the 11 episodes detected, 4 were AAEs and 7 PAEs, as shown in Table 4.

Table 1. Number and percentages of automatically and manually detected atrial arrhythmic episodes recorded with the implantable loop recorder (ILR) before atrial ablation

Patient no.	Automatically detected		Manually detected		Total number of episodes
	n	%	n	%	
1	2	100	0	0	2
2	6	60	4	40	10
3	30	94	2	6	32
4	10	50	10	50	20
5	43	61	28	39	71
6	17	85	3	15	20
7	16	70	7	30	23
Total	124	70	54	30	178

Table 2. Number and percentages of appropriate versus inappropriate activations among the patient-activated and the automatically activated detections of AF episodes before ablation

Patient no.	Appropriate		Inappropriate		Total number of episodes
	n	%	*n*	%	
Patient-activated episodes					
2	4	100	0	0	4
3	1	50	1	50	2
4	10	100	0	0	10
5	14	50	14	50	28
6	3	100	0	0	3
7	5	71	2	29	7
Total	37	69	17	31	54
Automatically activated episodes					
1	0	0	2	100	2
2	6	100	0	0	6
3	22	73	8	28	30
4	10	100	0	0	10
5	41	95	2	5	43
6	2	12	15	88	17
7	2	14	12	88	16
Total	83	67	41	33	124

Table 3. Reasons for inappropriate patient and automatic activations before ablation

Reason	Number of episodes	Percentage of episodes
Patient activations		
PAC	1	6
PAC–PVC	2	12
PACs–PVC–NSSVT	1	6
PVC	13	76
Total	17	
Automatic activations		
Bradycardia	1	2
Oversensing of T wave – PVC	1	2
Electrical cardioversion	4	10
Undersensing	35	85
Total	41	

PAC, premature atrial contraction; PVC, premature ventricular contraction; NSSVT, nonsustained supraventricular tachycardia

Table 4. Onset mechanisms as identified from the ILR stored recordings before ablation

Patient no.	Onset mechanism	Number of episodes with this onset mechanism
3	PAC	1
	Sudden	3
4	Short-long pattern	1
5	Short-long pattern	2
	PAC-PVC	1
7	PAC	1
	PAC-PVC	2
Total		11

Ablation Procedure

Six patients underwent ablation and one refused the procedure. In the six patients ablation was performed in SR; lines resulted in the appearance of fractionated potentials and an approximately 35% decrease (2.2±0.9 vs 1.37±0.6 mV) in the amplitude. Because of their fairly low amplitude, 11% of electrograms were not considered for analysis (major difficulties were represented for posteroseptal sites). The technique as described above allowed proper definition of the site and extension of ablation lines so that gaps in the lines could be avoided. In all patients each lesion was repeated at least twice to ensure closure of any gaps.

Spontaneous Episodes of AF After Ablation

After ablation, 167 episodes of arrhythmia were detected in the ablated patients over a mean follow-up period of 95.6±18.6 days. Of these, 29 were PAEs (17%) and 138 AAEs (83%; Table 5). Of 29 PAEs, 25 (86%) were appropriate detections and 4 (14%) were inappropriate detections, while for AAEs the numbers were 83 (67%) and 41 (33%), respectively (Table 6).

Based on ILR data and patient diaries, four patient showed clinical improvement and one patient no relevant change. Note that patient 1 did not have PAEs and that all this patient's AAEs were inappropriate detections, so he was not included in the analysis. In the remaining five patients, a mean number of 10.6±3.7 episodes per month were appropriately identified before the ablation; this number decreased to 4.9±1.8 episodes per month after ablation ($p<0.042$; Table 7, Fig. 1).

The reasons for and overall number of inappropriate detections are reported in Table 8. Their number per month and distribution did not change significantly after the ablation (Table 9).

Table 5. Number and percentages of automatically and manually detected atrial arrhythmic episodes recorded with the implantable loop recorder (ILR) after ablation

Patient no.	Automatically detected		Manually detected		Total number of episodes
	n	%	*n*	%	
1	3	100	0	0	3
2	12	67	6	33	18
3	55	100	0	0	55
4	7	33	14	67	21
5	43	93	3	7	46
6	18	75	6	25	24
Total	138	83	29	17	167

Table 6. Number and percentages of appropriate versus inappropriate activations among the patient-activated and the automatically activated detections after ablation

Patient no.	Appropriate		Inappropriate		Total number of episodes
	n	%	*n*	%	
Patient-activated episodes					
1	0	n.a.	0	n.a.	0
2	0	n.a.	0	n.a.	0
3	6	100	0	0	6
4	13	93	1	7	14
6	2	67	1	33	3
7	4	67	2	33	6
Total	25	86	4	14	29
Automatically activated episodes					
1	0	0	3	100	3
2	12	100	0	0	12
3	13	24	42	76	55
4	7	100	0	0	7
6	1	2	42	98	43
7	3	17	15	83	18
Total	83	67	41	33	124

Table 7. Incidence of arrhythmic episodes before and after ablation, measured as mean number of episodes

	Number of follow-up days		Episodes per month	
	Before ablation	After ablation	Before ablation	After ablation
2	22	118	14	6
3	48	117	14	6
4	47	85	13	7
6	23	72	7	2
7	36	86	6	4
Mean	35.2	95.6	10.8	5.0*
Standard deviation	11.2	18.6	3.5	1.8

*p= 0.042

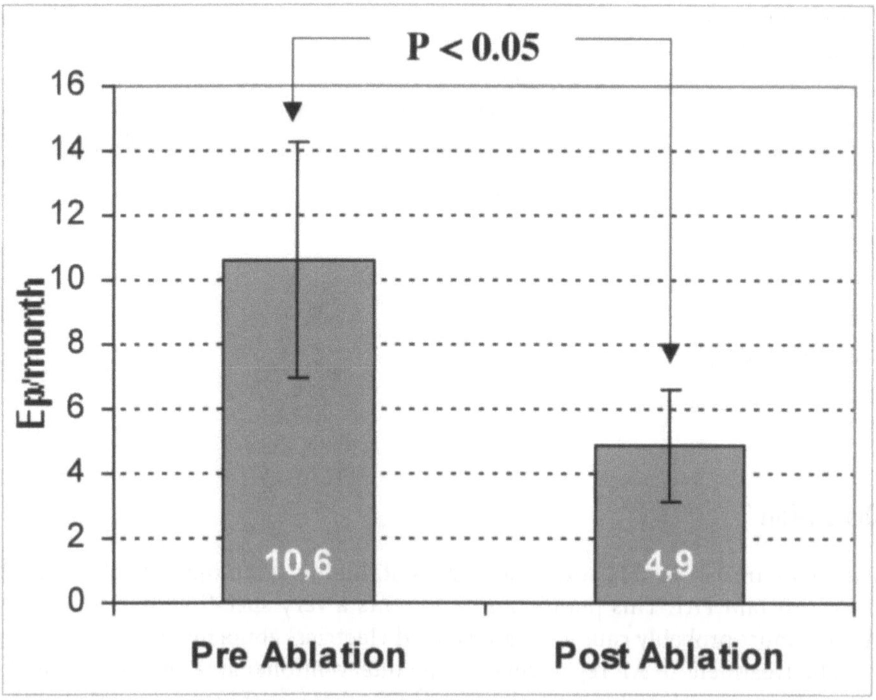

Fig. 1. Variation in the monthly rate of atrial tachyarrhythmia recurrences (episodes) in the study population before and after ablation

Table 8. Reasons for inappropriate patient and automatic activations after ablation

Reason	Number of episodes	Percentage of episodes
Patient activations		
NSSVT – frequent PACs	1	25
Sinus tachycardia	2	50
NSSVT	1	25
Total	4	
Automatic activations		
PAC	1	1
NSSVT – frequent PACs	1	1
Muscular noise	2	2
Undersensing	90	92
Sinus tachycardia	4	4
Total	98	

Table 9. Comparison among incidence and reasons for inappropriate activations before and after ablation

Reason	Inappropriate detections per month Before ablation	After ablation
Undersensing	30	39
Sinus tachycardia	0	2
EVC	4	0
Muscular noise	0	1
PACs PVC NSSVT	3	1.4
T wave oversensing	0	0.4

Discussion

Patients enrolled in this study had frequent, highly symptomatic episodes of drug-resistant PAF. This population represents a very specific group in which AF was most probably caused by an isolated electrical abnormality.

The treatment of AF represents a large interventional area, and assessment of its efficacy needs to be carefully monitored whatever therapy is applied. PAF is an arrhythmia with a high rate of recurrence, and although the patients usually enrolled in any sort of AF study are very symptomatic, the success rate of the treatment cannot be judged on the basis of symptoms alone because of the high rate of asymptomatic recurrences. So far as we know, this is the first study that extends the use of ILR to AF patients to evaluate the efficacy of right linear ablation.

The ILR provides a more reliable tool than mere symptoms by which to count AF recurrences and extend preliminary observations that right linear ablation may help to control AF in a certain population of patients [3-6]. It is worthy of note that, although the number of patients enrolled was small, a significant reduction in AF episodes was demonstrated ($p<0.042$). Therefore a different concept of "success rate" may be proposed which is more widely related to how the quality of life improves in the absence of any pharmacologic support rather than to whether or not AF episodes recur.

Of interest is that in all these patients the ECG, whenever recorded at the time of symptoms, always documented AF. Thus would have resulted in inappropriate treatment. On the other hand, the number of PAEs was considerably lower than that of AAE, demonstrating that symptoms may not be a good criterion by which to judge acute and long-term success. Thus, the "success rate" of any therapy may be misleading, so the accuracy with which recurrences are detected becomes very important in this subset of patients with a still unpredictable follow-up.

Technical Evaluation

The ILR was originally designed as an implantable device that would help to diagnose the causes of unexplained syncope by saving ECG information (close to the lead II ECG plot) about symptoms [8-15]. Patients were asked to activate the device just after the symptoms occurred, to store the information, and to attend follow-up for evaluation of the ECG. The ILR in the present study represents the second step of development of this device. In this model, an automatic detection capability has been added to improve clinicans' knowledge of asymptomatic events. This is made possible by allowing the loop recorder to sense the R waves, count them, and self-activate, saving the ECG in the device's memory when some programmable rules are satisfied. The programmable criteria are based on the rate (RR interval), with the chance to detect slow or fast ventricular rates or asystolic pauses. The Reveal Plus is the only device available with this set of characteristics, and it has been chosen as a monitoring tool for AF patients after selecting a set of programming options that could suit this rationale. It was known that some limitations could result from the absence of a specific set of options designed to detect supraventricular arrhythmias.

Conclusions

This study shows that to implant an ILR system helps to collect information on the frequency and/or the quality of the arrhythmic episodes with very minimal discomfort for the patient, which in our experience has led to very good compliance. Linear ablation performed in the right atrium may help to control AF recurrences.

References

1. Moe GK (1962) On the multiple wavelets hypothesis of atrial fibrillation. Arch Int Pharmacodyn Ther 140:183-188
2. Haïssaguerre M, Jaïs P, Shah DC et al (1998) Spontaneous initiation of atrial fibrillation by ectopic beats originating in the pulmonary veins. N Engl J Med 339:659-666
3. Haïssaguerre M, Jaïs P, Shah DC et al (1996) Right and left atrial radiofrequency catheter therapy of paroxysmal atrial fibrillation. J Cardiovasc Electrophysiol 7:1132-1144
4. Gaita F, Riccardi R, Calò L et al (1998) Atrial mapping and radiofrequency catheter ablation in patients with idiopathic atrial fibrillation: electrophysiological findings and ablation results. Circulation 97:2136-2145
5. Garg A, Finneran W, Mollerus M et al (1999) Right atrial compartmentalization using radiofrequency catheter ablation for management of patients with refractory atrial fibrillation. J Cardiovasc Electrophysiol 10:763-771

6. Montenero AS, Adam M, Franciosa P et al (2002) The linear ablation of atrial fibrillation in the right atrium: can the isthmus ablation improve its efficacy? J Interv Card Electrophysiol 6:251-265
7. Schneider MAE, Ndrepepa G, Zrenner B (2000) Noncontact mapping-guided catheter ablation of atrial fibrillation associated with left atrial ectopy. J Cardiovasc Electrophysiol 11:475-479
8. Krahn A, Klein G J, Yee R, Norris C (1997) Maturation of the sensed electrograms amplitude over time in a new subcutaneous implantable loop recorder. Pacing Clin Electrophysiol 20:1686-1690
9. Waktare J, Malik M (1997) Holter, loop recorder, and event counter capabilities of implanted devices. Pacing Clin Electrophysiol 20:2658-2669
10. Murdock C, Klein G, Yee R et al (1990) Feasibility of long-term electrocardiographic monitoring with an implanted device for syncope diagnosis. Pacing Clin Electrophysiol 13:1374-1378
11. Leitch J, Klein G, Yee R et al (1992) Feasibility of an implantable arrhythmia monitor. Pacing Clin Electrophysiol 15:2232-2235
12. Klein G, Krahn A, Yee R, Skanes A (2000) The implantable loop recorder: the herald of a new age of implantable monitors. Pacing Clin Electrophysiol 23:1456
13. Nierop P, Van Mechelen R, Van Elsacker A et al (2000) Heart rhythm during syncope and presyncope: results of implantable loop recorders. Pacing Clin Electrophysiol 23:1532-1538
14. Seidl K, Rameken M, Breunung S et al (2000) Diagnostic assessment of recurrent unexplained syncope with a new subcutaneusly implantable loop recorder. Europace 2:256-262
15. Futterman L, Lemberg L (2000) A novel device in evaluating syncope. Am J Crit Care 9:288-293

Cardioversion of Recent-Onset Paroxysmal Atrial Fibrillation to Sinus Rhythm in the Emergency Department: Comparison of Intravenous Drugs

G. Amatucci, G. De Luca, A. Palazzuoli, I. Signorini, G. Bova, A. Auteri, M.S. Verzuri

Introduction

Atrial fibrillation is the most common clinically significant arrhythmia encountered in the emergency department, occurring in 0.4% of the general population and in up to 5% of people older than 60 years [1]. Knowledge of the underlying heart disease is helpful in the critical evaluation and management of patients with atrial fibrillation. Coronary artery disease, cardiomyopathy, valvular disease, some kinds of congenital heart disease, hypertensive cardiovascular disease, and heart failure may all lead to atrial fibrillation. Occult or manifest thyreotoxicosis, alcohol abuse, and pulmonary embolism should be considered too, in patients with new-onset atrial fibrillation. The prognosis and treatment options of this arrhythmia may vary in these conditions, especially in patients who present new-onset arrhythmia [1, 2]. Loss of atrial contraction is not well tolerated by patients with impaired diastolic function or in the presence of systolic dysfunction, with hemodynamic consequences. Atrial fibrillation occurring in otherwise normal hearts or in the absence of an identifiable cause is called lone atrial fibrillation [3-6]. In critically ill patients the development of atrial fibrillation is often associated with significant hemodynamic impairment, generating the need for urgent cardioversion and the correction of treatable precipitating factors. When acute atrial fibrillation is associated with severe hemodynamic deterioration, electrical cardioversion is the treatment of choice. Electrical cardioversion is indicated when the ventricular response is greater than 130 beats/min in association with hypotension, an index of inadequate tissue perfusion. In a less urgent situation a less aggressive strategy and drug therapy can be considered [7-10]. Because systemic embolism is a complication of atrial fibrillation, electrical or drug-induced cardioversion can be performed without preceding anticoagulation up to 48 h after the onset of atrial fibrillation; when atrial fibrillation has started more than 2 days before, or its

Department of Internal Medicine, University of Siena, Italy

duration is uncertain, the current recommendation is to administer warfarin therapy to an INR of 2.0-3.0 for 3 weeks before attempting conversion, to prevent embolic events. However, the incidence of embolism appears to be similar with pharmacological and electrical cardioversion [9-11].

A great number of antiarrhythmic drugs including procainamide, amiodarone, flecainide, propafenone, sotalol, and ibutilide have been studied in patients with acute atrial fibrillation [10-13]. Although the use of antiarrhythmic drugs has been dramatically altered by the findings of the Cardiac Arrhythmia Suppression Trial (CAST), their role in the management of acute atrial fibrillation remains unquestionable [13-17].

Aim of the Study

The purpose of the present study is to evaluate pharmacological treatment of paroxysmal atrial fibrillation of recent onset in the emergency department with flecainide, propafenone, amiodarone, verapamil, and digoxin.

Patients and Methods

Two hundred two adult subjects (114 male and 88 female, mean age 75 years, range 19-95 years) admitted to the emergency room because of paroxysmal atrial fibrillation of recent onset (<48 h) between March 2000 and October 2002 were enrolled in this observational study. All patients without previously known severe cardiac dysfunction were included in this study group, whit heartburn as the only symptom. Exclusion criteria included the following conditions: heart surgery within the previous 6 months, severe uncontrolled heart failure (ejection fraction <30%), sick sinus syndrome, and history of second- or third-degree atrioventricular block. Patients who had taken any antiarrhythmic drug other than digoxin within a period of five half-lives of the drug prior to the study, and patients affected by cardiogenic shock, significant COPD, pulmonary embolism, pneumonia, liver or kidney failure, thyroid disease, electrolyte disturbances, pregnancy, and lactation were also excluded.

The patients were treated with various anti-arrhythmic drugs. The intravenous dosages of medication used for conversion of recent-onset atrial fibrillation and the maintenance of sinus rhythm were:

- Flecainide: 2 mg/kg over 20 min, then infusion at 1 mg/kg for 1 h
- Propafenone: 2 mg/kg over 10 min followed by infusion at 1 mg/kg in 2 h
- Amiodarone: 5 mg/kg over 20 min followed by infusion at 15 mg/kg over 24 h
- Verapamil: 5 mg over 2 min followed by a further 5 mg in 20 min
- Digoxin: 0.5 mg followed by 0.25 mg over 1 h

All the patients were monitored before and during drug infusion (ECG, blood pressure, Sat O_2). Restoration of sinus rhythm was registered by the physician reporting the exact time from the beginning of drug infusion to recovery of sinus rhythm.

Results

Our findings indicate a positive effect of class 1C anti-arrhythmic drugs in all patients without documented severe cardiac dysfunction. In particular flecainide, more than the other antiarrhythmic drugs, induces a significant rate of cardioversion in less than 1 h, 90% of patients have recovered sinus rhythm by 3 h (Table 1).

The intravenous administration of antiarrhythmic agents was effective and well tolerated; adverse effects were reported in only a low percentage of patients: only 5% of the treated patients showed transitory hypotension and/or bradyarrhythmia. These adverse effects did not require discontinuation of the drug infusion.

Table 1. Time to recovery of sinus rhythm

	<1 h	<3 h	>6 h
Flecainide (n = 50)	33 (66%)	12 (24%)	5 (10%)
Propafenone (n = 75)	32 (42%)	25 (33%)	18 (24%)
Amiodarone (n = 48)	7 (15%)	9 (19%)	32 (67%)
Verapamil (n =12)	0	0	3 (25%)
Digoxin (n = 17)	0	0	3 (18%)

Table 2. Number of dicharged patients and patients who were hospitalized because of the persistence of arrhythmia

	Discharged		Observation unit		Hospitalized	
	n	%	n	%	n	%
Flecainide (n=50)	45	(90)	3	(6)	2	(4)
Propafenone (n=75)	57	(76)	12	(16)	6	(8)
Amiodarone (n=48)	16	(33)	14	(29)	18	(38)
Verapamil (n=12)	0		3	(25)	9	(75)
Digoxin (n=17)	3	(18)	4	(24)	10	(59)

Conclusions

Our data indicate the effectiveness of flecainide in patients admitted to the emergency room with paroxysmal atrial fibrillation of recent onset without severe cardiac dysfunction. The primary outcome was cardioversion to sinus rhythm in a large number of patients within a few hours; therefore, the patients left the emergency room after some hours, reducing hospitalization and related costs. Under these circumstances prompt cardioversion of lone atrial fibrillation of recent onset prevents the risk of embolization (anticoagulantion therapy is not necessary) and the atrial electrophysiological remodeling that occurs with time ("atrial fibrillation begets atrial fibrillation").

References

1. Levy S, Breithardt G, Campbell RWF et al (1998) Atrial fibrillation: current knowledge and recommendations for manegement. Eur Heart J 19:1294-1320
2. Allessie MA, Rensma PL, Brugada J et al (1990) Patophisiology of atrial fibrillation. In: Zipes DP, Jalife J (eds) Cardiac Electrophysiology. From cell to bedside. Saunders, Philadelphia, pp 548-559
3. Allessie M et al (1990) Atrial fibrillation begets atrial fibrillation. Circulation 88 [Suppl 1]:1-18
4. Van Gelder IC, Crijns HIGM (1997) Cardioversion of atrial fibrillation ad subsequent maintenance of sinus rhythm. Pacing Clin Electrophysiol 20:2675-2683
5. Upshaw CB Jr (1997) Hemodynamic change after cardioversion of chronic atrial fibrillation. Arch Med Int 157:1070-1076
6. Falk RH (2001) Atrial fibrillation. N Engl J Med 344:1067-1078
7. Nattel S (1998) Mechanism of antiarrhythmic drug action. Card Electrophysiol Rev 2:115-118
8. Chakko S, Mitrani R (1998) Recognition and management of cardiac arrythmias: Part I. General principles and supraventricular tachyarrhythmias. J Intensive Care Med 13:15
9. Marik PE, Zaloga GP (2000) The management of Atrial Fibrillation in the ICU. J Intensive Care Med 15:181-190
10. Moeremans K, Aliot E, de Chillou C et al (2000) Second line pharmacological management of paroxysmal and persistent atrial fibrllation in France: A cost analysis. Value Health 3:407-416
11. Campbell TJ, Williams KM (1998) Therapeutic drug monitoring: antiarrhythmic drugs. British J Clin Pharm 46:307-319
12. Hilleman DE, Spinler SA (2002) Conversion of recent onset atrial fibrilation with intravenous amiodarone: a meta-analysis of randomized controlled trials. Pharmacotherapy 22:66-74
13. Martinez Marcos MJ, Garcìa-Garmendia JL, Ortega-Carpio A et al (2000) Comparison of intravenous flecainide, propafenone, and amiodarone for conversion of acute atrial fibrillation to sinus rhytm. Am J Card 86:950-953
14. Fauchier L, Babuty D, Autret ML et al (1998) Effect of flecainide on heart rate variability in subjects without coronary artery disease or congestive heart failure. Cardiovasc Drug Ther 12:483-486
15. Ruffy R (1998) Flecainide. Card Electrophysiol Rev 2:191-193
16. Khan IA (2001) Single oral loading dose of propafenone for pharmacological cardioversion of recent-onset atrial fibrillation. Am Coll Cardiol 37:542-47
17. Khand AU, Cleland JGF, Deedwania PC (2002) Prevention of and medical therapy for atrial arrhythmias in heart failure. Heart Fail Review 7:267-283

Is Fluoroscopic Electrode Positioning Improving the Clinical Efficacy of External Biphasic Cardioversion in Patients with Atrial Fibrillation?

P. Marconi, F. Sarro, C. Marioni, G. Castelli

Introduction

The use of external direct current (DC) transthoracic capacitor discharge to terminate atrial fibrillation (AF) was first reported in 1962 by Lown et al. [1]. However, external DC cardioversion with a monophasic damped sine waveform in patients with AF is ineffective in 6%-50% of cases [2-4]. An alternative when conventional DC cardioversion fails is low-energy internal cardioversion, performance of which carries increased risk because of the catheter insertion [5]. Recently, a biphasic shock waveform have been shown to be superior to monophasic shock in the treatment of AF patients. Mittal et al. [6] confirmed that rectilinear biphasic shock was more effective than monophasic shock for external atrial cardioversion in a prospective multicenter trial. The cumulative efficacy with the biphasic waveform was significantly greater than that with the monophasic waveform (94% vs 79%, p=0.005) [6].

The aim of the study was to compare the clinical efficacy of external cardioversion with rectilinear biphasic shock with fluoroscopy-guided electrode positioning versus standard electrode positioning (right anterior and left posterior) to increase the success rate of standard external cardioversion and avoiding the need of internal cardioversion in patients with AF.

Methods

Between December 2000 and October 2001, 70 consecutive patients with persistent AF (duration 14±13 months) were enrolled. Average age (±SD) among the patients was 64±9 years, mean weight was 72±31 kg, and there was a predominance of men (70%). The mean size of the left atrium was 45±6 mm and the left ventricular ejection fraction was 50%±14% (range 15%-75%).

Cardiologia 2, Azienda Ospedaliera Careggi, Florence, Italy

Structural heart disease was present in 63/70 of patients. Concomitant heart diseases were distributed as follows: coronary artery disease in 24/70 patients, cardiomyopathy (congestive or hypertrophic) in 9/70, valvular disease in 8/70, and arterial hypertension in 22/70.

Patients with hyperthyroidism were not enrolled in the study.

Informed written consent was obtained from every patient. In all patients a medical history was taken, followed by clinical examination. Conventional 12-lead ECG, chest X-ray, routine laboratory tests, conventional echocardiography (M- and B-mode and Doppler) were performed.

Of the 70 patients who underwent external cardioversion with rectilinear biphasic shocks, 35 were randomly assigned to a "conventional" technique group with electrodes in the standard (right anterior and left posterior) positions and 35 to an "optimized" technique group using fluoroscopy-guided pad placement and metallic markers. The anterior electrode was circular and had a diameter of 10 cm, which corresponded to an active surface area of 78 cm^2. The posterior electrode was rectangular and had a surface area of 113 cm^2. The two groups were similar with respect to age, sex, weight, left atrial size, left ventricular ejection fraction, underlying cardiac disease, duration of AF, and use of cardioactive drugs, including antiarrhythmic medications. Anticoagulation therapy was instigated using warfarin for patients with AF that had lasted longer than 48 h, with an international normalized ratio (INR) range of 2-3 for at least 3 consecutive weeks before and 4 weeks after cardioversion.

All patients with structural heart disease underwent transesophageal echocardiography 24 h before cardioversion to exclude thrombus formation and to measure of peak blood flow velocity in the left atrial appendage. Four hours after the procedure, creatine kinase (CK), myocardial bound creatine kinase (CK-MB), and troponin I were measured. At the time of attempted cardioversion 46 patients were taking amiodarone, 5 patients were taking β-blockers, 4 propafenone, and 3 were taking sotalol. Twelve patients were taking no antiarrhythmic medication before cardioversion.

Results

Cardioversion was performed in 70 patients. The amplitude of the energy of the rectilinear biphasic shocks was delivered as a function of the body surface area and varied from 70 J to 150 J (70 J in 5 patients, 100 J in 38 patients, 120 J in 22 patients, and 150 J in 5 patients).

The first shock with "conventional" cardioversion was successful in 32/35 (90.4%) patients. After a first unsuccessful shock the remaining 3 patients were immediately treated by fluoroscopic electrode positioning and successfully cardioverted using the same shock energy (respectively 100, 100, and 120 J) (Fig. 1). The first shock in the "optimized" group with fluoroscopic electrode positioning was successful in all patients (35/35). CK-MB and troponin I levels were unchanged 4 h after both transthoracic cardioversion strategies. Neither

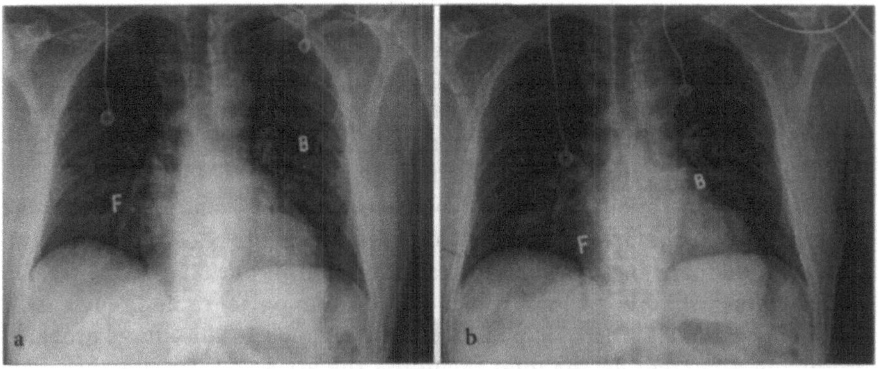

Fig. 1. Posteroanterior chest radiographs show by metallic markers (F, right anterior; B, left posterior): **a** conventional and **b** fluoroscopy-guided electrode positioning. Using the same shock energy (100 J), attempted cardioversion with electrode positioning in **a** failed; a later attempt with the positioning in **b** succeeded

thromboembolic complications or significant ST segment elevation was observed. After cardioversion a sinus bradycardia lasting less than 15 s was observed in 4 patients treated with amiodarone.

Discussion

Earlier studies have demonstrated that rectilinear biphasic shocks have a significantly greater efficacy than damped sine wave monophasic shocks for the external cardioversion of AF. Mittal et al. [6] in a prospective, randomized, multicenter trial evaluated patients undergoing external cardioversion of AF randomized to receive either damped sine wave monophasic or rectilinear biphasic shocks: 77 patients randomized to the monophasic protocol received sequential shocks of 100, 200, 300, and 360 J; 88 patients randomized to the biphasic protocol received sequential shocks of 70, 120, 150, and 170 J. The cumulative efficacy with the biphasic shock (83/88 patients, 94%) was significantly greater than that with the monophasic shock (61/77 patients, 79%, p=0.005). Ricard et al. [7] evaluated in 57 patients with AF whether biphasic shocks were superior to monophasic shocks using a similar study protocol: the first monophasic shock was effective in 16 patients (51%) and the first biphasic shock in 27 patients (86%) (p=0.02).

The success rate of external cardioversion depends on various factors, such as the duration of AF and pretreatment with low-dose oral amiodarone or with ibutilide [8, 9]. Success varies using electrode pads applied to the chest in the anteroapical position or the anteroposterior position [4]. Increasing the efficacy of external cardioversion and avoiding the need for internal cardioversion would be a valuable advance in the treatment of AF.

Consistent with a previous study by Mehdirad et al. [10], in our study fluoroscopic electrode positioning proved more effective (35/35 patients, 100%) than conventional (right anterior and left posterior) positioning (32/35 patients, 90.4%) for the first rectilinear biphasic shock for the transthoracic cardioversion of AF. It is important to note that in the three patients in whom the first shock with conventional electrode positioning failed, the subsequent successful cardioversion with fluoroscopic electrode positioning used only the same energy as the previous failure, i.e., the procedure was more effective. Moreover, the patients presented for cardioversion in our study were treated with rectilinear biphasic shock, which played an important role in increasing the success rate. Fluoroscopic pad location, as shown in this study, probably producing a current vector total including the atria, is very effective. This approach should be considered first in patients who fail to respond to shock using the conventional external electrode positioning.

References

1. Lown B, Amarasingham R, Neuman J (1962) New method for terminating cardiac arrhythmias-use of synchronised capacitor discharge. JAMA 182:548-555
2. Ewy GA (1994) The optimal technique for electrical cardioversion of atrial fibrillation. Clin Cardiol 17:79-84
3. Kerber RE, Jensen SR, Grayzel J et al (1981) Elective cardioversion: influence of paddle-electrode location and size on success rates and energy requirements. N Engl J Med 305:658-662
4. Mathew TP, Moore A, McIntyre M et al (1999) Randomized comparison of electrode positions for cardioversion of atrial fibrillation. Heart 81:576-579
5. Schmieder S, Schneider M, Karch MR et al (2001) Internal low energy cardioversion of atrial fibrillation using a single lead system. Comparison of a left and right pulmonary artery catheter approach. Pacing Clin Electrophysiol 24:1108-1112
6. Mittal S, Ayati S, Stein KM et al (2000) Transthoracic cardioversion of atrial fibrillation: comparison of rectilinear biphasic versus damped sine wave monophasic shocks. Circulation 101:1282-1287
7. Ricard S, Levy S, Boccara G et al (2001) External cardioversion of atrial fibrillation: comparison of biphasic vs monophasic waveform shocks. Europace 3:96-99
8. Capucci A, Villani GQ, Aschieri D et al (2000) Oral amiodarone increases the efficacy of direct-current cardioversion in restoration of sinus rhythm in patients with chronic atrial fibrillation. Eur Heart J 21:66-73
9. Oral H, Souza JJ, Michaud GF et al (1999) Facilitating transthoracic cardioversion of atrial fibrillation with ibutilide pretreatment. N Engl J Med 340:1849-1854
10. Mehdirad AA, Clem KL, Love CJ et al (1999) Improved clinical efficacy of external cardioversion by fluoroscopic electrode positioning and comparison to internal cardioversion in patients with atrial fibrillation. Pacing Clin Electrophysiol 22(Part II):233-237

Is Transesophageal Echocardiography Always Necessary Before Cardioversion of AF Patients After Conventional Anticoagulation Therapy?

G.L. Nicolosi

Cardioversion of patients from atrial fibrillation (AF) to normal sinus rhythm is frequently performed to relieve symptoms, improve cardiac performance, and decrease cardioembolic risk. However, the cardioversion procedure itself carries an inherent risk of stroke, presumably due to embolization of extant thrombus or postcardioversion thrombogenesis in the left atrium [1, 2].

To decrease this risk, patients with AF of more than 48 h or of unknown duration who undergo cardioversion are conventionally treated with therapeutic anticoagulation [international normalized ratio (INR) 2.0-3.0] for at least 3-4 weeks before and 4 weeks following cardioversion [1]. Screening for the presence of thrombus in the left atrial or left atrium appendage by transesophageal echocardiography (TEE) is an alternative to routine pre-anticoagulation in candidates for cardioversion of AF [1]. ACC/AHA/ESC guidelines recommend anticoagulation treatment of patients in whom no thrombus is identified with an initial bolus injection of intravenous unfractionated heparin before cardioversion, followed by continuous infusion at a dosage adjusted to prolong the activated partial thromboplastin time to 1.5-2 times the reference control value [1]. Next, the guidelines indicate provision of oral anticoagulation (INR 2.0-3.0) for a period of at least 3-4 weeks, as for patients undergoing elective cardioversion [1]. If a thrombus is identified by TEE, patients should be treated with oral anticoagulation for at least 3-4 weeks before and after restoration of sinus rhythm [1].

Since its introduction in the early 1990s, however, the use of TEE in the management of anticoagulation in patients with AF undergoing cardioversion has remained very controversial [3-5]. What is clear is that TEE cannot be used to avoid anticoagulant therapy, due to the risk of embolic events in patients with negative TEE findings [3, 5]. All patients must then be managed with adequate anticoagulation, regardless of the findings on TEE [3, 5, 6]. A recent observational cardioversion study comparing conventional strategy with the

Cardiology Department, ARC, Azienda Ospedaliera S. Maria degli Angeli, Pordenone, Italy

TEE-guided approach showed no differences in the rate of embolic events between the two treatment groups [7]. In patients with AF and effective anticoagulation, TEE-guided electrical cardioversion does not reduce the embolic risk [7]. However, TEE revealed left atrial thrombi in 7.7% of patients with AF and effective anticoagulation before direct-current cardioversion: thrombus resolution was found in 55% of patients after 1 month of adjusted-dose warfarin therapy (INR 3.0-3.5) [7]. A similar prevalence of thrombi would be expected in the conventional treatment group, but these patients were not excluded from cardioversion because they were not identified [7]. Nevertheless, the embolic rate was similar in the two groups. The authors [7] conclude that: (1) TEE before direct-current cardioversion is not needed in patients with effective anticoagulation at least 3 weeks before cardioversion; and (2) if TEE is performed early, more thrombi will be detected and more patients will be excluded from cardioversion. However, in patients with a normal TEE study, early cardioversion can be performed safely and the impact on the long-term prognosis of thrombi detected during TEE must be evaluated [7].

A national survey to assess the prevalence of the TEE-guided approach to cardioversion in the United States [8] showed that this approach was employed in approximately 12% of all the cardioversions performed in the 197 centers who returned the surveys. The data from this survey also reveal that nearly 75% of all clinical centers responding used the TEE-guided approach at least occasionally [8]. Thus, these data suggest that the relatively modest use of the TEE-guided approach is not a result of physicians' lack of familiarity with the procedure. The employment of the TEE-guided approach correlated positively with the total volume of TEE procedures and the volume of cardioversions performed at the institutions. Hence, institutions that performed a larger number of TEE procedures were also more likely to perform TEE-guided cardioversions [8]. This suggests that the TEE-guided approach may be dependent, at least to some degree, on physician preference and training, as well as the availability of a properly equipped echocardiographic laboratory. The survey also indicated that the use of TEE-guided cardioversion varied widely among institutions. There was also wide variation and lack of consensus on the most appropriate patient population for TEE screening before cardioversion, with either low-risk or high-risk patients, either inpatients or outpatients, selected for the TEE-guided approach to cardioversion [8].

A national ANMCO/SIC survey performed in Italy in the year 2000 among 772 out of 824 cardiological institutions indicated that each institution performed annually a mean number of 2362 transthoracic echocardiographic (TTE) examinations, actual numbers at the individual institutions varying widely from 69 to 12 342 [9]. Conversely, the mean number of TEE examinations for each institution was 112 (less than 5% of the total number of TTE examinations), with a similar astonishingly wide range from 1 to 1600. The total number of TEE studies performed in the year 2000 by all Italian institutions reached by the survey was 48 568. If the reported estimated prevalence of AF at 0.4%-1% of the general population [1, 10] is applied to Italy, this gives approximately 200 000-500 000 patients with AF, with a corresponding number of TEE studies needed if that approach were to be widely indicated.

All these data make it clear that the answer to the question of whether TEE should always be performed before cardioversion of AF patients after conventional anticoagulation therapy is definitely "no".

The problems seem in fact more the underuse of anticoagulation and the discrepancy between guideline recommendations and actual practice [10], which exposes patients to the risk of complications, than extensive use of TEE before cardioversion in all AF patients after conventional anticoagulant therapy.

It must be considered, however, that there is probably room for selective adjunctive indication for TEE in patients with AF undergoing cardioversion after conventional anticoagulant therapy, apart from the TEE-guided approach to cardioversion. TEE could in fact be suggested when subcutaneous administration of low-molecular-weight heparin is indicated, since limited data are available to support this type of therapy [1, 12]. TEE could also be considered in patients requiring urgent (not emergent) cardioversion in whom extended precardioversion anticoagulation is not desirable or is contraindicated; in patients who have had prior cardioembolic events thought to be related to intra-atrial thrombus; in patients with intra-atrial thrombus documented by previous TEE; and in patients in whom a decision about cardioversion could be influenced by TEE results [12, 13]. A new possible role for TEE should also be considered in conjunction with transesophageal electrical cardioversion of atrial fibrillation [15], when new TEE transducers equipped with built-in cardioversion electrodes will be fully developed.

References

1. Fuster V, Ryden LE, Asinger LW (2001) ACC/AHA/ESC guidelines for the management of patients with atrial fibrillation. Eur Heart J 22:1852-1923
2. Stoddard MF (2000) Risk of thromboembolism in acute atrial fibrillation or atrial flutter. Echocardiography 17:393-405
3. Grimm RA (2000) Transesophageal echocardiography-guided cardioversion of atrial fibrillation. Echocardiography 17:383-392
4. Becker ER, Culler SD, Shaw LJ, Weintraub WS (2000) Economic aspects of transesophageal echocardiography and atrial fibrillation. Echocardiography 17:407-418
5. Labovitz AJ, Bransford TL (2001) Evolving role of echocardiography in the management of atrial fibrillation. Am Heart J 141:518-527
6. Klein AL, Grimm RA, Murray D, Apperson-Hansen C, Asinger RW, Black IW, Davidoff R, Erbel R, Halperin JL, Orsinelli DA, Porter TR, Stoddard MF, for the ACUTE Investigators (2001) Use of transesophageal echocardiography to guide cardioversion in patients with atrial fibrillation. N Engl J Med 344:1411-1420
7. Seidl K, Rameken M, Drogemuller A et al (2002) Embolic events in patients with atrial fibrillation and effective anticoagulation: value of transesophageal echocardiography to guide direct-current cardioversion. J Am Coll Cardiol 39:1436-1442
8. Murray RD, Goodman AS, Lieber EA et al (2000) National use of the transesophageal

echocardiographic-guided approach to cardioversion for patients in atrial fibrillation. Am J Cardiol 85:239-244

9. Associazione Nazionale Medici Cardioligici Ospedalieri. www.anmco.it
10. Chug SS, Blackshear JL, Shen W-K, Hammil SC, Gersh BJ (2001) Epidemiology and natural history of atrial fibrillation: clinical implications. J Am Coll Cardiol 37:371-378
11. Frykman V, Beerman B, Ryden L, Rosenquist M (2001) Management of atrial fibrillation: discrepancy between guidelines recommendations and actual practice exposes patients to risk for complications. Eur Heart J 22:1954-1959
12. Klein AL, Murray DR, Grimm RA (2001) Role of transesophageal echocardiography-guided cardioversion of patients with atrial fibrillation. J Am Coll Cardiol 37:691-704
13. Chiettin MD, Alpert JS, Armstrong WF (1997) ACC/AHA guidelines for the clinical application of echocardiography: executive summary. J Am Coll Cardiol 29:862-879
14. Verhorst PMJ, Kamp O, Welling RC, Van Eenige MJ,Visser CA (1997) Transesophageal echocardiographic predictors for maintenance of sinus rhythm after electrical cardioversion of atrial fibrillation. Am J Cardiol 79:1355-1359
15. Zardo F, Brieda M, Hrovatin E et al (2002) Transesophageal electrical cardioversion of persistent atrial fibrillation: a new approach for an old technology. Ital Heart J 3:354-359

Anticoagulation Therapy of Atrial Fibrillation in the Elderly

G. Di Pasquale, E. Cerè, A. Lombardi, B. Sassone, S. Biancoli, R. Vandelli

Epidemiology

The prevalence of atrial fibrillation (AF) increases substantially with age. The most recent data come from a cross-sectional study of adults in California, dealing with a population of 1.89 million [1]. The overall prevalence of AF was 0.95%; prevalence increased from 0.1% among adults younger than 55 years to 4.0% in subjects older than 60 years and up to 9.0% in persons aged 80 years or older. The authors estimate that approximately 2.3 million adults in the United States currently have AF, and project that this figure will increase to more than 5.6 million by the year 2050, with more than 50% of affected individuals aged 80 years or older. The estimate for AF in Italy is about 500 000 subjects, with an incidence of 60.000 new cases per year.

Thromboembolic Risk

In the absence of any antithrombotic therapy the annual risk of stroke and systemic thromboembolism is 4.5%, rising to 8% in subjects older than 75 years. When the risk of transient ischemic attack (TIA) and silent cerebral infarction are also taken into account, the cerebral embolic risk exceeds 7% per year [2, 3]. Clinical features independently associated with a high risk of stroke in AF patients have been defined and integrated into several risk stratification schemes. High risk factors include age above 75 years, prior stroke/TIA or systemic embolism, history of hypertension, congestive heart failure or poor left ventricular systolic function, rheumatic mitral valve disease, and prosthetic heart valves. Moderate risk factors include age between 65 and 75 years, diabetes mellitus, and coronary artery disease with preserved left ventricular function.

Unità Operativa di Cardiologia, Ospedale di Bentivoglio, Bologna, Italy

It is evident from thromboembolic risk stratification that older age (>75 years) is per se a high risk factor for thromboembolism, and all patients older than 75 years should receive oral anticoagulant treatment (OAT) for effective prophylaxis. This represents a therapeutic dilemma because of the higher risk of life-threatenig hemorrhages, in particular cerebral hemorrhage, in these patients during OAT.

Indications for OAT

The effectiveness of OAT for the prevention of thromboembolism and stroke has been assessed by a number of randomized clinical trials [4, 5]. Six trials (AFASAK, SPAF, BAATAF, CAFA, SPINAF, and EAFT) compared adjusted-dose warfarin with placebo. Overall adjusted-dose warfarin reduced stroke by 62% (95% CI, range 48%-72%); absolute risk reductions were 2.7% per year for primary prevention [number needed to treat (NNT) for 1 year to prevent one stroke = 37] and 8.4% per year (NNT = 12) for secondary prevention.

The efficacy of aspirin for stroke prevention in AF patients is unclear and more disputed [4, 5]. Six trials (AFASAK, SPAF I, EAFT, ESPS II, LASAF, and UK TIA) compared antiplatelet therapy with placebo. Meta-analysis of all six trials showed that aspirin reduced the incidence of stroke by 22% (95% CI, 2%-38%). On the basis of these six trials, the absolute risk reduction was 1.5% per year (NNT = 67) for primary prevention and 2.5% per year (NNT = 40) for secondary prevention. Although all six trials showed trends toward reduced stroke with aspirin treatment, this result was statistically significant only in the SPAF I study.

Recommendations for treatment based on the evidence from the clinical trials and the thromboembolic risk stratification were reconfirmed at the Sixth Consensus Conference on Antithrombotic Therapy of the American College of Chest Physicians in 2001 [5] and in the 2001 ACC/AHA/ESC guidelines for the management of patients with AF [6]. OAT is mandatory in AF high-risk patients (those with any risk factor or with more than one moderate risk factor), provided that high-quality monitoring of OAT is possible and no risk factors for bleeding are present. These last two requirements are particularly important when deciding on OAT in patients older than 75 years.

Aspirin is a possible and acceptable alternative to OAT in moderate-risk patients (those with no high risk factors and with only one moderate risk factor). In this group of patients the choice between aspirin and OAT is based on the assessment of the risk/benefit ratio of OAT and also on the patient's preference [7]. Finally, aspirin is the treatment of choice in low-risk patients (those without high risk or moderate risk factors). This group is represented by patients with no clinical or echocardiographic evidence of cardiovascular disease.

Despite the strong evidence for the efficacy of OAT, the use of warfarin for stroke prevention in patients with AF is still low in general clinical practice [8, 9]. Paradoxically, underutilization of OAT is especially evident among elderly people with AF, in whom the thromboembolic risk is higher. Major reasons for this underuse are the difficulty of high-quality monitoring of OAT, especially in older patients, and the fear of bleedings. Therefore, new safer and effective thromboprophylactic strategies for AF are warranted, particularly for older patients, who represent a substantial proportion of the AF population.

Bleeding Risk of OAT

Bleeding is the most important complication of OAT, even though the incidence of bleeding in patients receiving OAT in the randomized clinical studies was quite low. The annual frequency of major bleeding events was 1.3% in warfarin-treated patients (vs 1.0% in patients receiving placebo or in controls, and 1.0% in aspirin-treated patients). However, the bleeding risk is probably higher in patients treated in general clinical practice. The patients in the clinical trials were carefully selected (representing only 7%-39% of the screened patients) and followed up carefully according to strict protocols. This may explain the low bleeding incidence during warfarin treatment. Moreover, the safety and tolerability of long-term anticoagulation to conventional levels has not been completely defined among patients older than 75 years. In the AFASAK study [10], which involved AF patients older than those enrolled in every other trial (mean age 75 years), the withdrawal rate from warfarin treatment was 38% after one year. In the SPAF II study [11] (INR 2.0 - 4.5, mean 2.7) the risk of major hemorrhage, mainly cerebral, was substantially higher among AF patients older than 75 years.

In the real world, bleeding is often a major concern related to anticoagulation for stroke prevention in elderly patients. In particular anticoagulation treatment at conventional intensities increases the risk of intracranial hemorrhage seven- to ten-fold, and the risk of cerebral bleeding is significantly higher in the elderly. The key issue in using warfarin to prevent stroke and systemic embolism in AF patients is whether the benefit of therapy outweighs the risk of bleeding in the individual patient.

Risk factors for bleeding during OAT include advanced age, high intensity of anticoagulation, recent initiation of warfarin therapy, and comorbid conditions. Patients of advanced age have been shown to be more prone to complications of OAT than younger patients [12, 13]. Only a few studies have shown that advanced age does not by itself increase the complication rate of OAT. A recent prospective Italian collaborative study (ISCOAT) investigated the frequency of bleeding complications in outpatients treated routinely in anticoagulation clinics [14]. The rate of fatal, major and minor bleeding events was quite low, 0.25, 1.1 and 6.2 per patient-years of follow-up respectively. The rate was higher in older patients and during the first 90 days of treatment than it was later. The risk of bleeding was related to the intensity of anticoagulation, although a fifth of the bleeding events occurred at INR < 2.0. Subsequent analysis performed in patients aged 75 years or more included in ISCOAT showed a nonsignificant trend toward a higher rate of both bleeding and thrombotic complications in elderly versus matched younger patients [15]. However, intracranial bleedings and fatal thrombotic events were more frequent in the elderly. The results of this analysis also indicate that an INR below 2.0 does not preclude bleeding in the elderly, nor does it offer adequate protection from thrombotic events. In the subset of patients with AF, major bleeding occurred more frequently in patients over 75 years of age (5.1% per year) than in younger patients (1.0% per year) [16]. Univariate analysis revealed a higher frequency of major bleeding in females, in diabetics, and in those who had suffered a previous thromboembolic event.

A clear correlation has been reported between intensity of anticoagulation and risk of bleeding. In the ISCOAT study in patients aged 75 years or over, the risk of bleeding increased markedly with INR values of 3.0-4.4, and became disproportionately high for INR values above 4.5 [15]. However, a substantial number of events (10%) occurred in association with very low INR values (< 2.0), confirming previous reports that bleeding during OAT is not always related to the intensity of OAT, but that OAT can unmask a local bleeding source.

A higher frequency of bleeding early in the course of OAT has been reported in a number of studies [14, 15, 17]. Several factors may contribute to the increased risk of bleeding within the first months of each OAT course. First, OAT can unmask a cryptic, often neoplastic, lesion. Second, dose adjustment may be less well-controlled at the start of treatment.

Several studies have evaluated the influence of additional drug intake on the complication rate of OAT. The use of multiple medications was identified as a risk factor for bleeding complications by several studies. A high number of additional drugs reflects a patient's morbidity. In a recent large study [18] in patients undergoing OAT for AF, patients taking >3 drugs had more bleeding or thromboembolic complications than patients who took ≤3 drugs (24.4% versus 4.3% per 100 patient-years; $p= 0.01$). Since the complication rate did not differ between patients taking drugs known to interact with OAT and those who did not take interacting drugs, it may be inferred that the increased complication rate of patients with multiple medications is a consequence of comorbidity rather than of drug interactions.

The quality of anticoagulation laboratory control is also affected by the mental ability of the patient. Palareti et al [19] found unsuspected reduction of mental ability or attention levels in a number of elderly patients receiving OAT; these patients presented longer periods of either under- or overanticoagulation and were therefore exposed to a higher risk of thrombotic or bleeding complications.

Recommendations

In the management of older patients with permanent AF, a risk/benefit assessment is warranted before initiating OAT. Major considerations should include:

- Decision for AF electrical cardioversion which, at least in some cases, could obviate the need of long-term OAT.
- Thromboembolic risk stratification in the individual patient: the prevalence of additional risk factors for thromboembolism besides advanced age (i.e., hypertension, prior stroke or TIA, heart failure or left ventricular dysfunction, diabetes mellitus) should reinforce the decision for OAT.
- Ability to provide high-quality monitoring of OAT through coordinated medical care (e.g., anticoagulation clinics).
- Patient's inherent risk of bleeding with OAT.
- Evaluation of risk factors for OAT-related bleeding complications.

When deciding to initiate OAT in older patients, patient education and optimal OAT monitoring are key to minimizing the risk of bleeding. High-quality monitoring of OAT is of the utmost importance. A systematic approach to anticoagulation management, as offered by anticoagulation clinics, can improve the safety and effectiveness of warfarin therapy by reducing related and unrelated complications. This coordinated care can be contrasted with that provided by a patient's own physician, without systematic coordination (routine medical care). Available data indicate that coordinated care, compared with routine medical care, reduces the incidence of adverse outcomes and also OAT-related financial costs [20-22].

References

1. Go AS, Hylek EM, Phillips KA et al (2001) Prevalence of diagnosed atrial fibrillation in adults. National implications for rhythm management and stroke prevention: the Anticoagulation and Risk Factors In Atrial Fibrillation (ATRIA) Study. JAMA 285:2370-2375
2. Atrial Fibrillation Investigators (1994) Risk factors for stroke and efficacy of antithrombotic therapy in atrial fibrillation: analysis of pooled data from five randomized controlled trials. Arch Intern Med 154:1449-1457
3. Hart RG, Pearce LA, McBride R et al, on behalf of the Stroke Prevention in Atrial Fibrillation (SPAF) Investigators (1999) Factors associated with ischemic stroke during aspirin therapy in atrial fibrillation. Analysis of 2012 participants in the SPAF I-III clinical trials. Stroke 30:1223-1229
4. Hart RG, Benavente O, McBride R, Pearce LA (1999) Antithrombotic therapy to prevent stroke in patients with atrial fibrillation: a meta-analysis. Ann Intern Med 131:492-501
5. Albers GW, Dalen JE, Laupacis A, Manning WJ, Petersen P, Singer DE (2001) Antithrombotic therapy in atrial fibrillation. Sixth ACCP Consensus Conference on Antithrombotic Therapy. Chest 119 [Suppl]:194S-206S
6. Fuster V, Ryden L et al (2001) ACC/AHA/ESC guidelines for the management of patients with atrial fibrillation: executive summary. Am J Cardiol 38:1231-1265
7. Di Pasquale G, Cerè E, Biancoli S et al (2002) Antiplatelet agents for prevention of thromboembolism in atrial fibrillation: when, why, and which one? In: Raviele A (ed) Cardiac Arrhythmias 2001. Springer, Milan, pp 422-435
8. Bungard TJ, Ghali WA, Teo KK, Mc Alister FA, Tsuyuki RT (2000) Why do patients with atrial fibrillation not receive warfarin? Arch Intern Med 160:41-46

9. Cohen N, Sarafian DA, Alon I et al (2000) Warfarin for stroke prevention still underused in atrial fibrillation. Stroke 31:1217-1222
10. Petersen P, Boysen G, Godtfredsen J et al (1989) Placebo-controlled, randomised trial of warfarin and aspirin for prevention of thromboembolic complications in chronic atrial fibrillation. The Copenhagen AFASAK Study. Lancet 1:175-179
11. Stroke Prevention in Atrial Fibrillation Investigators (1994) Warfarin versus aspirin for prevention of thromboembolism in atrial fibrillation: Stroke Prevention in Atrial Fibrillation II Study. Lancet 343:687-691
12. Sebastian J, Tresch DD (2000) Use of oral anticoagulants in older patients. Drugs Aging 16:409-435
13. Beyth RJ, Landefeld S (1995) Anticoagulants in older patients: a safety perspective. Drugs Aging 6:45-54
14. Palareti G, Leali N, Coccheri S et al, on behalf of the Italian Study on Complications of Oral Anticoagulant Therapy (1996) Bleeding complications of oral anticoagulant treatment: an inception-cohort, prospective collaborative study (ISCOAT). Lancet 348:423-28
15. Palareti G, Hirsh J, Legnani C et al (2000) Oral anticoagulation treatment in the elderly: a nested prospective, case-control study. Arch Intern Med 160:470-478
16. Pengo V, Legnani C, Noventa F, Palareti G, on behalf of the ISCOAT Study Group (2001) Oral anticoagulant therapy in patients with nonrheumatic atrial fibrillation and risk of bleeding. Thromb Haemost 85:418-422
17. Landefeld CS, Goldman L (1989) Major bleeding in outpatients treated with warfarin. Incidence and prediction by factors known at the start of outpatient therapy. Am J Med 87:144-152
18. Wehinger C, Stollberger C, Langer T, Schneider B, Finsterer J (2001) Evaluation of risk factors for stroke/embolism and of complications due to anticoagulant therapy in atrial fibrillation. Stroke 32:2246-2252
19. Palareti G, Poggi M, Guazzaloca G et al (1997) Assessment of mental ability in elderly anticoagulated patients: its reduction is associated with a less satisfactory quality of treatment. Blood Coagul Fibrinolysis 8:411-417
20. Ansell JE, Hughes R (1996) Evolving models of warfarin management: anticoagulation clinics, patient self-monitoring, and patient self-management. Am Heart J 132:1095-1100
21. Chiquette E, Amato MG, Bussey HI (1998) Comparison of an anticoagulation clinic with usual medical care: anticoagulation control, patient outcomes, and health care costs. Arch Intern Med 158:1641-1647
22. Fitmaurice DA, Hobbs FD, Delaney BC, Wilson S, McManus R (1998) Review of computerized decision support system for oral anticoagulation management. Br J Hematol 102:907-909

Is There Still a Role for Right Atrial Ablation in Patients with Atrial Fibrillation?

M.L. Loricchio, L. Calo', F. Lamberti, A. Castro, A. Boggi, C. Pandozi, M. Santini

Background

Radiofrequency (RF) transcatheter ablation has been recently proposed to cure atrial fibrillation (AF). Initial studies tried to replicate the surgical "maze" procedure, performing linear lesions in the right atrium (RA) and/or the left atrium [1-5]. The first report of RF catheter ablation suggested that linear lesions in the RA are able to cure AF [1]. Additional studies have been done using only right atrial ablation to prevent AF recurrence, with varying results but without serious complications [2-5]. More recently, several reports have pointed to the importance of the posterior region of the left atrium, particularly the pulmonary veins, as a critical area in the initiation and maintenance of AF [6-10]. However, the approaches used vary, the reproducibility of the results is uncertain, and the studies are not controlled. Furthermore, these ablative therapies are not without risks [11]. Haïssaguerre et al. [7] reported a success rate of 71% with a 3% incidence of pulmonary vein stenosis in patients with paroxysmal AF who underwent focal ablation in the pulmonary veins. A different approach, circumferential pulmonary vein ablation, proved to be effective in 80% of patients, with an 0.8% incidence of major complications [8]. Nowadays, the low efficacy of right atrial ablation procedures is generally accepted, but some issues remain to be clarified. Can we increase the efficacy of the linear lesions in the RA with new mapping systems? What is the most effective lesion design in the RA, and what is the effect of these lesions on quality of life?

Patients

We performed RF ablation in the RA in 78 symptomatic patients with paroxysmal (n=51) or permanent (n=27) AF. Sixty-five patients had structural heart disease.

Department of Cardiology, Ospedale San Filippo Neri, Rome, Italy

Methods

A nonfluoroscopic electroanatomic mapping system (Carto, Biosense-Webster) was used to perform four linear lesions, as follows: intercaval line from the superior vena cava (SVC) to the inferior vena cava (IVC) in the posterior wall; septal line through the fossa ovalis and behind the coronary sinus ostium; a transverse lesion connecting the previous two lines; and an isthmic line across the tricuspid-IVC isthmus. The electrophysiological effects of the linear lesions were evaluated using (1) the *activation map* to analyze the distribution of local activation times in relation to the linear lesions and (2) the *voltage map* to determine the peak-to-peak amplitude of the local bipolar electrograms at each sampled site. Complete conduction block across a linear lesion was defined by the presence of double potentials separated by an isoelectric interval across the line, a local activation time difference greater than 50 ms between adjacent points on opposite sites of the lesion (<10 mm apart), and opposite orientation of the wave fronts on the two sides of the line. The low-voltage area (bipolar amplitude <0.1 mV) inside and around the lesions, the total right atrial surface area, and ratio of the low-voltage area to the total right atrial surface area were determined. Quality of life was assessed with a self-administered questionnaire before ablation and at each scheduled outpatient visit after the ablation, using an Italian translation of the 36-item Short-Form Health Survey questionnaire. The patient's perception of the frequency and severity of arrhythmia-related symptoms was evaluated with the Symptom Checklist Frequency and Severity Scale.

Results

Postablation line validation was performed in all patients. Twenty percent of patients showed a complete pattern of ablation lines. Of the remaining patients with incomplete lesions, all showed complete isthmus line block, 92% had a totally blocked intercaval posterior line, and 19% had complete block along the septal line. In all patients, the postablation voltage maps revealed the absence of discrete electrical activity (voltage <0.1 mV) in a large area between the posterior line and the septal line. There were no complications. During follow-up (19±8 months) sinus rhythm was maintained in 63 patients (81%): 50 (64%) were totally asymptomatic and 13 (17%) had a dramatic reduction in symptoms. The majority of these patients continued previously ineffective antiarrhythmic drug treatment. Arrhythmia-related symptom frequency and severity improved significantly after ablation. Quality of life before ablation was significantly lower on all scales than among the general population. After ablation all scores increased significantly, reaching the levels of the general Italian population. Univariate predictors of AF recurrence included were a lower ejection fraction, a lower extension of low-voltage area, and a lower low-voltage area/total right atrial surface area ratio.

Discussion

The rationale for our approach was to create electrical barriers in the posterior wall and the septum and to extend our lesions in the SVC and behind the coronary sinus ostium. These areas have been shown to be critical for the maintenance and/or induction of AF [11-16]. Furthermore, the coronary sinus ostium and the SVC are in some cases the source of ectopic acitivity triggering AF [14-16]. It is also possible that the linear lesions performed in the posterior wall, inside the SVC, and behind the coronary sinus ostium affected vagal innervation, given that these areas contain the largest populations of cardiac ganglia, and catheter ablation of the atrial parasympathetic nerve system has been shown to abolish vagally mediated AF in dogs [17]. The isthmus line was created to prevent the reentrant circuit of atrial flutter. In the postablation map, the area between the septal and posterior lesions showed the absence of discrete electrical activity in all patients and, interestingly, the extent of this low-voltage area was a univariate predictor of AF recurrence. Thus, it is possible that the efficacy of ablation is at least in part related to the extent of electroanatomic remodeling of the posteroseptal atrial wall. In conclusion, our experience suggests that right atrial ablation, in combination with previously ineffective antiarrhythmic drug treatment, prevents recurrences of AF and improves quality of life in patients with refractory AF.

References

1. Haïssaguerre M, Jaïs P, Shah DC et al (1996) Right and left atrial radiofrequency catheter therapy of paroxysmal atrial fibrillation. J Cardiovasc Electrophysiol 7:1132-1144
2. Gaita F, Riccardi R, Calò L et al (1998) Atrial mapping and radiofrequency catheter ablation in patients with idiopathic atrial fibrillation. Electrophysiological findings and ablation results. Circulation 97:2136-2145
3. Pappone C, Oreto G, Lamberti F et al (1999) Catheter ablation of paroxysmal atrial fibrillation using a 3D mapping system. Circulation 100:1203-1208
4. Garg A, Finneran W, Mollerus M et al (1999) Right atrial compartimentalization using radiofrequency catheter ablation for management of patients with refractory atrial fibrillation. J Cardiovasc Electrophysiol 10:763-771
5. Natale A, Leonelli F, Beheiry S et al (2000) Catheter ablation approach on the right side only for paroxysmal atrial fibrillation therapy: long-term results. Pacing Clin Electrophysiol 23:224-233
6. Haïssaguerre M, Jaïs P, Shah DC et al (1998) Spontaneous initiation of atrial fibrillation by ectopic beats originating in the pulmonary veins. N Engl J Med 339:659-666
7. Haïssaguerre M, Jaïs P, Shah DC et al (2000) Electrophysiological end point for catheter ablation of atrial fibrillation initiated from multiple pulmonary venous foci. Circulation 101:1409-1410
8. Pappone C, Rosanio S, Oreto G et al (2000) Circumferential radiofrequency ablation of pulmunary vein ostia: a new approach for curing atrial fibrillation. Circulation 102:2619-2628

9. Pappone C, Oreto G, Rosanio S et al (2001) Atrial electroanatomic remodeling after circumferential radiofrequency pulmonary vein ablation. Efficacy of an anatomic approach in a large cohort of patients with atrial fibrillation. Circulation 104:2539-2544
10. Marrouche NF, Dresing T, Cole C et al (2002) Circular mapping and ablation of the pulmonary vein for treatment of atrial fibrillation. J Am Coll Cardiol 40:464-474
11. Yu WC, Hsu TL, Tai CT et al (2001) Acquired pulmonary stenosis after radiofrequency catheter ablation of paroxysmal atrial fibrillation. J Cardiovasc Electrophysiol 12:887-89
12. Gaita F, Calò L, Riccardi R et al (2001) Different patterns of atrial activation in idiopathic atrial fibrillation: simultaneous multisite atrial mapping in patients with paroxysmal and chronic atrial fibrillation. J Am Coll Cardiol. 37:534-534
13. Tondo C, Scherlag BJ, Otomo K et al (1997) Critical atrial site for ablation of pacing-induced atrial fibrillation in the normal dog heart. J Cardiovasc Electrophysiol 8:1255-1265
14. Tsai C, Tai C, Hsieh M et al (2000) Initiation of atrial fibrillation by ectopic beats originating from the superior vena cava: electrophysiological characteristics and results of radiofrequency ablation. Circulation 102:67-74
15. Goya M, Ouyang F, Ernst S et al (2002) Electroanatomic mapping and catheter ablation of breakthroughs from the right atrium to the superior vena cava in patients with atrial fibrillation. Circulation 106:1317-1320
16. Chen YJ, Chen CY, Yeh HI et al (2002) Electrophysiology and arrhythmogenic activity of single cardiomyocytes from canine superior vena cava. Circulation 105: 2679-2685
17. Schauerte P, Scherlag BJ, Pitha J et al (2000) Catheter ablation of cardiac autonomic nerves for prevention of vagal atrial fibrillation. Circulation 102:2774-2780

Present Role and Future Perspectives of Radiofrequency Ablation of Atrial Fibrillation

M. Scaglione, D. Caponi, P. Di Donna, M. Bocchiardo

Transcatheter ablation of atrial fibrillation has been recently developed and is part now of the armamentarium in the treatment of atrial fibrillation. The ablation of atrial fibrillation started out from the experience of the surgical maze procedure, which showed very encouraging results but at a high price because it required open chest surgery. In the following years the attempt has been made to produce similar results using transcatheter ablation. Different approaches have been used: linear lesions mimicking the surgical maze operation, linear lesions in the right or left atrium using different schemes, or a sequential approach ablating first in the right and then in the left atrium.

What we have learned from all this is that it is extremely difficult to obtain a complete transmural lesion with the transcatheter approach, and this reduces the chances of success of the procedure. In addition, it has been shown that right atrial linear ablation alone is less effective but safer, whereas linear lesions in the left atrium carry a higher success rate but with the disadvantage of an increased rate of complications (pericardial effusion, pericardial tamponade, and thromboembolism).

A major breakthrough has been the recognition of a focal mechanism in the initiation of many cases of idiopathic atrial fibrillation. The foci are mainly localized in the pulmonary veins (PVs). The exact mechanism of the focal activity is not clear, but it seems to be due to triggered activity. The presence of these foci can be suspected when Holter monitoring documents the presence of early atrial extrasystoles ("P on T" phenomenon) or evidence of high-frequency organized atrial activity in the initiation of atrial fibrillation or the presence of brief self-terminating episodes of atrial fibrillation.

Based on this evidence, Haïssaguerre proposed ablation of these foci located inside the PV involved in the initiation of atrial fibrillation, looking for the "PV spike" expression of the automatic activity. Using this approach it has been possible to eliminate the focal extrasystoles and atrial fibrillation in a

Centro Aritmologico, Ospedale Civile di Asti, Italy

high number of patients. Unfortunately, stenosis of the PVs occurred in a small percentage of patients, and very often more than one PV was involved in triggering atrial fibrillation, so that multiple procedure sessions were required. To eliminate these problems, a different technique has been developed: using special multipolar catheters it is possible to map the ostium of each PV and thus identify the electrical connections between the PV and the left atrium, which can then easily be targeted and ablated.

Using this technique with the application of radiofrequency energy at selected ostial sites, stenosis of the pulmonary vein has been almost eliminated. Moreover, using this technique it is also possible to electrically disconnect all the PVs in one session in the majority of cases, allowing the possibility of treating multiple PV foci in one session. Analyzing the clinical results of the centers that use this technique, it may be seen that the rate of success (elimination of atrial fibrillation) is about 65%–70%. The failure in the other 30%–35% of cases can be explained by the fact that in some cases the trigger points are located outside the PVs, and in other cases the substrate plays an important role in the genesis and maintenance of the arrhythmia. Alternative sites of initiation of atrial fibrillation may be the superior vena cava, Marshall's ligament, the posterior region of the left atrium, and the epicardial surface of the coronary sinus. It is sometimes difficult to localize them because this requires extensive electrical mapping of both the atria and, above all, the presence of the focal discharge during the ablation procedure.

As mentioned earlier, this approach has shown higher success rates in idiopathic atrial fibrillation, whereas in the case of persistent or chronic atrial fibrillation associated with organic heart disease, in which the substrate seems to play a more important role, it has demonstrated less efficacy.

Our experience in ablating atrial fibrillation dates to the mid-1990s. At that time we performed linear ablation in the right atrium in patients affected by "vagal" idiopathic atrial fibrillation. No complications occurred with this approach, but the success rate was 55% at 1-year follow-up and dropped to 25% at 3-year follow-up. For this reason we moved to PV foci ablation, and for the last two years we have performed electrical disconnection of the PVs. Our clinical results using electrical PV disconnection (Figs. 1, 2) show a 70% success rate with no major complications (pericardial tamponade, pulmonary vein stenosis) in patients with atrial fibrillation of focal origin.

Electrical disconnection of the PVs in patients affected by persistent atrial fibrillation or chronic atrial fibrillation associated with organic heart disease has a lower success rate in our experience, confirming the literature data. Since in this population the substrate plays a more important role in the genesis and maintenance of atrial fibrillation, as shown by the surgical experience, some centers have decided to perform left linear lesions in addition, improving the success rate at the expense of a higher rate of complications.

On the basis of this experience we have decided to reevaluate the safe right atrial linear approach to modify the substrate combined with PV disconnection in this group of patients.

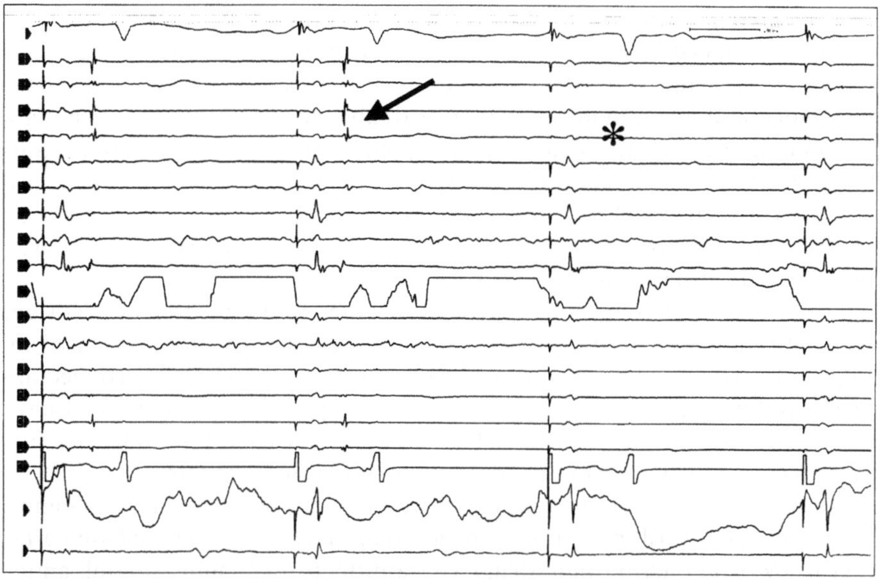

Fig. 1. Endocardial recordings from left superior pulmonary vein using a basket catheter to map the electrical connections during pacing from coronary sinus. The *arrow* indicates the pulmonary vein potential and the * its disappearance during radiofrequency application at the ostial site, demonstrating electrical disconnection of that vein

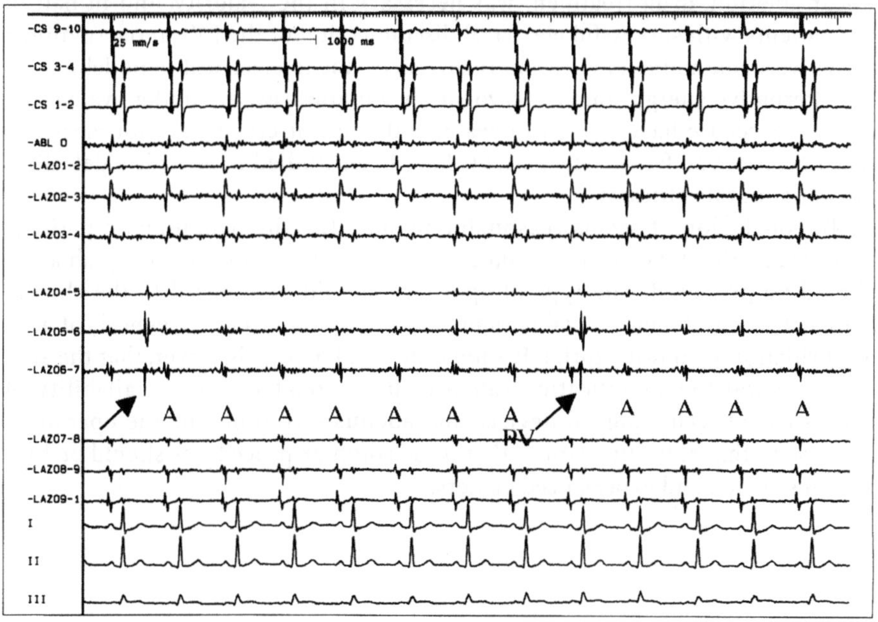

Fig. 2. Endocardial recordings from left superior pulmonary vein using a "lasso" catheter to map the electrical connections of the pulmonary vein. Arrows indicate pulmonary vein potential (PV) dissociated from left atrial activity (A) after disconnection of the targeted vein. CS, coronary sinus recordings; ABL, distal bipole ablation catheter recording

Our current linear lesions scheme includes an intercaval posteroseptal linear lesion associated with ablation of the inferior vena cava–tricuspid annulus isthmus. The endpoint of the procedure is demonstration of a complete isthmus block and a continuous corridor of double atrial potentials indicating a transmural lesion in the posteroseptal region. We were able to achieve isthmus block in 100% of cases and the electrophysiological endpoint of the intercaval posteroseptal line in 93% of cases. By these criteria we achieved a success rate of about 50% at a mean 6-month follow-up maintaining antiarrhythmic drug therapy. Only minor complications have occurred.

This approach has been designed as a first step in the ablation of persistent atrial fibrillation or in the absence of clinical evidence of a focal mechanism. In patients who do not respond, the next step is to add electrical disconnection of the pulmonary veins. The group of nonresponding patients who have undergone the second step is small so far, but the second procedure has further increased the number of patients maintaining sinus rhythm.

Despite these encouraging results, however, in our opinion pharmacological treatment should still have a prominent role; in fact we propose ablation after inefficacy of antiarrhythmic drugs (flecainide, propafenone, sotalol, amiodarone) has been demonstrated. In our experience the best results are seen using amiodarone and/or flecainide plus sotalol. In addition, pharmacological treatment improves the success in maintaining normal sinus rhythm when employed together with ablation. Among our patients who underwent right linear ablation, drug treatment was necessary in the majority, and in half of the patients with successful electrical disconnection of the PVs antiarrhythmic drugs were maintained to prevent recurrences due to electrical remodeling.

Alternative energy sources (cryoenergy, microwaves) are under evaluation. In our center we have started to evaluate the use of cryoenergy for electrical disconnection. So far too few patients have been studied to provide a definitive answer about its efficacy.

In conclusion, it seems reasonable to state that in symptomatic patients with drug-refractory atrial fibrillation, transcatheter radiofrequency ablation should be proposed. The type of approach should be tailored to the clinical presentation of the individual patient, bearing in mind that the genesis of atrial fibrillation is multifactorial. It should be emphasized, however, that the success rate and the complication rate are closely related to the availability of sophisticated technological devices and adequate training for the operators. Because of this, it is our opinion that these complex procedures should be limited to selected and experienced centers.

Atrial Pacing Algorithms for the Prevention of Atrial Fibrillation

E. CRYSTAL[1-2], I.E. OVSYSHCHER[1]

Background

Atrial fibrillation (AF) is by far the most common form of sustained cardiac arrhythmia. Primary and secondary prevention of AF is an important clinical goal. The idea of preventing recurrence of AF by different location of the lead(s) and different modes and/or algorithms of pacing has been under evaluation for the last decade. The ability of pacing mode to affect the occurrence of AF was first noted from observational studies [1, 2]. During the past several years it was confirmed in four randomized pacing trials [3]. Recent large trials of rhythm control versus rate control in AF - such as the Pharmacological Intervention in Atrial Fibrillation (PIAF) [4], AF Follow-up Investigation in Rhythm Management (AFFIRM)[5], and Rate Control vs Electrical Cardioversion for Persistent Atrial Fibrillation (RACE) trials [6] - suggest that suppression of AF has no effect on the traditional hard outcomes like stroke and cardiovascular death. Reduced frequency and duration of AF, however, is still an important clinical goal in patients with symptomatic AF. The aim of this paper is to review the accumulated data on the pacing algorithms for secondary prevention of AF.

Table 1 presents the types of algorithms available in modern pacemakers.

Fixed Overdrive Algorithms

Early observations that patients with sinus bradycardia frequently experienced AF resulted in attempts to prevent the appearance and recurrence of AF by increasing the lower cardiac rate by pacing.

[1]Department of Cardiology, Soroka University Medical Center, Faculty of Health Sciences, Ben-Gurion University, Israel; [2]Division of Cardiology, Sunnybrook and Women's College Health Science Center, Faculty of Health Sciences, University of Toronto, Canada

Table 1. Available prophylactic pacing algorithms in pacemakers

Manufacturer	Name of algorithm	Device	Description of algorithm	Reference randomized clinical trial
Medtronic	Atrial preference pacing	AT 500	Dynamic overdrive algorithm	[22] [22]
	Atrial rate stabilization	AT 500	Post-atrial extrasystole pacing with gradual increase in pacing cycling	[22]
	Post-mode-switch overdrive	AT 500 Kappa 900	Decrease in pacing cycling after every episode of atrial arrhythmia detected	
	DDDR+ or consistent atrial pacing	Thera DR	Flexible overdrive algorithm	[13, 18]
Vitatron	Pace conditioning	Selection 900E/9000	Flexible overdrive algorithm	[14, 15]
	PAC suppression	Selection 900E/9000	Post-atrial extrasystole pacing at higher rate with gradual increase in pacing cycling	
	Post PAC response	Selection 900E/9000	Shortens the escape interval for a beat after a PAC	
	Post exercise response	Selection 900E/9000	The post-exercise intervention rate slowly drifts upwards until just below the underlying intrinsic rate, and limits the rate deceleration during recovery	
	Post-AF response	Selection 9000	Increases the pacing rate after cessation of a previous AF episode	
	Rate soothing	Selection 9000	Dynamic adaptation of the pacing rate to a rate slightly above the intrinsic rate, aiming at simultaneous atrial depolarization from two sites (pacing lead and sinus beat)	
Guidant/CPI	Atrial preference pacing	Pulsar MAX II Discovery II	Flexible overdrive algorithm	
	Atrial rate smoothing	Pulsar MAX II Discovery II	Pacing to help smooth out the response to extrasystole	
Ela Medica	Automatic rest rate	Talent DR	Pacing at preprogrammed rate during resting cardiovascular conditions as detected by device	[11]
	Post-extrasystole overdrive supression	Chorus	Post-atrial extrasystole pacing with gradual increase in pacing cycling	[21]
St. Jude	Dynamic atrial overdrive	TrilogyDR+ IntegrityAF DR IdentityDR	Flexible overdrive algorithm	[16, 17]
	Rest rate, or circadian overdrive pacing	TrilogyDR AffinityDR IntegrityAF DR IdentityDR	Increases base rate during the day and decreases it during the night	[23]
Biotronik	DDD+	Philos, INOS^2	Flexible overdrive algorithm	[20]

The incidence of atrial arrhythmia was prospectively evaluated in 22 patients with DDDR pacemakers (Chorus, Ela Medical) [7]. A three-phase protocol of 1 month each was used. During the initial phase arrhythmia data were collected after discontinuation of antiarrhythmic therapy. During the second phase the pacemaker was programmed at the lower rate of 55 bpm and arrhythmia data again analyzed. During the third phase atrial "overdrive" was activated by programming the atrial rate 10 bpm above the average rate analyzed throughout a prior 24-h period (mean pacing rate at this stage was 75±5 bpm). In phase 3, episodes of arrhythmia were completely eliminated in 65% (14) of the patients, and the number and duration of episodes were considerably reduced in the rest.

In another study the same overdrive protocol [8] was evaluated in 27 patients with paroxysmal AF and the same DDD pacemaker in a randomized, single-blinded crossover study. Contrary to the observations just mentioned [7], in this study there was no significant difference in the number of AF episodes. In an earlier report from the same group [9], pacing at a base rate of 70 bpm showed a trend to an AF-preventive effect compared with pacing at 40 bpm.

In another study [10], 18 patients with pacemakers who had a history of paroxysmal AF were randomly assigned for three 2-month periods of pacing at 60, 75, or 90 bpm and the burden of AF was prospectively assessed. There was no significant difference in the burden of AF between periods of pacing at different rates. A third of the patients did not tolerate pacing at 90 bpm.

The initial results of the AF Prevention by Overdriving (PROVE) trial were recently published [11]. Patients receiving a Talent DR 213 pacemaker (Ela Medical) were grouped according to AF burden and randomly assigned, in a crossover design, to standard DDDR mode or a combination of fixed overdrive pacing (10 bpm above the detected spontaneous rate), and a rest rate algorithm, each programmed for a 3-month period. "Automatic rest rate" is a specific modifier of the low pacing rate during resting conditions when detected by pacemaker sensors. Preliminary results reported for 78 patients show a 34% reduction in the mean number of mode switches, and a mean 48% shortening of the overall duration of episodes by overdrive pacing ± automatic rest rate algorithm. This combination was well tolerated and associated with a slight improvement in quality of life.

In the most recent study [12], 42 patients with DDD pacemakers and a history of paroxysmal AF were randomly assigned to overdrive atrial pacing at rates of 10-19 bpm or 20-29 bpm above the spontaneous rate, or to no pacing. The pacing site was the right atrial appendage. The number of symptomatic AF episodes verified by the event recorder was an end-point of the study. Both overdrive pacing groups in this study demonstrated a statistically significant decrease in the number of AF episodes.

Thus, the data as to the effect of fixed overdrive atrial pacing on the prevention of AF are limited to a very few small studies with contradictory results. Larger randomized trials with longer follow-up will be needed to evaluate whether fixed overdrive algorithms have any effect in the secondary prevention of AF.

Dynamic Overdrive Algorithms

Consistent atrial pacing or dynamic atrial overdrive (DAO) is another group of algorithms based on pacing just above the sensed atrial rate. Most of these algorithms also have upper overdriving rate limitation to improve pacing tolerability. After sensing a somewhat lower atrial rate, this algorithm activates the pacing rate, with a period of overdrive pacing at the higher rate and later rate smoothing. This kind of algorithm has been investigated in 15 pacemaker (Thera, Medtronic Inc) patients with sick sinus syndrome and AF [13]. No change in the burden of AF was found. After a 2-month follow-up period there was a significant decrease in the number of atrial premature beats, but not of AF episodes.

The AF*therapy* study by Vitatron, NL, randomized 372 patients with drug-refractory AF and dual-chamber pacemakers to crossover periods of atrial pacing at different low rates and activated DAO algorithms. The anti-AF strategy included four algorithms (see Table 1) [14, 15]. The burden of symptomatic atrial arrhythmia was significantly decreased in the treatment period, and the percentage of days during which AF occurred decreased by 67%. The anti-AF algorithms also included Atrial Premature Contraction (APC)-suppression and prevention of APC-induced pauses [14].

The Atrial Dynamic Overdrive Pacing Trial (ADOPT-A) evaluated the DAO algorithm available in the TrilogyDR and IntegrityDR devices from St. Jude Medical in a randomized controlled trial in 400 patients [16]. The burden of AF (measured in this trial as the percentage of days when symptomatic AF occurred) decreased from 2.5% to 1.9% (p<0.05). Significant improvement in the quality of life was measured. The need for cardioversion showed a trend to decrease as well. Total mortality increased with DAO pacing from 6 patients in the control group to 11 in the treatment group, but the deaths were unrelated to the DAO feature of the device. ADOPT-ALL is an ongoing European randomized study of the DAO algorithm available in devices from St Jude Medical. Initial results from the Austrian center (44 patients followed for 6 months) demonstrated a 54% reduction in AF burden in patients randomized to activated DAO pacing [17].

Another dynamic atrial pacing algorithm (consistent atrial pacing, or CAP) was evaluated in a randomized cross-over trial of 61 patients with sick sinus node and paroxysmal AF [18]. The crossover period was 30 days, and 25% of patients had symptomatic AF. During CAP implementation the mean number of mode switches per day was reduced by 80%, with a significant reduction of the atrial premature beats associated with AF. The algorithm implementation was not associated with side effects.

The initial results from the Pacing in Prevention of AF (PIPAF) trial were presented at North American Society of Pacing and Electrophysiology (NASPE) 2002. In this report on 91 patients, the overdrive pacing algorithm was activated in patients with single- and dual-site atrial pacing. Activation of the algorithm was not associated with significant decrease in the burden of AF [19].

Interim results regarding the first 41 patients in the Inos[2] CLS study (Biotronik GmbH) were recently reported [20]. The study is randomized with a crossover trial of DAO pacing. The mean burden of AF, number of episodes, and time to first AF recurrence showed a trend to decrease. However, only the length of time to the first event changed significantly (from 0.5±0.2 to 1.4±0.5 weeks).

Thus, the data accumulated in the trials of DAO algorithms for AF prevention are mostly unimpressive or incomplete. Based on some preliminary results, the magnitude of the prophylactic effect of DAO-type algorithms on the total burden of AF may be characterized as moderate, but the trials have still to be completed.

Other Available Prophylactic Pacing Algorithms

An atrial rate stabilization algorithm is available in several devices (see Table 1). The rationale behind the idea is the observation that in some patients premature atrial beats are frequent immediately before an AF recurrence. Only two studies evaluating this algorithm have been performed [21]. Despite a significant decrease in premature beats, there was no change in the overall frequency of AF. In another trial this algorithm was evaluated along with two additional algorithms [22]. All three algorithms jointly significantly reduced the mean number of atrial tachyarrhythmia episodes without decreasing of the time during which patients were in atrial tachyarrhythmia.

A circadian variant of the fixed overdrive algorithm (circadian overdrive pacing) was evaluated in patients with implanted TrilogyDR pacemakers [23]. By comparison with a fixed overdrive pacing rate, this algorithm decreased the number of AF episodes significantly.

Post-mode-switch overdrive pacing is based on the observation of clustering of paroxysms of AF. After the resumption of sinus rhythm after the mode switch due to atrial tachyarrhythmia, the patient's atrium is paced at an increased programmable rate. No study evaluating the efficacy of this specific algorithm has been published. It was one of three evaluated algorithms in the report of Israel et al. [22].

The rationale of the automatic rest rate algorithm (Ela Medical) is observational data on the increased propensity to AF in the rest condition with low heart rates. The efficacy of this algorithm has been evaluated in the PROVE study and is mentioned above [11].

Combined Pharmacological and Pacing Therapy

The data on combining pharmacological and pacing intervention on the prevention of AF is very limited. It should, however, be noted that during most of the pacing evaluation trials complete drug discontinuation was rare, and because of this the results of the above-mentioned trials of pacing algorithms are mixed.

Garrigue et al. [24] reported the effect of adding propafenone to the atrial overdrive approach for the prevention of atrial arrhythmia episodes in 22 patients with DDD pacemakers in a randomized crossover study. The authors used the above-mentioned overdrive pacing at rate of 10 bpm above previously observed sinus rhythm. The arrhythmia burden was compared in the same patients randomly assigned to overdrive pacing alone or overdrive and propafenone. Drug therapy added nothing to the benefits of overdrive pacing. However, in the subgroup of patients with brady-tachycardia syndrome the combination of atrial overdrive and propafenone reduced the cumulative duration of atrial arrhythmia and the number of atrial arrhythmia episodes.

Pacing Algorithms in the Prevention of Postoperative Atrial Fibrillation

A detailed meta-analysis of trials on the efficacy of overdrive pacing in reducing total AF burden in patients after cardiac surgery has recently been published [25]. In ten trials of varying size the treatment protocols used various locations for the pacing electrodes (right atrial, left atrial, bi atrial pacing). Pacing algorithms were either fixed rate overdrive or dynamic overdrive algorithms. Patients in the control groups received atrial demand pacing at rates of 30-45 bpm. A decrease in the AF occurrence was shown for all three pacing locations, with some superiority of biatrial pacing. Both groups of overdriving algorithms (fixed and dynamic) showed a similar efficacy: respectively Odds Ratio (OR) 0.58 (95%CI 0.32, 1.07) vs OR 0.62 (95%CI 0.38, 1.01).

Conclusions

In patients with paroxysmal AF, the use of preventive pacing algorithms can reduce the overall burden of AF. The effect of these algorithms is mild to moderate, especially in patients with long-standing and drug-refractory AF. In patients with recent-onset AF (AF after cardiac surgery), pacing algorithms are more effective. Large randomized controlled studies are needed to demonstrate the influence of these algorithms (used alone as well as in combination with other approaches) on the standard outcomes such as stroke, cardiovascular death, and health-related quality of life.

References

1. Connolly SJ, Kerr C, Gent M et al (1996) Dual-chamber versus ventricular pacing. Critical appraisal of current data. Circulation 94:578-583
2. Ovsyshcher IE, Hayes DL, Furman S (1998) Dual-chamber pacing is superior to ventricular pacing: fact or controversy? Circulation 97:2368-2370
3. Cooper JM, Katcher MS, Orlov MV (2002) Implantable devices for the treatment of atrial fibrillation. N Engl J Med 346:2062-2068
4. Hohnloser SH, Kuck KH (2001) Randomized trial of rhythm or rate control in atrial fibrillation: the Pharmacological Intervention in Atrial Fibrillation Trial (PIAF). Eur Heart J 22:801-802
5. Wyse DG (2002) Atrial Fibrillation Follow-up Investigation in Rhythm Management. Annual Scientific Sessions of the American College of Cardiology
6. Crijns HJ (2002) Rate Control vs Electrical Cardioversion. Annual Scientific Sessions of the American College of Cardiology
7. Garrigue S, Barold SS, Cazeau S et al (1998) Prevention of atrial arrhythmias during DDD pacing by atrial overdrive. Pacing Clin Electrophysiol 21:1751-1759
8. Levy T, Walker S, Rex S et al (2000) Does atrial overdrive pacing prevent paroxysmal atrial fibrillation in paced patients? Int J Cardiol 75:91-97
9. Levy T, Walker S, Rochelle J et al (1999) Evaluation of biatrial pacing, right atrial pacing, and no pacing in patients with drug refractory atrial fibrillation. Am J Cardiol 84: 426-429
10. Ward KJ, Willett JE, Bucknall C et al (2001) Atrial arrhythmia suppression by atrial overdrive pacing: pacemaker Holter assessment. Europace 3:108-114
11. Funck RC, Adamec R, Lurje L et al (2000) Atrial overdriving is beneficial in patients with atrial arrhythmias: first results of the PROVE Study. Pacing Clin Electrophysiol 23:1891-1893
12. Wiberg S, Lonnerholm S, Jensen S et al (2001) Effect of right atrial overdrive pacing on symptomatic attacks of atrial fibrillation: a multicenter randomized study. Pacing Clin Electrophysiol 24:A554
13. Lam CT, Lau CP, Leung SK et al (2000) Efficacy and tolerability of continuous overdrive atrial pacing in atrial fibrillation. Europace 2:286-291
14. Remmen JJ, Verheugt FW (2001) The hotline sessions of the 23rd European congress of cardiology. Eur Heart J 22:2033-2037
15. Camm AJ (2002) AFtherapy study: preventive pacing for paroxysmal atrial fibrillation. Pacing Clin Electrophysiol 24:A125
16. Carlson MD, Gold MR, Messenger JC et al (2001) Dynamic atrial overdrive pacing decreases symptomatic atrial arrhythmia burden in patients with sinus node dysfunction. Circulation 104:383
17. Beinhauer A, Vock P, Nobis H et al (2002) Significant reduction of AF burden by the AF supression algorithm DAO™. Europace 3[Suppl A]:A194
18. Ricci R, Santini M, Puglisi A et al (2001) Impact of consistent atrial pacing algorithm on premature atrial complex number and paroxysmal atrial fibrillation recurrences in brady-tachy syndrome: a randomized prospective crossover study. J Interv Card Electrophysiol 5:33-44
19. Seidl K, Cazeau S, Gaita F et al (2002) Dual-site pacing vs mono-site pacing in prevention of atrial fibrillation. Pacing Clin Electrophysiol 25(4 pt 1):568 (Abstract)

20. Attuel P, El Allaf D, Konz I et al (2001) Is overdrive pacing useful for the prevention of paroxysmal atrial fibrillation? In: Raviele A (ed) Cardiac arrhythmias Springer, Milan, pp 492-497
21. Murgatroyd FD, Nitzsche R, Slade AK et al (1994) A new pacing algorithm for overdrive suppression of atrial fibrillation. Chorus Multicentre Study Group. Pacing Clin Electrophysiol 17:1966-1973
22. Israel CW, Lawo T, Lemke B et al (2000) Atrial pacing in the prevention of paroxysmal atrial fibrillation: first results of a new combined algorithm. Pacing Clin Electrophysiol 23:1888-1890
23. de Vusser P, Mairesse GH, Van Mieghem W et al (2001) Significant reduction in atrial fibrillation using circadian overdrive pacing at 80/65 ppm. Pacing Clin Electrophysiol 24:663A
24. Garrigue S, Barold SS, Cazeau S et al (2000) Is there a synergic effect of propafenone associated with atrial overdrive pacing for atrial arrhythmia prevention? A randomised crossover study. Heart 83:172-177
25. Crystal E, Connolly SJ, Sleik K et al (2002) Interventions on prevention of postoperative atrial fibrillation in patients undergoing heart surgery: a meta-analysis. Circulation 106:75-80

Treatment of Atrial Fibrillation in Patients Affected by Sick Sinus Syndrome: Role of Prevention and Antitachycardia Pacing Algorithms. Preliminary Results from PITAGORA Study

M. GULIZIA[1], S. MANGIAMELI[2], P. GAMBINO[3], V. BULLA[4], V. SPADOLA[5], G. CHIARANDÀ[6], L. VASQUEZ[7], G.M. FRANCESE[1], E. CHISARI[8], A. GRAMMATICO[8], ON BEHALF OF THE PITAGORA STUDY INVESTIGATORS

Introduction

With a prevalence rising with age from 0.05% at age 25-35 years to more than 5% among people aged 69 years or more, atrial fibrillation (AF) and in general atrial tachyarrhythmias (AT) are now the single most common sustained arrhythmia [1]. Once considered a benign disease, AF is increasingly being recognized as a significant cause of morbidity and mortality. AT can be treated by a vast array of pharmaceutical and nonpharmacological therapies, suggesting that no single treatment is sufficiently simple, successful, and cheap to exclude other therapies. Many new therapies are presently being developed, among which are electrical therapies designed to prevent and convert AT. Clinical experience indicates that monotherapeutic approaches (drug, ablation, or device) are often associated with unsatisfactory results in the treatment of AT patients [1-12]. Because all therapies have poor efficacy when considered alone, interest in the role of combinations of therapies (hybrid therapy) has recently increased. The rationale underlying hybrid therapy is that a combination of modalities of intervention in AT might have a synergistic effect, with the efficacy of each intervention building upon that of the others [12]. At present this concept is being considered particularly in the prevention of AT recurrence, but hybrid therapy has also been utilized both in facilitating restoration to sinus rhythm and in control of heart rate.

Drug therapy has poor long-term efficacy when used alone, with 50%–70% of patients eventually progressing to chronic AT [1, 2]. It also carries a risk for proarrhythmia and may increase mortality, especially in patients with left ven-

[1]Cardiology Department, San Luigi - S. Currò Hospital, Catania; [2]Cardiology Department, Garibaldi Hospital, Catania; [3]Cardiology Department, Civili Hospital, Sciacca; [4]Cardiology Department, Cannizzaro Hospital, Catania; [5]Cardiology Department, Civile Hospital, Ragusa; [6]Cardiology Department, Di Maria Hospital, Siracusa; [7]Cardiology Department, Civile Hospital, Milazzo; [8]Medtronic Italy, Rome, Italy

tricular dysfunction [2, 3]. It has been suggested [13-15] that antiarrhythmic drugs may improve the efficacy of cardiac pacing in preventing AF, by increasing the percentage of paced beats and by impacting on the factors that initiate AF. Several noncontrolled studies of this hybrid therapy approach have been reported. Two randomized studies have shown that daily maintenance doses of 200 mg amiodarone prevent AF recurrences better than sotalol [16] and sotalol or propafenone [17]. Some researchers have shown that overdrive pacing is effective in the reduction of premature atrial contractions and atrial arrhythmia recurrences [18]. Many authors have shown that antitachy pacing therapies are safe and effective in terminating supraventricular atrial arrhythmias. Efficacy has been reported in the range between 30% and 99% [19-25]. Recently the efficacy of the pacing therapies in terminating AT and reducing AT burden has been proved in patients also affected by ventricular arrhythmias [26, 27] and in patients affected by atrial arrhythmia associated with bradycardia [28]. Permanent overdrive atrial pacing is believed to have a palliative effect on the incidence of AT. Increases in the temporal dispersion of atrial refractoriness may increase atrial vulnerability [29]. It is hypothesized that chronic atrial pacing may prevent slow conduction in abnormal myocardium and suppress ectopic activity by effecting change in the effective refractory period, dispersion of refractoriness, conduction velocity, and the length of the excitation wave.

Methods

Study Design

Despite advances in drug treatment, many patients with AT have severe recurrences. The effectiveness of both antiarrhythmic drugs and electrical therapies is highly variable and patient-specific, but a direct comparison among different antiarrhythmic drugs used in conjunction with electrical therapies would be important to establish long-term care continuum. The PITAGORA study is a multicenter, prospective, randomized, nonblinded trial proposed to compare class III vs class IC antiarrhythmic drug therapy in preventing AT recurrences in patients suffering from AT in the setting of bradycardia. PITAGORA patients are also enrolled in a single-blind crossover evaluation with the prevention algorithms (PrAl) and antitachycardia pacing (ATP) therapies Off in the first period and On in the second. Patients give written informed consent according to a protocol approved by the local Human Subjects Committee. The study is performed in conformance with the Code of Federal Regulations, the ICH Guideline for Good Clinical Practice, and EN 540. At implant only the AT detection algorithm is enabled while PrAl and ATP features are programmed Off. A 1-month run-in period has been designed to allow for any lead fixation problems or pharmacological adjustment: a waiting period allows physicians to adjust drug therapy that has a primary antiarrhythmic effect and to reach a stable drug level. In addition, patients need time to recover from the pacemaker implant procedure, return to normal daily activities, and return to a baseline state for quality of life evaluation. Data analysis will not take into account the first month and a 1-month period after each programming change. At the 5-month follow-up, PrAl and ATP therapies are enabled according to protocols specific for the two study groups. Follow-up visits are programmed at 5, 9,13 and 18-months. At each follow-up, clinical data are collected, the quality of life (QoL) EUROQOL questionnaire and Symptom Checklist questionnaire are administered, and data from the device memory are saved on floppy disks for further analysis.

Antiarrhythmic drug therapy is maintained stable after implant. Recommended drug doses are the following: amiodarone 200 mg per day, sotalol 160-240 mg per day, propafenone 450-750 mg per day, flecainide 200 mg per day. The amiodarone loading procedure is as follows: amiodarone will be given at a dose of 600 mg per day for 10 days, followed by 400 mg per day for 10 days, after which a daily maintenance dose of 200 mg per day will be administered.

Patient Selection

To be eligible for study participation patients have to have class I or II pacemaker indication, age higher than 18 years, at least three episodes of symptomatic (paroxysmal or persistent [30]) AT in the 12 months before enrollment, at least one episode in the last 3 months, atrial arrhythmia episodes which terminate spontaneously, and at least one AT episode documented by ECG or Holter recording. Other eligibility conditions are that it must be possible to implant both atrial and ventricular bipolar leads, and that patients are expected to remain on a stable regimen of drugs that have a primary antiarrhythmic effect (this includes patients who are not expected to take any such medications) throughout the duration of follow-up. Exclusion criteria are as follows: permanent AF, left ventricular dysfunction (LVEF <40%), intolerance to class IC or III antiarrhythmic drugs, AF due to a reversible cause, pacemaker already implanted, indication for an implantable cardioverter defibrillator (ICD), cardiac surgery within the last month before implantation, life expectancy of less than 2 years, mechanical right heart valve, anticoagulation therapy that cannot be interrupted, pregnancy, thyroid disease, or inability to attend follow-up visits.

Study Endpoints

Main endpoint is the length of time to a first persistent AT recurrence, or first symptomatic paroxysmal AT recurrence which causes a hospital visit. Secondary endpoints are AT burden, AT frequency, the proportion of patients with AT recurrences, the proportion of patients with AT recurrences which require electrical or pharmacological cardioversion and/or hospital admission, number of hospital days, the proportion of patients with drug-related or device-related adverse events, and QoL scores.

Statistical Methods

We estimated that the enrollment of 160 patients with symptomatic AF would be necessary in order for the study to achieve a power of more than 0.80 to detect a reduction of 40 percentage points in the rate of recurrence of AF in the amiodarone group with a two-sided α level of 0.05, assuming a recurrence rate of 70% at one year in the group assigned to class IC drugs and a 15% loss to follow-up. Categorical variables are expressed in terms of percentages with associated standard deviations (SD). Continuous variables are expressed in terms of means with SD if the quantity was normally distributed; skewed variables are expressed as medians with ranges. Statistical significance of the difference between continuous variables is assessed by using a Student *t*-test of the means of normally distributed variables and a Wilcoxon rank sum test for skewed distribution. For the statistical analysis SPSS software (SAS Institute Inc., Cary, NC) has been used.

Device Characteristics

The Medtronic AT500TM (model 7253) device can treat each AT episode by a programmable set of automatic atrial ATP therapies. It is possible to program three different therapies, selecting between "burst+" (constant drive coupled with up to two extrastimuli) and "ramp" (decremental drive). Each therapy may be released up to ten times if the episode fails to terminate. The device software includes three pacing algorithms dedicated to prevent AT occurrence. These consist of an atrial overdrive algorithm for maintenance of a pacing rate just above the intrinsic rate [atrial pacing preference (APP)], an atrial overdrive mode designed to avoid short-long intervals [atrial rate stabilization (ARS)] following a premature atrial contraction (PAC), and an algorithm designed to inhibit early recurrence of AF following a mode-switching episode [post-mode-switching overdrive pacing (PMOP)].

Preliminary Results

We studied 59 consecutive patients treated with AT500 DDDRP pacemakers (Medtronic Inc., Minnesota, USA) in 20 medical centers (see Appendix). Data collection started in January 2001.

Patients' characteristics are described in Table 1. The arrhythmia at implantation was defined as paroxysmal in 53 patients (89.8%) and persistent in 6 patients (10.2%). A bipolar atrial lead was positioned in the right atrial appendage in 53 patients (89.8%), in atrial lateral free wall in 5 (8.5%), and in the interatrial septum in 1 (1.7%). So far 59 patients have been randomized to be treated by class IC (26 patients) or class III (33 patients) antiarrhythmic drugs. We have considered for data analysis 54 patients being treated with the assigned drug. Twenty-two take amiodarone, average dose 210±44 mg per day;

Table 1. Clinical data on the 59 patients enrolled in the study

Gender (n,%)	
☐ Male	25 (42.3%)
☐ Female	34 (57.6%)
Age (years)	
☐ Mean± standard deviation	70±9
☐ Range	61 - 82
Primary indication (n,%)[a]	
☐ Sinus node dysfunction	56 (94.9%)
☐ Acquired AV block	1 (1.7%)
☐ Other	2 (3.4%)
Primary cardiovascular history (n,%)[b]	
☐ Normal	16 (27.1%)
☐ Ischemic heart disease	6 (10.2%)
☐ Coronary artery disease	1 (1.7%)
☐ Myocardial infarction	4 (6.8%)
☐ Cardiomyopathy	8 (13.6%)
☐ Valvular disease	5 (8.5%)
☐ Hypertension	30 (50.8%)
Atrial tachyarrhythmia history (n,%)[b]	
☐ Atrial fibrillation	55 (93.2%)
☐ Typical atrial flutter	8 (13.6%)
☐ Atrial tachycardia	6 (10.2%)
☐ Atypical atrial flutter	3 (5.1%)
☐ Junctional tachycardia	1 (1.7%)
Left ventricular ejection fraction	
☐ Mean± standard deviation	54±7%
☐ Range	40 - 62
Left atrium dimensions (mm)	
☐ Mean± standard deviation	48±12
☐ Range	35 - 75
New York Heart Classification (n,%)	
☐ Class I	11 (18.6%)
☐ Class II	44 (74.6%)
☐ Class III	4 (6.8%)

[a]Mutually exclusive categories
[b]Nonexclusive categories

10 patients take sotalol, average dose 145±86 mg per day; 13 patients take flecainide, average dose 158±49 mg per day; and 9 patients take propafenone, average dose 478±212 mg per day.

Sixteen patients have reached 9-month follow-up and have been analyzed in terms of number of patients with symptomatic episodes, number of symptoms, and QoL scores. Results are shown in Table 2.

Table 2. Preliminary results of the study

	Baseline	PrAl & ATP Off	PrAl & ATP On
Number of patients with symptomatic episodes	16	12	7
Number of symptoms	2.5±0.9	1.3±1.1 (*p*<0.005 vs baseline)	1.0±0.0 (*p*<0.005 vs baseline and Off)
Quality of life	49±17	66±19 (*p*<0.01 vs baseline)	75±10 (*p*<0.001 vs baseline) (*p*<0.03 vs Off)

PrAl, prevention algorithm; ATP, antitachycardia pacing

Conclusions

Preliminary results of the PITAGORA study show that, in patients with SB and AT, prevention and antitachycardia pacing algorithms significantly reduce the number of patients with symptomatic episodes and the number of symptoms, and significantly improve QoL.

Acknowledgments: The authors express their gratitude to Giuseppe Scardace for technical assistance, Tiziana De Santo for statistical analysis, and Daniela Fabrizi and Massimiliano Pepe for data management support.

Appendix

Steering Committee of the PITAGORA Study: M. Gulizia, Chairman; S. Mangiameli, Co-chairman; A. Grammatico.
Investigators and Study Sites of the PITAGORA Study: A. Battaglia, O. Pensabene, Villa Sofia Hospital, Palermo; O. Bramanti, Policlinico Hospital, Messina; V. Bulla, Cannizzaro Hospital, Catania; G. Butera, Noto-Pasqualino Hospital, Palermo; G. Chiarandà, Muscatello Hospital, Augusta; A. Circo, V. Emanuele Hospital, Catania; N. Di Giovanni, V. Guzzo, Aiello Hospital, Mazara del Vallo; R. Evola, G. Galvagna, S. Vincenzo Hospital, Taormina; R. Ferrante, Paternò-Arezzo Hospital, Ragusa; P. Gambino, Civile Hospital, Ribera; S. Giglia, S.Elia Hospital, Caltanissetta; R. Grassi, G. Busà, Papardo Hospital, Messina; M. Gulizia, G.M. Francese, S. Luigi-S. Currò Hospital, Catania; V. Indelicato, Civili Riuniti Hospital, Sciacca; S. Mangiameli, Garibaldi Hospital, Catania; E. Mossuti, Umberto I Hospital, Siracusa; S. Orazi, Civile Hospital, Rieti; L. Pavia, Piemonte Hospital, Messina; V. Spadola, Civile Hospital, Ragusa; I. Vaccaro, G.

Caramanno, S. Giovanni di Dio Hospital, Agrigento; C. Vasco, Umberto I Hospital, Enna; L. Vasquez, Civile Hospital, Milazzo.

References

1. Narayan SM, Cain ME, Smith JM (1997) Atrial fibrillation. Lancet 350:943-950
2. Pritchett ELC, McCarthy EA, Wilkinson WE (1991) Propafenone treatment of symptomatic paroxysmal supraventricular arrhythmias. A randomized, placebo-controlled, crossover trial in patients tolerating oral therapy. Ann Intern Med 114:539-544
3. Coplen SE, Antman AM, Berlin JA, Hewitt P, Chaimers TC (1990) Efficacy and safety of quinidine therapy for mantenance of sinus rhythm after cardioversion: a meta-analysis of randomized control trials. Circulation 82:1106-1116
4. Flaker GC, Blackshear JL, McBride R, Kronmal RA, Halperin JL, Hart RG, on behalf of the Stroke Prevention in AF Investigators (1992) Antiarrhythmic drug therapy and cardiac mortality in AF. J Am Coll Cardiol 20:527-532
5. Cox JL, Canavan TE, Schuessler RB et al (1991) The surgical treatment of AF. II. Intraoperative electrophysiologic mapping and description of the electrophysiologic basis of atrial flutter and AF. J Thorac Cardiovasc Surg 101: 408-426
6. Jais P, Haïssaguerre M, Shah DC et al (1997) A focal source of AF treated by discrete radiofrequency ablation. Circulation 95:572-576
7. Haïssaguerre M, Jais P, Shah DC et al (1996) Right and left atrial radiofrequency catheter therapy of paroxysmal AF. J Cardiovasc Electrophysiol 12:1132-1144
8. Ching Man K, Daoud E, Knight B et al (1996) Right atrial radiofrequency catheter ablation of paroxysmal AF. J Am Coll Cardiol 27:188A (Abstract)
9. Rosenqvist M, Brandt J, Schuller H (1988) Long-term pacing in sinus node disease: effect of stimulation mode on cardiovascular mortality and morbidity. Am Heart J 116:16-22
10. Sgarbossa EB, Pinski SL, Maloney JD et al (1993) Chronic AF and stroke in paced patients with sick sinus syndrome. Relevance of clinical characteristics and pacing modalities. Circulation 88:1045-1053
11. Jung W, Wolpert C, Esmailzadeh B et al (1998) Specific considerations with the automatic implantable atrial defibrillator. J Cardiovasc Electrophysiol 9(8 Suppl):S193-201
12. Timmermans C, Levy S, Ayers GM et al (2000) Spontaneous episodes of atrial fibrillation after implantation of the Metrix Atrioverter: observations on treated and non-treated episodes. Metrix Investigators. J Am Coll Cardiol 35(6):1428-1433
13. Capucci A, Villani GQ (2000) Combined approach of pharmacological and non-pharmacological treatment of atrial fibrillation. In: Bloch-Thomsen PE, Clement DL Everyday problems in cardiology. Excerpta Medica, Amsterdam, vol II, no 2, pp 3-8
14. Default P, Saksena S, Prakash A et al (1998) Long-term outcome of patients with drug-refractory atrial flutter and fibrillation after single-dual-site right atrial pacing for arrhythmia prevention. J Am Coll Cardiol 32:1900-1908
15. Saksena S, Prakash A, Michael H et al (1996) Prevention of recurrent AF with chronic dual-site right atrial pacing. J Am Coll Cardiol 28:687-694
16. Vardas PE et al (1998) Low-dose amiodarone versus sotalol for suppression of recurrent symptomatic AF. Am J Cardiol 81: 995-998
17. Roy D, Talajic M, Dorian P et al (2000) Amiodarone to prevent recurrence of atrial fibrillation. N Engl J Med 342:913-920

18. Ricci R, Santini M, Puglisi A et al (1999) Intermittent or continuous overdrive atrial pacing significantly reduces paroxysmal atrial fibrillation recurrences in brady-tachy syndrome. Pacing Cling Electrophysiol 22:A175 (abstract)
19. Barold S et al (1987) Implanted atrial pacemakers for paroxysmal atrial flutter. Ann Intern Med 107:144-149
20. Connelly DT, de Belder MA, Cunningham D et al (1993) Long-term follow-up of patients treated with a software-based antitachycardia pacemaker. Br Heart J 69:250-254
21. den Dulk K, Brugada P, Smeets J et al, (1990) Long-term antitachycardia pacing experience for supraventricular tachycardia. Pacing Clin Electrophysiol 13:1020-1030
22. den Dulk K et al (1983) A versatile pacemaker system for termination of tachycardias. Am J Card 52(7):731-738
23. Fromer M, Gloor H, Kus T (1990) Clinical experience with the Intertach pulse generator in patients with recurrent supraventricular and ventricular tachycardia. Pacing Clin Electrophysiol 13:1955-1959
24. Kappenberger L, Valin H, Sowton E (1989) Multicenter long-term results of antitachycardia pacing for supraventricular tachycardias. Am J Cardiol 64:191-193
25. McComb JM, Jameson S, Bexton R (1990) Atrial antitachycardia pacing in patients with supraventricular tachycardia: clinical experience with the Intertach pacemaker. Pacing Clin Electrophysiol 13:1948-1954
26. Adler SW, Wolpert C, Warman EN et al (2001) Efficacy of pacing therapies for treating atrial tachyarrhythmias in patients with ventricular arrhythmias receiving a dual-chamber implantable cardioverter defibrillator. Circulation 104: 887-892
27. Friedman PA, Dijkman B, Warman EN et al (2001) Atrial therapies reduce atrial arrhythamias burden in defibrillator patients. Circulation 104:1023-1028
28. Disertori M, Padeletti L, Santini M et al (2001) Antitachycardia pacing therapies to terminate atrial tachycardia: the AT500 Italian Registry. Eur Heart J Suppl 3[Suppl. P]P16-P24
29. Tsuji H, Fujiki A, Tani M et al (1992) Quantitative relationship between atrial refractoriness and the dispersion of refractoriness in atrial vulnerability. Pacing Clin Electrophysiol 15:403-410
30. Gallagher MM, Camm AJ (1997) Classification of atrial fibrillation. Pacing Clin Electrophysiol 20:1603-1605

Recent and Ongoing Trials on Device Therapy of Atrial Fibrillation

P. DELISE

Atrial fibrillation is a complex arrhythmia from both an electrophysiologic and a clinical point of view. As to its electrophysiologic mechanism, three main factors are at work: triggers, initiators, and perpetuators [1, 2]. Several triggers have been identified [3-6]: supraventricular reentry tachycardias, atrial extrasystoles, and, more recently, pulmonary vein foci. Possible initiators are Bachmann's bundle [7] and other critical atrial areas. Finally, the perpetuators are atrial electrophysiologic and anatomic alterations (atrial dilatation, fibrosis, and/or fatty degeneration) which represent the substrate of sustained atrial fibrillation [8, 9].

Preventing atrial fibrillation is not easy, and, at present no single effective therapy has been identified. Many therapeutic options are available (drugs, ablation of triggers, ablation of the substrate), but none of them is successful in all patients. The most probable reason for this is that in different patients the prevailing electrophysiologic mechanisms (trigger, substrate) are not the same, and the various therapies frequently are not able to act on all the factors producing atrial fibrillation.

Atrial fibrillation can be interrupted by drugs or by electrical cardioversion. For the latter, intracardiac defibrillation has the highest success rate [10, 11].

In recent years sophisticated devices have been produced with the double purpose of preventing and terminating atrial fibrillation. Some devices are targeted to only prevent atrial fibrillation, others to terminate atrial fibrillation, and, finally, some devices are designed both to prevent and to interrupt atrial fibrillation.

Prevention of Atrial Fibrillation with Conventional Pacemakers in Patients with Bradycardia

Patients with sick sinus syndrome have a high incidence of atrial arrhythmias including atrial fibrillation. This fact derives from various reasons. First, the

Operative Unit of Cardiology, Hospital of Conegliano, Treviso, Italy underlying pathology affecting the sinus node may also in many patients involve the atria. Second, bradycardia in itself favors the discharge of ectopic foci, the dispersion of atrial refractoriness, and delayed conduction of premature atrial beats. In consequence, it facilitates the occurrence of multiple atrial reentries which initiate and perpetuate sustained atrial fibrillation. It follows that, at least theoretically, preventing bradycardia by atrial pacing should prevent atrial fibrillation.

Both retrospective [12-14] and prospective [15-19] randomized studies have demonstrated the superiority of physiologic pacing (AAI or DDD pacing) over ventricular pacing in patients with the sick sinus syndrome. All of these studies have demonstrated a reduction both in the incidence of paroxysmal atrial fibrillation and in the risk of chronic atrial fibrillation. The benefit of physiologic pacing in patients with atrioventricular (AV) block is less clear. For example, the Canadian Trial of Physiologic Pacing [19] showed that atrial fibrillation was reduced by implantation of a physiologic pacemaker both in the sick sinus syndrome and in AV block, although the effect was evident only after 2 years. In contrast, Lamas et al. [16], in another trial, suggested that, in comparison to VVI pacing, physiologic pacing leads to a lower incidence of atrial fibrillation in sick sinus syndrome but not in patients with AV block.

All these studies suggest that in patients with the sick sinus syndrome an AAI/DDD physiologic pacemaker should be implanted whereas a VVI pacemaker should be avoided. However, they do not demonstrate that atrial pacing prevents atrial fibrillation. In fact, these results may depend not on the beneficial effect of pacing the atrium, but on the deleterious effect of retrograde activation of the atria due to the ventricular pacing. To clarify this point, a study should be performed in patients with recurrent atrial fibrillation comparing two groups randomly treated with and without physiologic pacing. Unfortunately such a study has never been published.

Prevention of Atrial Fibrillation by Pacing the Interatrial Septum and/or by Dual-Site Pacing

Delayed conduction in the atria facilitates atrial fibrillation. This condition is present particularly in patients with a long P wave. Theoretically, by shortening P wave duration, the dissynchrony of atrial activation should diminish and consequently atrial fibrillation should be prevented.

Many authors [20-25] have studied the effects of pacing the atria at various sites in an effort to promote more synchroinized atrial activation in patients with atrial fibrillation. For example, some [20, 22, 25] suggest that attaching a pacing lead to the interatrial septum or to the opening of the coronary sinus results in a narrower P wave. A similar result can be achieved by pacing at Bachmann's bundle [23], which is a band of tissue that electrically connects the right and left atria. Others have demonstrated that in patients with recurrent atrial fibrillation in whom pacemaker implantation was required, those in whom the atrial lead was placed in Bachmann's bundle [24] or in the interatrial septum [25] had a lower incidence of paroxysmal and chronic atrial fibrillation than those in whom the lead was positioned in the right atrial appendage.

Another way to resynchronize the atria is to pace two sites simultaneously [26-29]. The most common configuration is a lead attached to the right atrial appendage and a lead placed in the coronary sinus, in order to stimulate both the right and the left atria. The clinical value of this pacing strategy has been assessed, in randomized studies of patients who have undergone cardiac surgery [26-29] and of patients with a prolonged P wave [30]. In three of four studies, conducted in patients with a coronary artery bypass graft [27-29], dual-site pacing compared to single-site pacing or to no pacing showed a significant reduction of the incidence of atrial fibrillation. In a study conducted in patients with sick sinus syndrome, a history of atrial fibrillation, and prolonged P wave, significant reduction of both paroxysmal and permanent atrial fibrillation was demonstrated.

In conclusion, a limited number of reports suggest the possibility that synchronization of the atria by pacing the interatrial septum, the region around Bachman's bundle, or both atria simultaneously can help in preventing atrial fibrillation. Patients who may benefit from these strategies appear to be those with a long P wave and/or in whom the substrate appears more important than the trigger in the development of the arrhythmia.

Prevention of Atrial Fibrillation with Complex Overdrive Atrial Pacing Algorithms

Theoretical benefits deriving from overdrive pacing include elimination of bradycardia periods, atrial pauses, and short-long atrial cycles and suppression/reduction of atrial premature beats by producing exit block. Such effects should prevent the onset of triggers and also of dispersion of conduction/refractoriness in the atria - all mechanisms which can facilitate atrial fibrillation.

Several prospective studies suggest that increasing the atrial pacing rate results in a higher percentage of paced beats and a lower atrial fibrillation burden. For example, Garrigue et al. [31], in a small study in which the lower rate of atrial pacing was programmed at 10 bpm faster than the mean spontaneous heart rate, observed a significant reduction of episodes of recurrent atrial fibrillation. Defaye et al. [32] demonstrated that patients who had a higher percentage of paced beats had a lower incidence of atrial fibrillation. These observations, however, were not confirmed by Levy et al. [33]. In any case, a major problem of overdrive atrial pacing is that the use of excessive rates of pacing is badly tolerated by some patients.

In an attempt to obtain the objective of overdrive atrial pacing without the use of excessive rates of pacing, complex algorithms have been developed. Three main algorhithms have been introduced: atrial preference pacing (also called consistent atrial pacing), atrial rate stabilization, and post-mode-switching overdrive pacing. The more recent devices generally include all three algorithms.

Atrial preference pacing (APP) has the goal of using a pacing rate that is slightly faster than spontaneous atrial activity. This approach advocates continuous monitoring of native atrial activity. After every sensed atrial event the atrial escape interval of the pacemaker is shortened by a programmable value (Δ deceleration). After a programmable number of paced atrial beats (plateau beats) the atrial escape interval is lengthened by a programmable value (ARS Δ) until a sinus beat arises. When atrial fibrillation occurs the APP algorithm is switched off.

Atrial rate stabilization (ARS) has the goal of avoiding short - long intervals after an atrial premature beat. Thus, after a premature atrial beat the atrium is paced after an interval slightly longer than the length of the premature beat and thereafter the pacing rate progressively decreases until the reonset of spontaneous rhythm.

Post-mode-switching overdrive pacing (PMOP) has been designed to inhibit early reinitiation of atrial fibrillation following a mode-switching episode. It allows stimulation of the atria at a higher rate than the "lower rate" after the termination of atrial fibrillation. The atrial rate and duration of DDI stimulation are programmable.

Several studies [34-38] have demonstrated the ability of these algorithms to increase the percentage of atrial pacing by more than 80%.

Ricci et al. [38], in a randomized study conducted in patients with the sick sinus syndrome, compared patients with DDDR APP versus DDDR, that is with and without algorithms to prevent atrial fibrillation. With the DDDR AAP they observed a significant reduction in atrial premature beats and a significant reduction in mode-switch episodes/day, but only in comparison to patients with DDDR who had less than 90% paced beats. In contrast, in comparison to patients with DDDR who had more than 90% paced beats no additional benefit was observed. Furthermore, no difference was observed between the two stimulation modalities with regard to the number of asymptomatic patients.

The recent ADOPT-A trial [38], which has not yet been extensively reported on, evaluated the efficacy of atrial fibrillation prevention algorithms in patients with sick sinus syndrome. It showed that the use of preventing algorithms decreased by 25% the burden of symptomatic atrial fibrillation in comparison to DDDR pacing alone.

The AF therapy study too, not yet published, and whose results were reported by Camm in ESC Stockolm, showed a reduction of atrial fibrillation burden by activation algorithms in patients with DDD pacemaker who had drug-refractory atrial fibrillation and no conventional pacing indications. In contrast, Israel et al. [35] in patients with conventional pacemaker implantation (66% for sick sinus syndrome) did not find a benefit of preventive pacing algorithms in respect of either the number or the duration of atrial tachycardia or atrial fibrillation episodes. Murgatroyd et al. [34] in a short-term multiple crossover study, observed a reduction of atrial fibrillation burden but only in a subgroup of patients with a high prevalence of atrial fibrillation at baseline

In conclusion, there is a sufficient evidence that new preventive algorithms are able to increase the number of paced beats, to reduce the number of premature atrial beats, and, at least in some studies, to reduce atrial fibrillation burden in patients with recurrent atrial fibrillation. There is no proof that they can eliminate symptomatic atrial fibrillation. As to the quality of life, no benefit has been demonstrated either by Ricci et al. [38] nor by the AF therapy study. Lastly, no data are available about their effect on morbidity and mortality.

Other trials are ongoing. In particular, the PIPAF (Pacing in Prevention of Atrial Fibrillation) studies [39], which are examining the synergistic effects of overdrive pacing combined with various single and multiple pacing sites.

Atrial Defibrillators and Antitachycardia Devices

The first two defibrillators which became available in recent years were the Metrix (InControl, Redmond, Wa.) [40] and the Jewel 7250 AF (Medtronic, Minneapolis, Minn.) [41].

The first, Metrix, was implanted in 1995. This unit is a pure atrial defibrillator which has sensing and defibrillator capability in the atrium and sensing and pacing capability in the ventricle. The device employs a right atrial, a coronary sinus, and a right ventricular bipolar lead. The bipolar right ventricular lead is used for R wave synchronization and post-shock pacing. Graded shock therapy is available for up to eight shocks (at each level) for each episode of atrial fibrillation. Biphasic shocks are programmable in 20-V increments up to 300 V. The shock is delivered between the electrodes in the right atrium and the coronary sinus. As the Metrix system did not have the possibility of defibrillating the ventricles, it was built to minimize the risk of inducing ventricular arrhythmias. The device can be programmed into any of the following operating modes: fully automatic, patient-activated, monitor mode, bradycardia pacing only, and off. In the automatic mode the device is only intermittently active in detecting and treating atrial fibrillation, and this "sleep-awake interval" is programmable. At the end of the "sleep" interval it "awakens" and runs its detection algorithm. If atrial fibrillation is not detected it returns to sleep mode for another cycle. The patient-activated mode differs from the automatic mode in that the device "awakens" only when a magnet is placed briefly over it. The sleep mode significantly reduces energy consumption and prolongs the device's life.

The device has some limitations, and for this reason its production has been discontinued. First, it is unable to distiguish atrial fibrillation from other rapid atrial tachycardias such as atrial flutter. Second, owing to the sleep mode, the device cannot differentiate continuous/persistent from intermittent/self-terminating atrial fibrillation. Third, in the automatic mode the device cannot be programmed to delay interventions. This is a limitation because atrial fibrillation is not a life-threathening arrhythmia and frequently terminates spontaneously within minutes or hours, so that it is not always necessary to interrupt it at once. Furthermore, the device permits only the delivery of shocks and not of atrial bursts. Finally, the low energy available (maximum 6 J) allows the device to be used in no more than two-third of eligible patients [40].

The Jewel 7250 AF became available next [41]. The Jewel AF has dual-chamber sensing and pacing as well as defibrillator capability in both the atrium and ventricle with a maximum output of 27 J. This unit is basically a ventricular defibrillator with atrial capability as well. It also has the capacity to treat atrial and ventricular arrhythmias with paced termination modalities before low-energy shocks [41].

The device is connected to two or three catheters: two catheters are positioned in the right atrium and in the right ventricle, respectively. Another catheter may be positioned in the coronary sinus if the atrial defibrillator threshold during implantation is high (about 7% of cases). The device is able to discriminate atrial tachycardia from atrial fibrillation, permitting antitachycardia pacing for fast regular atrial arrhythmias [41]. Atrial tachycardia and atrial fibrillation are identified on the basis of atrial cycle length within programmable detection zones. The detection zones for the two arrhythmias may overlap. If the atrial cycle length is in this overlap zone, the rhythm is classified as atrial tachycardia if it is regular and as atrial fibrillation if it is not.

The device is able to deliver burst pacing, ramp pacing, or 50-Hz burst pacing, it can treat atrial tachycardia or atrial flutter without delivering shocks. The device can also prevent recurrent atrial tachycardia/fibrillation by atrial pacing both during bradycardia periods and with overdrive atrial pacing and/or post-extrasystolic pacing by means of specific algorithms. It can be set to automatic mode, patient- or physician-activated mode, or to monitor mode. In the automatic mode the intervention delay is programmable.

Clinical Results of Implantable Atrial Defibrillators and Antitachycardia Devices

Both Metrix and Jewel AF have been demonstrated to be efficacious and safe. The Metrix system has a sensitivity of 92% and a specificity of 100% in detecting atrial fibrillation [41]. The Jewel AF device has a sensitivity of 100% and a specificity of 99.9% in detecting atrial tachycardia/fibrillation [41]. In particular, among detected episodes of atrial tachycardia/fibrillation, 98% of atrial fibrillation episodes are correctly identified, while 88% of atrial tachycardia episodes are correctly identified (98% for atrial cycle lengths <300 ms). The main cause of false-positive detections of atrial tachycardia is intermittent sensing for brief periods (lasting 2.6±2 min) of far-field R waves during sinus tachycardia.

The efficacy of the Metrix system in converting atrial fibrillation is 96% (using a mean of three shocks). Taking into account, however, that atrial fibrillation recurs early (within 1 min) in 27% of cases, and that only in some cases can the sinus rhythm be definitely restored, the overall success rate is 86% [40].

The efficacy of the Jewel AF in converting atrial tachycardia is 87%-89% with bursts, 23%-31% with 50 Hz, and 75%-100% with shock. Its efficacy in converting atrial fibrillation is 17%-40% with 50 Hz and 88%-92% with shock [42, 43].

In patients with an ICD implanted for ventricular arrhythmias, some authors [44] reported the termination of 48% of atrial tachycardia/fibrillation episodes. In addition, other authors [45] reported a decrease in the mean atrial tachycardia/fibrillation burden by 87%, in a crossover study of an algorithm programmed to be off or on. No ventricular proarrhythmia has been reported either for the Metrix system or for the Jewel AF.

As to long-term complications, among 187 patients with Metrix devices implanted, during a follow-up of 19.9 months no coronary sinus perforation or death has been observed [46]. Complications include lead dislodgement (0.5%), high defibrillation threshold (1.1%), infections (0.5%), pericarditis (1.1%), etc. The complication-free rate is 94.4%±2.0% at 2 years.

Shocks can be self-administered by patients. In 51 selected patients the Metrix system has been tested in the patient-controlled mode. Patients administering treatment outside hospital successfully terminated 81% of spontaneous episodes, versus 84% in hospital. No inappropriate shock was discharged [47]. Similar good results results were also obtained with the Jewel AF [48].

An unresolved problem of the atrial defibrillator is the tolerability of shocks [49, 50]. Any defibrillator shock between 1 and 3 J produces discomfort and any shock above 3 J produces pain in most patients. The mean defibrillator threshold is generally higher than 3 J. For example, in the Jewel AF the threshold at the time of implantation was 5.3±4.4 J. In a recent report Ricci et al. [51], grading the discomfort produced by shock on a scale ranging from 1 (not perceived) to 5 (severe discomfort), found that in the case of a single successful shock the discomfort score was 2.9±0.7, while in the case of multiple/unsuccessful shock the discomfort score was 3.9±1.

In the case of regular atrial arrhythmias, the Jewel AF is able to obtain the restoration of sinus rhythm in a significant number of patients by atrial bursts without pain. The Metrix system can only deliver shocks. In both devices, however, in most instances the device eliminates a symptom by producing another symptom. As a consequence, Geller J et al. [52] reported that after a follow-up of about 2 years, only 42% of patients with the Metrix system continued to use the device to deliver shocks, while in 26% it was explanted. In contrast, however, Gold et al. [53] suggested that with the Jewel AF the number of patients self-administering shock therapy does not reduce over time.

In conclusion, the atrial defibrillator is efficacious, safe, and sometimes well tolerated by patients. Further, it is able to reduce atrial tachycardia/fibrillation burden. Unfortunately, no data are available about its effect on quality of life and on morbidity and mortality.

Possible Alternative Strategies in Atrial Fibrillation and the Role of Implantable Devices

The AFFIRM study [54] has recently suggested that the strategy of rate control has no worse results than serial cardioversion and drug prophylaxis in terms of both survival and quality of life. The AFFIRM study contains two important messages: (1) abandoning sinus rhythm is not necessarily a losing strategy; (2) the effort to maintain sinus rhythm at any cost is not necessarily a winning strategy. The AFFFIRM results further support the hypothesis that when treating atrial fibrillation there is no "best strategy" which must be applied to any patient; but the best strategy must be tailored to each patient individually.

At present many therapeutic options are available in atrial fibrillation: (1) rate control, (2) serial conventional cardioversions followed by drug prophylaxis, (3) pill in the pocket, (4) ablate and pace, (5) ablation of the substrate, (6) ablation of triggering foci, and (7) implantable devices.

The role of implantable devices is not clearly defined. Devices with prevention algorithms should theoretically be of benefit to patients in whom the substrate (slow conduction, dispersion of refractoriness) has a predominant role in the occurrence of the arrhythmia. In contrast, in patients with rapidly firing foci no rationale for these devices can be identified. The available scientific data suggest that in some patients they may reduce the burden of atrial fibrillation. Also in these patients, however, their real clinical usefulness must be better defined. Their impact on quality of life, morbidity and mortality are uncertain.

The implantable atrial defibrillator is a palliative device which interrupts but does not prevent atrial tachycardia/fibrillation. Prompt defibrillation of atrial fibrillation, avoiding atrial remodeling, may reduce atrial fibrillation burden, but there is no proof that it may eliminate atrial fibrillation recurrences. In addition, in patients with recurrent atrial fibrillation the superiority of prompt intracardiac defibrillation over conventional cardioversion delivered after a delay of some hours has yet to be demonstrated.

The patients in whom an atrial defibrillator is primarily indicated are few. In contrast, the patients in whom an implantable atrial defibrillator is not primarily indicated are many: patients with paroxysmal (self-limiting) atrial fibrillation; those with frequent episodes which would require multiple shocks; those with persistent atrial fibrillation whose episodes are not very frequent (i.e., 1-2/year) and can be treated by conventional methods; those with a high threshold and/or who do not easily tolerate shocks; those who can derive benefit from other procedures (ablate and pace, ablation, etc.); and, finally, patients in whom conservative treatment (rate control and anticoagulants) is well tolerated.

In contrast, patients in whom ICD implantation is indicated and who may benefit from algoritms that can electrically interrupt atrial arrhythmias probably are not so rare. About 25%-50% of patients who receive an ICD for primary or secondary prevention of malignant arrhythmias develop atrial arrhythmias

[51, 55] which can cause various problems: angina, hypotension, cardiac insufficiency. Furthermore, in these patients, who frequently have a low ejection fraction, many antiarrhythmic drugs may be contraindicated. In such conditions, where a device is already implanted, the possibility of treating atrial tachycardias (by bursts in addition to shocks) with prompt restoration of sinus rhythm, in hospital or at home by the patient himself, may be a useful option that would probably favor a reduction of costs and of hospitalizations.

References

1. Allessie MA, Konings KTS, Kirchof CJHJ et al (1996) Electrophysiologic mechanisms of perpetuation of atrial fibrillation. Am J Cardiol 77:10A-23A
2. Allessie MA, Boyden PA, Camm AJ et al (2001) Pathophysiology and prevention of atrial fibrillation. Circulation 103:769-777
3. Waktare J, Hnatkova K, Sopher S et al (2001) The role of atrial ectopics in initiating paroxysmal atrial fibrillation. Eur Heart J 22:333-339
4. Pristowsky EN (1995) Tachycardia-induced tachycardia: a mechanism of initiation of atrial fibrillation. In: Di Marco JP, Prystowsky EN (eds) Atrial arrhhythmias: state of the art. Futura, Armonk, NY, pp 81-95
5. Delise P, Gianfranchi L, Paparella N et al (1997) Clinical usefulness of slow pathway ablation in patients with both paroxysmal atrioventricular nodal reentrant tachycardia and atrial fibrillation. Am J Cardiol 79:1421-1423
6. Jais P, Haïssaguerre M, Shah DC et al (1997) A focal source of atrial fibrillation treated by discrete radiofrequency ablation. Circulation 95: 572-576
7. Ogawa S, Dreyfus L, Osmick M (1977) Longitudinal dissociation of Bachmann's bundle as a mechanism of paroxysmal supraventricular tachycardia. Am J Cardiol 40: 915-922
8. Wang J, Liu L, Feng J et al (1996) Regional and functional factors determining induction and mainteinance of atrial fibrillation in dogs. Am J Physiol 273:H148-H158
9. Ausma J, Wijffels M, van Eys G et al (1997) Differentiation of atrial cardiomyocits as a result of chronic atrial fibrillation. Am J Pathol 151:985-997
10. Murgatroyd FD, Slade AKB, Sopher SM et al (1995) Efficacy and tolerability of transvenous low energy cardioversion of paroxysmal atrial fibrillation in humans. J Am Coll Cardiol 25:1347-1353
11. Corò L, Delise P, Bertaglia E et al (2001) The duration of atrial fibrillation influences the long-term efficay of low-energy internal cardioversion. Ital Heart J 2:388-393
12. Hesselson AB, Parsonnet V, Bernstein AD, Bonavita GJ (1992) Deleterious effects of long-term single chamber ventricular pacing in sick sinus syndrome: the hidden benefits of dual-chamber pacing. J Am Coll Cardiol 19:1542-1549
13. Stangl K, Seitz K, Wirzfeld A, Alt E, Blomer H (1990) Differences between atrial single chamber pacing (AAI) and ventricular single chamber pacing (VVI) with respect to prognosis and antyarrhythmic effects in patients with sick sinus syndrome. Pacing Clin Electrophysiol 13:2080-2085
14. Sgarbossa EB, Pinski SL, Maloney JD et al (1993) Chronic atrial fibrillation and stroke in paced patients with sick sinus syndrome: relevance of clinical characteristics and pacing modalities. Circulation 88:1045-1053
15. Anderson HR, Nielsen JC, Thomsen PEB et al (1997) Long-term follow-up of patients from a randomized trial of atrial versus ventricular pacing for sick-sinus syndrome.

Lancet 350:1210-1216
16. Lamas GA, Orav J, Stambler BS et al (1998) Quality of life and clinical outcomes in elderly patients treated with ventricular pacing compared with dual-chamber pacing. N Engl J Med 338:1097-1104
17. Gillis AM, Wyse DG, Connolly SJ et al (1999) Atrial pacing periablation for prevention of atrial fibrillation. Circulation 99:2553-2558
18. Gillis AM, Connolly SJ, Lacombe P et al (2000) Randomized crossover comparison of DDDR versus VDD pacing after atrioventricular junction ablation for prevention of atrial fibrillation. Circulation 102:736-741
19. Skanes AC, Krahn AD, Yee R et al (2001) Progression to chronic atrial fibrillation after pacing: the Canadian Trial of Physiologic Pacing. J Am Coll Cardiol 38:167-182
20. Spencer WH, Zhu DW, Markovitz T, Badruddin SM, Zoghbi WA (1997) Atrial septal pacing: a method for pacing both atria simultaneously. Pacing Clin Electrophysiol 20:2739-2745
21. Papageorgiou P, Anselme F, Kirchof CJ et al (1997) Coronary sinus pacing prevents induction of atrial fibrillation. Circulation 96:1893-1898
22. Katsivas A, Manolis AG, Lazaris E, Vassilopoulos C, Louvros N (1998) Atrial septal pacing to synchronize atrial depolarization in patients with delayed interatrial conduction. Pacing Clin Electrophysiol 21:2220-2225
23. Roithinger FX, Abou-Harb M, Pachinger O, Hintringer F (2001) The effect of the atrial pacing site on the atrial activation time. Pacing Clin Electrophysiol 24:316-322
24. Bailin SJ, Adler S, Giudici M (2001) Prevention of chronic atrial fibrillation by pacing in the region of Bachmann's bundle: results of a multicenter randomized trial. J Cardiovasc Electrophysiol 12:912-917
25. Padeletti L, Pieragnoli P, Ciapetti C et al (2001) Randomized crossover comparison of right atrial appendage pacing versus interatrial septum pacing for prevention of paroxysmal atrial fibrillation in patients with sinus bradycardia. Am Heart J 142:1047-1055
26. Gerstenfeld EP, Hill MR, French SN et al (1999) Evaluation of right and biatrial temporary pacing for the prevention of atrial fibrillation after coronary bypass surgery. J Am Coll Cardiol 33:1981-1988
27. Fan K, Lee KL, Chiu CSW et al (2000) Effects of biatrial pacing in prevention of postoperative atrial fibrillation after coronary artery bypass surgery. Circulation 102:755-760
28. Daoud EG, Dabir R, Archanbeau M, Morady F, Strickberger SA (2000) Randomized, double-blind trial of simultaneous right and left atrial epicardial pacing for prevention of post-open heart surgery atrial fibrillation. Circulation 102:761-765
29. Levy T, Fotopoulos G, Wallker S et al (2000) Randomized controlled study investigating the effect of biatrial pacing in prevention of atrial fibrillation after coronary bypass grafting. Circulation 102:1382-1387
30. Leclerq JF, De Sisti A, Fiorello P et al (2000) Is dual site better than single site right atrial pacing in the prevention of atrial fibrillation? Pacing Clin Electrophysiol 23:2101-2107
31. Garrigue S, Barold S, Cazau S et al (1998) Prevention of atrial arrhythmias during DDD pacing by atrial overdrive. Pacing Clin Electrophysiol 21:1751-1759
32. Defaye P, Dournaux F, Mouton E (1998) Prevalence of supraventricular arrhythmias from the automated analysis of data stored in the DDD pacemakers of 617 patients: the AIDA study. Pacing Clin Electrophysiol 21:250-255
33. Levy T, Walker S, Rochelle J, Paul V (1999) Evaluation of biatrial pacing, right atrial pacing and no pacing in patients with drug refractory atrial fibrillation. Am J Cardiol

84:426-429
34. Murgatroyd FD, Nitzche R, Slade AKB et al (1999) A new pacing algorithm for overdrive suppression of atrial fibrillation. Pacing Clin Electrophysiol 17:1966-1973
35. Israel CW, Lawo T, Lemke B, Gronefeld G, Hohnloser SH (2000) Atrial pacing in the prevention of paroxysmal atrial fibrillation: first results of a new combined algorithm. Pacing Clin Electrophysiol 23:1888-1890
36. Funk RC, Adamec R, Lurje L et al (2000) Atrial overdriving is beneficial in patients with atrial arrhythmias: first results of the PROVE study. Pacing Clin Electrophysiol 23:1891-1893
37. Carlson MD et al (2001) Dinamic atrial overdrive pacing decreases symptomatic atrial arrhythmia burden in patients with sinus node dysfunction. Circulation 104 [Suppl]:II-383
38. Ricci R, Santini M, Puglisi A et al (2001) Impact of consistent atrial pacing algorithm on premature atrial complex number and paroxysmal atrial fibrillation recurrences in brady-tachy syndrome: a randomized prospective cross over study. J Interv Cardiac Electrophysiol 5:33-44
39. Anselme F, Saoudi N, Cribier A (2000) Pacing in prevention of atrial fibrillation: the PIPAF studies. J Cardiovasc Electrophysiol 4:177-184
40. Wellens HJJ, Lau CP, Luderitz B et al (1998) Atrioverter: an implantable device for the treatment of atrial fibrillation. Circulation 98:1651-1165
41. Swerdlow CD, Schsls W, Dijkman B et al (2000) Detection of atrial fibrillation and flutter by a dual-chamber implantable cardioverter-defibrillator. Circulation 101: 878-885
42. Wharton M (1998) Treatment of spontaneous atrial tachyarrythmias with the Medtronic 7250 Jewel AF: worldwide clinical experience. Circulation 98 [Suppl]: I-190
43. Sulke N, Bailin SJ, Swerdlow CD et al (1999) Worldwide clinical experience with a dual chamber defibrillator in patients with atrial fibrillation and flutter. Eur Heart J 20:114
44. Adler SW, Wolpert C, Warman EN et al (2001) Efficacy of pacing therapies for treating atrial tachyarrhythmias in patients with ventricular arrhythmias receiving a dual-chamber implantable cardioverter defibrillator. Circulation 104:887-892
45. Friedman PA, Dijkman B, Barman E et al (2001) Atrial therapies reduce atrial arrhythmia burden in defibrillator patients. Circulation 104:1023-1028
46. Timmermans C, Wellens H, Lau CP et al (2000) Chronic safety of an implanted coronary vein lead in atrial defibrillator patients. Europace Suppl 1:D275
47. Jung W, Wolpert C, Herwig S, Lüderitz B (1999) Implantable atrial defibrillator: what are the future perspectives? In: Raviele A (ed) Cardiac arrhythmias 1999. Springer, Milan pp 125-130
48. Hoyt RH, Ben Jomson W, Bailin S et al (2001) Long term results with the implantable atrial defibrillator. Pacing Clin Electrophysiol 24:684-689
49. Cannom DS (2000) Atrial fibrillation: nonpharmacologic approaches. Am J Cardiol 85:25D-35D
50. Timmermans C, Wellens HJ (1998) Effect of device-mediated therapy on symptomatic episodes of atrial fibrillation. J Am Coll Cardiol 31:331
51. Ricci R, Pignalberi C, Disertori M et al (2002) Efficacy of a dual chamber defibrillator with atrial antitachycardia functions in treating spontaneous atrial tachyarrhythmias in patients with life-threathening ventricular tachyarrhythmias. Eur Heart J 23:1471-1479
52. Geller CJ, Reek S, Timmermans C et al (2001) Treatment of atrial fibrillation with an implantable defibrillator: long term results. Pacing Clin Electrophysiol 24:225

53. Gold MR, Sulke N, Schwartzman DS et al (2001) Clinical experience with a dual-chamber implantable cardioverter defibrillator to treat atrial tachyarrhythmias. J Cardiovasc Electrophysiol 12:1247-1253
54. The AFFIRM Investigators (2002) Atrial fibrillation follow up investigation of rhythm management. Am Heart J 143:991-1001
55. Schmitt C, Montero M, Melichercik J et al (1998) Significance of supraventricular tachyarrhythmias in patients with implanted pacing cardioverter defibrillators. Pacing Clin Electrophysiol 17:295-302

Criteria for Selection of Patients with Atrial Fibrillation to Receive a Dual-Site ICD

E. Occhetta[1], F. Paltrinieri[2], C. Vassanelli[1]

Atrial fibrillation is the most common sustained tachyarrhythmia and is increasing in prevalence as the population ages [1, 2]. It causes symptoms such as palpitations and dyspnea, but is also associated with stroke, heart failure, and an increasing risk of hospitalization and death. Over one-third of hospital admissions for arrhythmias are secondary to atrial fibrillation [3]. Restoration and maintenance of normal sinus rhythm by means of cardioversion is the first treatment option for clinicians. The choice of therapeutic intervention is generally guided by the severity and duration of the patients' symptoms and their tolerance or response to intervention.

There have been several review articles discussing atrial fibrillation and outlining the existing treatment options for atrial fibrillation. Wijffels et al. [4] have introduced the concept that "atrial fibrillation begets atrial fibrillation". Previous studies have shown that paroxysmal atrial fibrillation can, over time, transform into chronic atrial fibrillation. Wijffels's group demonstrated this phenomenon in the experimental laboratory, increasing the frequency of atrial fibrillation and the duration of each episode.

Current treatment of atrial fibrillation consists of pharmacological therapy, the surgical Maze procedure, ablative procedures, and internal/external electrical cardioversion. Drug therapy consists of rate control plus anticoagulation or rhythm control with antiarrhythmic medications. Neither of these two strategies is ideal: anticoagulation does not eliminate the risk of stroke, and the antiarrhythmic drugs often do not maintain sinus rhythm [5, 6]. Both approaches also entail a risk of side effects and complications.

Surgical treatment of atrial fibrillation requires an open chest procedure. Ablative procedures for ventricular rate control cause pacemaker dependency and require subsequent implementation of a permanent pacemaker ("ablate and pace"). Ablative procedures for treatment of atrial fibrillation (linear lesions and/or pulmonary veins ablation) are still under investigation.

[1]Divisione Clinicizzata di Cardiologia, Facoltà di Medicina e Chirurgia di Novara, Università degli Studi del Piemonte Orientale, Novara; [2] Guidant Italia, Milan, Italy

Internal cardioversion of atrial fibrillation is a promising treatment for recurrent persistent atrial fibrillation. New electrical therapeutic options (pacing and/or defibrillation) will influence the management of atrial fibrillation. The fundamental function of the pacemaker is to prevent a fall in the heart rate. The actual percentage of pacing depends on the relationship between the programmed lower rate limit and the native heart rate. The faster the setting of the pacemaker, the more it will override the heart ("overdrive" pacing). In addition to influencing the pattern of atrial depolarization, atrial pacing most likely suppresses premature atrial beats, which precede and trigger episodes of atrial fibrillation [7, 8]. Both of these effects reduce the chance of atrial fibrillation starting, particularly when atrial pacing predominates over native atrial activity.

Several prospective studies have demonstrated that a faster atrial pacing rate results in a higher percentage of paced beats and fewer episodes of atrial fibrillation. In one small trial in which the atrial pacing rate was 10 beats per minute higher than the mean heart rate [9], the incidence of atrial arrhythmias was significantly reduced over a 30-day period, and atrial fibrillation was eliminated in 14 of the 28 patients. A recent trial achieved a rate of atrial pacing of 93% of the recorded time with the use of the dynamic atrial overdrive algorithm and decreased by 25% the number of days on which atrial fibrillation occurred [10].

Although aggressive atrial pacing may help to prevent atrial fibrillation, it has no effect on atrial fibrillation once it has occurred. Sinus rhythm should be restored soon after the onset of atrial fibrillation in order to minimize the risk of stroke, to rapidly reestablish physiological hemodynamics, and to avoid the electrical changes in the atria that tend to maintain a fibrillatory substrate [4,11]. In the past the available devices were used exclusively to treat supraventricular tachycardias that are electrically organized, such as atrioventricular node reentry and atrial flutter, and therefore amenable to termination by rapid atrial pacing [12, 13]. However, rapid pacing did not interrupt atrial fibrillation.

Advances in technology, such as the Metrix implantable atrial defibrillator (Inontrol Inc., USA), have now demonstrated proof-of-concept for implantable defibrillators to treat atrial fibrillation patients. Data obtained from clinical testing of the Metrix demonstrate that automatic internal cardioversion of atrial fibrillation is safe and effective, as summarized in the May 2000 Metrix implantable atrial defibrillator annual progress report [14]: 5,616 atrial defibrillation shocks have been delivered (in 65 patients), with no incidence of ventricular proarrhythmia. Successful atrial fibrillation conversion to normal sinus rhythm was evaluated in the hospital and ambulatory settings. The observed therapy phase, where commanded cardioversion was monitored by health care professionals, reported atrial fibrillation conversion acutely (device shock efficacy) and 1 h after atrial fibrillation (clinical conversion). In the observational period, device shock efficacy was reported to be 95.3% (302/317 episodes) and clinical conversion was 84.9% (265/312 episodes). In the ambulatory setting (the out-of-hospital therapy phase), where atrial fibrillation conversion was evaluated without external monitoring, the reported clinical conversion was 90% (557/619 episodes).

Other implantable devices [15] which treat atrial arrhythmia have reported 24% (74/308 episodes) conversion efficacy in converting atrial fibrillation to normal sinus rhythm using burst pacing methodologies, and an 80% (86/108 episodes) conversion efficacy rate of atrial defibrillation. Updated versions of these devices are currently in use.

The Prizm AVT (Guidant Inc., USA) is a multifunctional device designed to provide ventricular cardioversion/defibrillation therapy as well as ventricular antitachycardia pacing (ATP) and dual-chamber adaptive-rate bradycardia therapy (DDDR). In addition to the ventricular detection and therapy features available, this device can deliver rapid atrial pacing to treat atrial arrhythmias. The shocks for atrial defibrillation can be activated automatically or by the patient himself, who is allowed to also program them to discharge automatically in the early morning while he is asleep.

Theoretically, prompt cardioversion may prevent the risk of thrombus formation and stroke, although this outcome has not yet been studied.

These various therapies for atrial arrhythmias have been very safe, with no reported instances of ventricular proarrhythmia. Special pacing functions, such as ventricular rate regulation for the reduction of ventricular cycle length variability, and atrial pacing preference, are implemented in the devices to reduce the occurrence of ventricular and atrial tachyarrhythmias.

Atrial defibrillator therapy is currently indicated only for a small subgroup of patients with symptomatic, drug-refractory atrial fibrillation, since there is no evidence that treating asymptomatic episodes of atrial fibrillation might give a clinical benefit. The frequency of atrial fibrillation is another important variable. The ideal patient population for this invasive antiarrhythmic strategy has not yet been defined. Because approximately 45% of patients who receive an implantable defibrillator for ventricular arrhythmias also have atrial fibrillation [16], a combined treatment device may also be appropriate.

Recent studies have shown that these devices can significantly decrease the incidence of atrial fibrillation and improve the quality of life [17]. Although the current guidelines for the management of atrial fibrillation predominantly encompass pharmacological strategies, implantable devices are likely to have an increasing role in the near future, particularly when they are used in combination with other treatments [18].

References

1. Benjamin EJ, Wolf PA, D'Agostino RB, Silbershatz H, Kannel WB, Levy D (1998) Impact of atrial fibrillation on the risk of death: the Framingham Heart Study. Circulation 98:946-952
2. Wolf PA, Mitchell JB, Baker CS, Kannel WB, D'Agostino RB (1998) Impact of atrial fibrillation on mortality, stroke, and medical costs. Ann Intern Med 158:229-234

3. Baily D, Lehmann MH, Schumacher DN, Steinman RT, Meissner MD (1992) Hospitalization for arrhythmias in the United States: importance of atrial fibrillation. Am J Cardiol 19:14A
4. Wijffels M, Kirschhof C, Boersma L, Allessie M (1994) Atrial fibrillation begets atrial fibrillation. In: Atrial fibrillation: mechanisms and therapeutic strategies. Futura, Armonk, pp 195-201
5. Nattel S, Hadjis T, Talajic M (1994) The treatment of atrial fibrillation: an evaluation of drug therapy, electrical modalities and therapeutic consideration. Drugs 48:345-371
6. Ganz LI, Antman EM (1997) Antiarrhythmic drug therapy in the management of atrial fibrillation. J Cardiovasc Electrophysiol 8:1175-1189
7. Cosio FG, Palacios J, Vidal JM, Cocina EG, Gomez-Sanchez MA, Tamargo L (1983) Electrophysiologic studies in atrial fibrillation: slow conduction of premature impulses: a possible manifestation of the background for reentry. Am J Cardiol 51:122-130
8. Waktare JE, Hnatkova K, Sopher SM et al (1992) The role of atrial ectopics in initiating paroxysmal atrial fibrillation. J Am Coll Cardiol 19:1531-1535
9. Garrigue S, Barold SS, Cazeau S et al (1998) Prevention of atrial arrhythmias during DDD pacing by atrial overdrive. Pacing Clin Electrophysiol 21:1751-1759
10. Carlson MD (2001)The atrial dynamic overdrive pacing trial. North American Society of Pacing and Electrophysiology, Boston, May 2001
11. Goette A, Honeycutt C, Langberg JJ (1996) Electrical remodeling in atrial fibrillation: time course and mechanisms. Circulation 94:2968-2974
12. Fromer M, Gloor H, Kus T, Shenasa M (1990) Clinical experience with a new software based antitachycardia pacemaker for recurrent supraventricular and ventricular tachycardias. Pacing Clin Electrophysiol 13:890-899
13. Connelly DT, De Belder MA, Cunningham D et al (2000) Long-term follow up of patients treated with a software based antitachycardia pacemaker. Circulation 102:1407-1413
14. Guidant METRIX Implantable Atrial Defibrillator Annual Progress Report. Guidant Inc., USA, May 2000
15. Medtronic Jewel AF 7250 Dual-Chamber Implantable Cardioverter Defibrillator System Summary of Safety and Effectiveness. Medtronic Inc., USA, 14 June 2000
16. Best PJ, Hayes DL, Stanton MS (1999) The potential usage of dual chamber pacing in patients with implantable cardioverter defibrillators. Pacing Clin Electrophysiol 22:79-85
17. Friedman PA, Dijkman B, Warman EN et al (2001) Atrial therapies reduce atrial arrhythmia burden in defibrillator patients. Circulation 104:1023-1028
18. Cooper JM, Katcher MS, Orlov MV (2002) Implantable devices for the treatment of atrial fibrillation. N Engl J Med 346:2062-2068

Pacing, ICD, or Both for the Hybrid Therapy of Atrial Arrhythmias?

G. BORIANI[1], M. BIFFI[1], C. MARTIGNANI[1], C. CAMANINI[1], C. VALZANIA[1], I. CORAZZA[1], G. CALCAGNINI[2], P. BARTOLINI[2], A. BRANZI[1]

Introduction

Atrial fibrillation (AF) is the most common cardiac arrhythmia, and its prevalence is expected to increase further in the coming years [1]. The treatment of recurrent paroxysmal AF is frustrating in clinical practice, due to the high rate of recurrences and the lack of uniformly effective treatments [2-4]. Antiarrhythmic drugs are classically the first approach to preventing AF recurrences, but no more than 50% of patients respond to drug therapy within 1 year [2-4]. In view of this limited efficacy and the risk of proarrhythmia, especially in patients with left ventricular dysfunction, new, nonpharmacological treatments for AF are being developed [5, 6]. These treatments may be classified as: rescue (catheter-based atrial cardioversion), curative (focal ablation), suppressive (atrial pacing algorithms), and palliative (ablate and pace strategy). No definite algorithms for choosing the most appropriate treatment in the individual patient have been developed. The therapeutic approach for patients with AF remains clinical and is primarily guided by the clinical presentation of the AF. A series of important questions regarding nonpharmacological treatments are still open; they relate to the selection of candidates for any of these treatments or particular combinations of treatments, the true efficacy, the patient acceptance, the risk-benefit and cost-benefit ratios, and the related social costs.

Atrial Pacing for Atrial Tachyarrhythmias and AF Prevention

The effects of conventional atrial pacing in preventing AF recurrences need to be evaluated in patients with sick sinus syndrome at low risk of AF, in patients

[1] Institute of Cardiology, University of Bologna; [2] Department of Biomedical Engineering, Istituto Superiore di Sanità, Rome, Italy

with brady-tachy syndrome at high risk of AF, and in patients with paroxysmal AF without significant bradycardia.

In the last 10 years, a series of retrospective studies [7-12] showed that patients with sick sinus syndrome paced in the VVI mode were at higher risk of developing AF than were those paced in the AAI or DDD mode. Sgarbossa et al. [13] in a retrospective study found that VVI pacing was associated with a risk of developing chronic AF in patients with preimplantation AF but not in those without. The prospective randomized study reported by Andersen et al. [14], involving 225 patients, showed that more patients (23%) randomized to VVI pacing developed AF over a 40-month period than patients randomized to AAI pacing (14%). This difference, however, did not reach statistical significance. A prospective trial (CTOPP) recently confirmed these findings, showing that dual-chamber pacing decreased the incidence of both AF and progression to chronic AF, with a beneficial effect appearing 2 years after the implant [15]. In patients with sick sinus syndrome with a high risk of AF (brady-tachy syndrome), DDDR pacing achieved a reduction of AF episodes in comparison with both baseline and DDD pacing [16].

In patients with AF without symptomatic bradycardia, the possible mechanisms supporting a beneficial effect of pacing in AF prevention are: (1) prevention of bradycardia, (2) better adaptation of heart rate to exercise, (3) overdrive suppression of ectopic beats, and (4) shortening of long interatrial conduction due to atrial ectopic beats. The ways to positively influence the risk of AF relate to: (1) pacing mode, (2) pacing rate, (3) pacing site (single site or multisite), (4) the use of novel, dedicated pacing algorithms (consistent atrial pacing, CAP; atrial rate stabilization, ARS; dynamic atrial overdrive, DAO) and, finally, (5) the use of pacing to stop AF episodes.

Great interest has developed in recent years on the effect of pacing site on the risk of AF. The site of atrial pacing can impact on the development of AF in pacemaker patients. Multisite atrial pacing may favorably modify the atrial electrophysiological substrate in patients with paroxysmal AF [17, 18]. These findings had important implications for the application in the clinical setting of pacing techniques aimed to reduce inhomogeneities in atrial conduction and refractoriness and normalize atrial activation.

The incidence of AF appears to be higher with a pacing site in the right auricular lateral wall compared with the right auricular appendage [19], whereas pacing from the interatrial septum can reduce the interatrial conduction time and possibly prevent AF [20].

The search for better clinical results in terms of AF prevention led to the testing of pacing in alternative sites (coronary sinus, coronary sinus os, interatrial septum) and of dual/multisite atrial pacing. Clinically, multisite atrial pacing has been achieved by means of biatrial pacing (one lead in the right auricular appendage and the other in the coronary sinus to pace the left atrium) and by dual-site right atrial pacing (one lead in the appendage and the other in the interatrial septum just outside the coronary sinus os).

To date, the translation of these observations into the clinical setting has shown that multisite atrial pacing or pacing from alternative sites is more effective than single-site right auricular pacing when AF was associated with bradycardia [20, 21], but disappointing results were found in controlled studies when AF was not associated with bradycardia [22]. This finding stresses the need for further knowledge of the complex interaction between atrial pacing and the electrophysiological substrate favoring the onset of AF in specific subgroups of patients.

New pacing modalities for preventing AF recurrences include special algorithms to increase the rate of atrial pacing, leading to continuous overdrive pacing or to suppress of the pauses that follow an atrial ectopic beat [23]. These algorithms (CAP, ARS, DAO, and similar algorithms for atrial overdrive) have been evaluated or are currently under evaluation [24]. The ADOPT trial of DAO pacing showed that use of this algorithm achieved a rate of atrial pacing of 93% and decreased the number of days during which AF occurred by 25% [25]. In the AF therapy trial four overdrive pacing algorithms were used and compared with standard DDDR pacing and AAI pacing. In this trial, use of the overdrive algorithms was associated with reduction of the AF burden and an increase in sinus rhythm duration. However, many patients in the trial were excluded from analysis and this may reduce the relevance of the findings [26].

Atrial Cardioversion/Defibrillation for Atrial Tachyarrhythmias and Termination of AF

Delivery of intracardiac shocks can convert different forms of AF, even those of long duration and resistant to external cardioversion, at relatively low energies (<6-10 J) [27]. Both animal and human studies showed that catheter-based atrial defibrillation is safe and highly effective in restoring sinus rhythm. In view of the technical improvements in catheter-based atrial defibrillation, the concept of an implantable device for atrial defibrillation ("atrial defibrillator") has become a real therapeutic possibility, tested in selected groups of patients [27]. Two different devices have become available in recent years for defibrillation therapy in selected groups of patients with AF: a stand-alone atrial defibrillator (Metrix, InControl) and a dual defibrillator (Jewel AF or GEM III AT, Medtronic, or Prizm AVT, Guidant) for patients with ventricular tachyarrhythmias associated with AF or for selected patients with AF [27]. These two devices have major differences with regard to diagnosis and treatment. The most important differences are the ability of the dual defibrillator to deliver shock therapy for ventricular tachyarrhythmias and, at the atrial level, to deliver painless therapy to treat atrial tachyarrhythmias (antitachycardia pacing including 50-Hz bursts).

A number of factors may influence the choice of a device for atrial defibrillation and the treatment of selected patients. The problem of shock-induced discomfort remains one of the major limitations for a widening of the indications for these devices. Acceptance of this type of therapy could be improved in different ways: by improving atrial defibrillation thresholds, by reducing the occurrences of AF episodes in combination with other preventive interventions (drugs, pacing algorithms, etc.), and by reducing early recurrences of AF after shocks, thus minimizing the need for multiple shocks. Using antiarrhythmic drugs in combination with devices for pacing/shock therapy may have several advantages because of the possibility that these drugs may reduce AF recurrences, at least as a result of partial prophylactic efficacy, and because of the possibility that the antiarrhythmic agents may lengthen the atrial tachyarrhythmia cycle length, thus increasing the efficacy of antitachycardia pacing, or reduce the atrial defibrillation threshold and/or reduce early AF recurrences after shock delivery.

In 51 patients with atrial tachyarrhythmias (atrial tachycardias–AF) but without previous ventricular tachyarrhythmias, who underwent implantation of a Jewel AF device [27], painless therapies were effective in a high proportion of atrial tachyarrhythmias (antitachycardia pacing effective in 89% of slow atrial tachycardias), but even in arrhythmias occurring in the AF zone, (50-Hz bursts were effective in 40% of the cases). In another series [27], the efficacy of 50-Hz bursts on AF episodes occurring in the AF zone was only 27%.

Rationale for a Hybrid Approach to AF Treatment

Awareness of the limitations of pharmacological treatment has led in recent years to the development of a wide spectrum of electrical, nonpharmacological treatments. Despite a number of limitations, nonpharmacological techniques of treating AF may confer significant benefit in appropriately selected groups of patients. However, so far it has not been possible to identify a single procedure that will cure drug-refractory AF in a large percentage of patients with the best guarantees of safety and efficacy. The limitations in terms of efficacy rate of AF management based on a single treatment has led to the concept of combined or hybrid treatment. The rationale of combined or hybrid treatment is to combine different therapeutic modalities in an attempt to achieve a synergistic effect, to improve efficacy over single approaches by acting on different targets (the electrophysiological substrate, the anatomical substrate, the triggers, the modulating factors), and also to have a rescue treatment in case of failure. Given the potential effects on different targets (AF terminations, atrial conduction and refractoriness, frequency of atrial premature beats, atrial electrophysiological remodeling, atrial size), a series of treatments (antiarrhythmic drugs, internal cardioversion, atrial pacing with or without specific pacing algorithms, focal ablation, linear ablation) may be combined with the aim of achieving a synergetic effect. This approach is therefore justified by two expectations: (1) some nonpharmacological treatments may render AF responsive to previously ineffective drugs and (2) the combined use of more than one nonpharmacological treatment is expected to be required, alone or in combination with drugs, in some patients, to obtain a synergetic effect.

Prospective studies are required to evaluate the risk-benefit profile of these strategies in appropriately selected patients. Moreover the capabilities of atrial defibrillators may be associated with preventive pacing algorithms (DAO, CAP, ARS) active during sinus rhythm, and with pacing for regional entrainment during AF, in order to organize AF and reduce the atrial defibrillation threshold.

Conclusions

AF is a difficult arrhythmia to treat given the multiple factors involved in the initiation and maintenance of the arrhythmia and given the great variability of the underlying substrate, both structural (underlying heart disease) and electrophysiological. Overall, conventional treatment based on use of drugs is characterized by limited efficacy. Implantable devices for pacing and cardioversion/defibrillation are undergoing very rapid evolution and in selected patients may reduce the incidence of AF and improve the quality of life.

In view of the limitation of the conventional approach based on only a single treatment aimed at controlling AF and atrial tachyarrhythmias, a hybrid approach has been proposed. The hybrid approach is based on the use of different therapeutic modalities (pharmacological and non-pharmacological), in an attempt to achieve synergetic effects and increase overall efficacy while decreasing adverse effects. In line with this trend, the use of devices that can provide dual chamber pacing and atrial and ventricular defibrillation in combination with drugs or other treatments, including ablation in appropriately selected cases, is probably one way towards treatment of appropriately selected groups of patients in the future. What we need is to define the subset of patients for which this complex and expensive approach seems to be cost-effective. Finally, it must be considered that multipurpose devices will be available in the near future. These devices will be able to treat a series of arrhythmic problems such as bradyarrhythmias, tachyarrhythmias, ventricular tachycardia, and ventricular fibrillation, and also to improve and monitor hemodynamics.

References

1. Kannel WB, Wolf PA, Benjamin EJ, Levy D (1998) Prevalence, incidence, prognosis and predisposing conditions for atrial fibrillation: population-based estimates. Am J Cardiol 82:2N-9N
2. Waktare J, Camm A (1998) Acute treatment of atrial fibrillation: why and when to mantain sinus rhythm. Am J Cardiol 81:3C-15C
3. Van Gelder I, Crijns HJGM (1998) Cardioversion of atrial fibrillation and subsequent maintenance of sinus rhythm. Pacing Clin Electrophysiol 20:2675-2683
4. Boriani G, Biffi M, Branzi A, Magnani B (1998) Pharmacological treatment of atrial fibrillation: a review on prevention of recurrences and control of ventricular respon-

se. Arch Gerontol Geriatr 27:127-139
5. Lesh MD, Kalman JM, Roithinger FX, Karch MR (1997) Potential role of hybrid therapy for atrial fibrillation. Semin Interv Cardiol 2:267-271
6. Krol RB, Saksena S, Prakash A (2000) New devices and hybrid therapies for treatment of atrial fibrillation. J Interv Card Electrophysiol 4:163-169
7. Feuer J, Shalding A, Messeguer J (1989) Influence of cardiac pacing mode on long-term development of atrial fibrillation. Am J Cardiol 64:1376-1379
8. Grimm W, Langfeld H, Maisch B, Kochsiek K (1990) Symptom, cardiovascular profile and spontaneous ECG in paced patients: a five year follow-up study. Pacing Clin Electrophysiol 13:2086-2090
9. Hesselson A, Parsonnet V, Bernstein A, Bonavita G (1992) Deleterious effects of long-term single chamber ventricular pacing in patients with sick sinus syndrome: the hidden benefits of dual-chamber pacing. J Am Coll Cardiol 19:1542-1549
10. Rosenqvist M, Brandt J, Schuller H (1988) Long-term pacing in sinus node disease: effects of stimulation mode on cardiovascular morbidity and mortality. Am Heart J 116:16-22
11. Stangl K, Seitz K, Wirtzfeld A, Alt E, Blomer H (1990) Differences between atrial single chamber pacing (AAI) and ventricular single chamber pacing (VVI) with respect to prognosis and antiarrhythmic effect on patients with sick sinus syndrome. Pacing Clin Electrophysiol 13:2080-2085
12. Zanini R, Facchinetti A, Gallo G, Cazzamalli L, Bonandi L, Dei Cas L (1990) Morbidity and mortality of patients with sinus node disease: comparative effects of atrial and ventricular pacing. Pacing Clin Electrophysiol 13:2076-2079
13. Sgarbossa E, Pinsky S, Maloney J, Simmons T, Wilkoff B, Castel L, Trohman R (1993) Chronic atrial fibrillation and stroke in paced patients with sick sinus syndrome. Circulation 88:1045-1053
14. Andersen H, Thuesen L, Bagger J, Vesterllund T, Thomsen P (1994) Prospective randomised trial of atrial versus ventricular pacing in sick sinus syndrome. Lancet 344:1523-1528
15. Cooper JM, Katcher MS, Orlov MV (2002) Implantable devices for the treatment of atrial fibrillation. N Engl J Med 346:2062-2068
16. Boriani G, Botto G, Frabetti L, Biffi M, Bellocci F, Bernabò D, Capucci A, Dini P, Leoni G, Lisi F, Marchini A, Morocchini P, Nicotra G, Nipro P, Puglisi A, Ricci R, Spampinato A, Cavaglia S, De Seta F (1998) Does dual chamber pacing prevent paroxysmal atrial fibrillation in brady-tachy patients? G Ital Cardiol 28:121-124
17. Papageorgiou P, Anselme F, Kirchhof C, Monahan K, Rasmussen C, Epstein L, Josephson M (1997) Coronary sinus pacing prevence induction of atrial fibrillation. Circulation 96:1893-1898
18. Yu W, Chen S, Tai C, Feng A, Chang M (1997) Effects of different atrial pacing modes on atrial electrophysiology: implicating the mechanism of biatrial pacing in prevention of atrial fibrillation. Circulation 96:2992-2996
19. Siedl K, Hamer B, Schwick N (1995) Is the site of atrial lead implantation in dual chamber pacing of importance for preventing atrial fibrillaton? The hidden benefit of lead implantation in the right atrial appendage (abstract). Pacing Clin Electrophysiol 18:1820
20. Padeletti L, Porciani M, Michelucci A, Colella A, Ticci P, Vena S, Costoli A, Ciapetti C, Pieragnoli P, Gensini G (1999) Interatrial septum pacing: a new approach to prevent recurrent atrial fibrillation. J Interv Card Electrophysiol 3:35-43
21. Delfaut P, Saksena S (2000) Electrophysiological assessment in selecting patients for multisite atrial pacing. J Interv Card Electrophysiol 4:81-85

22. Levy T, Walker S, Rochelle J, Paul V (1999) Evaluation of biatrial pacing, right atrial pacing, and no pacing in patients with drug refractory atrial fibrillation. Am J Cardiol 84:426-429
23. Boriani G, Biffi M, Padeletti A, Spampinato A, Pignalberi C, Botto G, Grammatico A, Piana M, De Seta F, Branzi A (2000) Evaluation of consistent atrial pacing and atrial rate stabilisation algorithms for suppressing recurrent paroxysmal atrial fibrillation in brady-tachy syndrome (abstract). Eur Heart J 21:604
24. Boriani G, Biffi M, Padeletti L, Spampinato A, Botto G, Pignalberi C, Grammatico A, Piana M, Cavaglià S, De Seta F, Branzi A (1999) Consistent atrial pacing (CAP) and atrial rate stabilisation (ARS): new algorithms to suppress recurrent paroxysmal atrial fibrillation. G Ital Cardiol 29:88-90
25. Carlson MD (2001) The Atrial Dynamic Overdrive Pacing Trial. Presented at the late breaking clinical trials session of the 22nd Annual Scientific Meeting of the North American Society of Pacing and Electrophysiology, Boston, 2-5 May 2001
26. Daubert JC, Mabo P (2002) Implantable devices to treat atrial fibrillation: real prospects or just new gimmicks? Europace 4:161-164
27. Boriani G, Biffi M, Martignani C, Luceri R, Bartolini P, Branzi A (2002) Current clinical perspectives on implantable devices for atrial defibrillation. Curr Opin Cardiol 17:82-89

Surgical Treatment of Atrial Fibrillation During Mitral Valve Surgery

A. Cavallaro, L. Patanè

Introduction

Chronic atrial fibrillation (AF) is the most common arrhythmia in mitral valve (MV) disease, occurring in 30%-85% of all patients. It is associated with excessive morbidity and mortality [1]. Up to 80% of these patients will remain in AF after surgical correction of the underlying cardiac disease. The goal for patients with MV surgery and permanent AF is not only restoration and optimal function of the MV but also return to permanent normal sinus rhythm (SR), restoration of biatrial transport function, and prevention of thromboembolism.

Physiopatology

The pathogenesis of AF associated with MV disease is uncertain. In opposition to the multiple reentrant circuits hypothesis, recent electrophysiological study suggests that in many patients AF may be caused by reentry circuits limited to specific areas (focal activation). This critical zone is present at the junction of the left atrium (LA) with the pulmonary veins (PVs). It contains stable reentrant circuits, houses foci that trigger AF, and contains critical fibers involved in AF maintenance such as the ligament of Marshall [2]. The "critical zone" hypotesis explains why the LA is so important for the ablation to be successful, and why more limited procedures aimed at the electrical isolation of discrete atrial regions, utilizing atriotomy, radiofrequency ablation, cryoablation, or other energy sources.

Surgical Ablation Procedures

The Cox Maze III procedure (Fig.1) is the culmination of multiple surgical approaches (LA isolation, "corridor" procedure, and Maze I and II) for the

Centro Cuore Morgagni, Pedara (CT), Italy

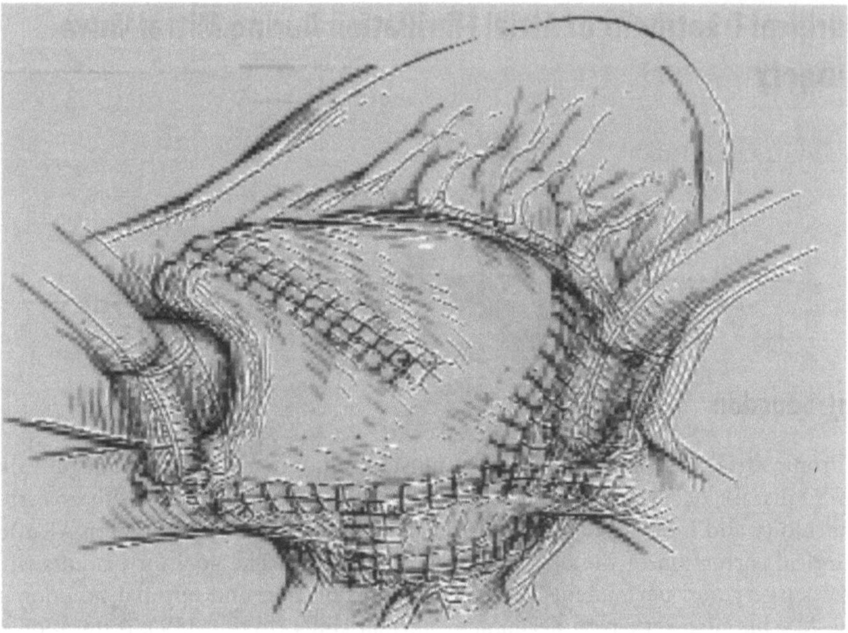

Fig. 1. Appearance of the completed Maze III procedure

treatment of supraventricular arrhythmias [3]. The success of the Maze procedure in curing AF has generated multiple modifications in the attempt to simplify the operation, particularly when associated MV disease is present. The procedure is based on the concept that multiple precise incisions and suture lines in the right and left atria, may be used to reduce atrial critical mass, interrupt all possible macro-reentrant circuits responsible for this arrhythmia, and direct normal sinus impulses to travel to the atrioventricular (AV) node as they normally should. Although reported results indicate that 75% [4] to 82% [5] of patients who undergo the Maze III procedure are relieved of AF, this procedure is nevertheless invasive, requiring median sternotomy, long cardiopulmonary bypass, cardioplegic arrest, extensive cardiac dissection, and multiple atrial incisions, and is associated with significant mortality and morbidity [5]. The relative success of the Maze procedures and the notion that isolation of the PVs and portions of the LA can eliminate AF encouraged surgeons to perform partial Maze procedures, where the incisions are made only on the LA, or to seek out other methods of isolation rather than "cutting and sewing". Three alternative energy sources are used to treat AF surgically: radiofrequency, cryothermy, and microwave. Two others, laser and ultrasound, are not completely proven at this point. The goal of all five procedures is to develop controlled lesions of coagulative necrosis and, ultimately, scar tissue to block the abnormal electrical impulses from being conducted through the heart and promote the normal conduction of impulses through the proper pathway [6].

Radiofrequency Ablation

A special radiofrequency energy catheter is used to heat the tissue and produce epicardial and/or endocardial lesions on the heart similar to the lesions of the Maze procedure. A variety of surgical techniques exist related to the type of catheter used (original multipolar, bipolar, or unipolar), the amount of energy employed (100 W, ± 65-80 °C for 80-120 s), and the types of lesions created (Melo PV encirclings, Alfieri set, etc.).

Cryoablation

Very cold temperatures (- 80°C for 2 min) are applied through a cryoprobe to create lesions. This technique is commonly used during arrhythmia surgery to complete or replace the incisions made during the Cox Maze III procedure.

Microwave Technology

A special wand-like catheter (the Flex-4 catheter) is used to direct microwave energy to create several lesions on the heart. The lesions block the conduction of abnormal electrical beats and restore a normal heartbeat. These three surgical ablation procedures (radiofrequency, cryothermy, microwave) cure AF in about 80% of patients [2].

Laser Ablation

The device, a 980-nm-diode laser, produces harmonic oscillation of water, with the production of kinetic energy and subsequent heat that causes the ablation.

The 980 nm device has a 4-mm penetration of just the laser energy, so it is quite efficient and provides a uniform distribution of the energy. This device produces lesions in 36 s and is adaptable to minimally invasive approaches because of its fiberoptics technology, but the lesions are generally a little shorter than with radiofrequency energy.

Ultrasound Ablation

Ablation by ultrasound is at a very early stage of development; it uses mechanical hyperthermia resulting from ultrasound wave propagation. The energy causes compression/refraction of the tissue, resulting in motions that produce heat. Both focused (very short lesion times) and nonfocused ablation are possible with ultrasound. It has the potential advantages of producing lesions very rapidly, tuning the depth, and monitoring the lesion by imaging as it is created. It has the disadvantages of transducers: they are less flexible and the apparatus is expensive and difficult to manufacture.

Patients and Methods

From July 1999 to August 2002, we performed a modified Maze procedure during MV surgery in 36 patients, with a mean age of 62.0 years (range 35-82 years; 57% female, 43% male) who had suffered from either intermittent or chronic AF for more than 6 months (range 9 months to 18 years, mean 41.4±48.7 months). MV disease was rheumatic in 22 patients (61.1%) and degenerative in 14. Twenty-six patients (72.2%) had MV repair. Mean LA size was 58±1.6 mm. The ablations were performed using a temperature-controlled multipolar radiofrequency probe (Therma Line, Boston Scientific). Encircling lesions around the right and left PVs were carried out epicardially (65%) before cardiopulmonary bypass or endocardially through a conventional left atriotomy. The ablation procedure was completed with two endocardial lesions, one connecting the two encircling lesions and one connecting the MV annulus (Fig. 2). After the MV procedure was performed, the left appendage was sutured. The mean cardiopulmonary bypass and aortic cross-clamp time were, respectively, 123±28.1 and 86±26.0 min. No reexploration for bleeding was necessary, and one patient needed permanent pacemaker implantation.

No patients died. Mean postoperative hospital stay was 9.2±6.4 days. At follow-up (mean 19.5±11.8 months), 27/36 (75.0%) of the patients were in stable SR, and 86% of the patients in SR 3 months after the operation had recovered biatrial contractility at echocardiographic control (Santa Cruz score 4).

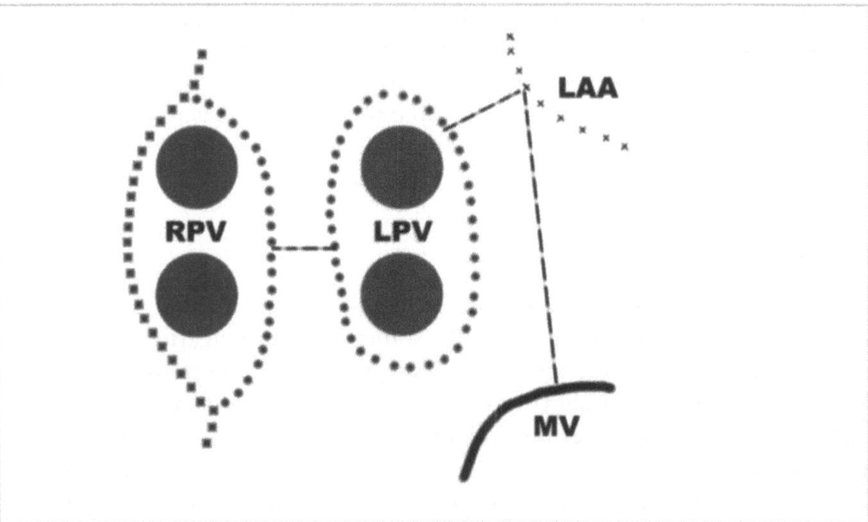

Fig. 2. Epicardial and endocardial line in radiofrequency ablation. LAA, left atrial appendage; RPV, right pulmonary veins; LPV, left pulmonary veins; MV, mitral valve. ■, incision line; •, epicardial ablations; –, endocardial ablations; x, suture line

Discussion

Persistent AF leaves patients symptomatic and at increased risk of thromboembolism even after otherwise successful MV surgery. In the last several years, ablation of atrial tissue has been accomplished using a variety of energy source devices [2, 7] as alternative to the traditional "cut and sew" approach. In order to choose the best energy source for creating atrial lesions with these alternative methods, one must consider among other factors the speed of the ablation method, confinement of the lesion to the target atrial tissue with minimum collateral damage to adjacent atrial tissue, and avoidance of damage to surrounding vital structures, e.g. esophageal injury [8]. Regardless of the method used, the goal is that the lesions should ideally be transmural and appropriate to the variable thickness and characteristics of the tissues. The atrium of a patient with rheumatic atrial pathology will be much more difficult to ablate than the atrium of a coronary bypass patient. A longer time is required to assess the end result of these techniques, because complete healing of the ablation lesions takes 3-6 months [2]. This explains the differences between early and late results of each procedure (Fig. 3). Computerized intraoperative atrial activation mapping should help and guide the surgeon in deciding on the appropriate surgical procedure for chronic AF associated with MV disease. With the new noninvasive multidetector helical computed tomographic technology [7], which provides an unprecedented level of detail concerning the dimensions and morphology of the LA and distal PVs, probably, will be possible designing interventions or deploying tools for interventions involving these structures. To evaluate the mid-term rate of success of the different procedures, a five-point (0-4) scoring system named the Santa Cruz score, based upon the postoperative atrial rhythm and effective atrial contraction, is used [9]. A score of 4 corresponds to SR and biatrial contraction. Today, the indications for ablation of chronic AF during MV surgery are extensive, except for enlarged and heavily calcified LA. This to reduce thromboembolic events and the use of anticoagulant or antiarrhythmia medications.

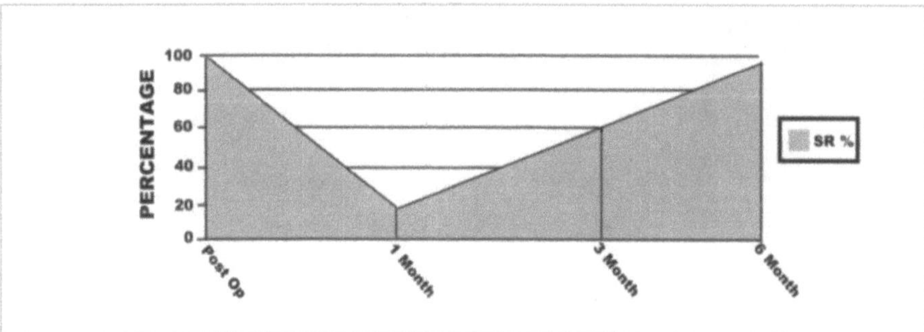

Fig. 3. Time line of sinus rhythm in patients with chronic AF after radiofrequency ablation

Conclusions

Intraoperative application energy from various sources (catheter ablation) is a valid alternative to surgical incisions to perform AF surgery. These modified "left side only" Maze procedures or mini-Maze procedures are simple, quick, efficient, safe, and reproducible methods for the treatment of chronic AF with MV disease. The various energy sources will enable development of a minimally invasive procedure for AF and will extend ablation to several cardiac diseases associated with AF. More reports are needed to evaluate their efficacy and cost/benefit ratio.

References

1. Benjamin EJ, Wolf PA, D'Agostino RB, Silbershatz H, Kannel WB, Levy D (1998) Impact of atrial fibrillation on the risk of death. The Framingham Study. Circulation 98:946-952
2. Pappone C, Rosanio S et al (2002) Theory and practice of catheter ablation of atrial fibrillation-syllabus. San Raffaele University Hospital, Milan (in Italian)
3. Cox JL, Schuessler RB et al (1991) The surgical treatment of atrial fibrillation. Development of a definitive surgical procedure. J Thorac Cardiovasc Surg 101:569-583
4. Cox JL, Jaquiss RDB et al (1995) Modification of the Maze procedure for the treatment of atrial flutter and fibrillation. Rationale and surgical results. J Thorac Cardiovasc Surg 110:485-495
5. Kosakai Y, Kawaguchi AT, Isobe F et al (1995) Modified Maze peocedure for patients with atrial fibrillation undergoing simultaneous open heart surgery. Circulation 92[Suppl 9]:II359-364
6. Benussi S, Pappone C et al (2000) A simple way to treat chronic atrial fibrillation during mitral valve surgery: the epicardial radiofrequency approach. Eur J Cardiothorac Surg 17:524-529
7. Heart Surg Forum Rev (2002) 1:1-14
8. Gillinov AM, Pettersson G et al (2001) Esophageal injury during radiofrequency ablation for atrial fibrillation. J Thorac Cardiovasc Surg 122:1239-1240
9. Melo JQ, Neves J et al (1997) When and how to report results of surgery on atrial fibrillation. Eur J Cardiothorac Surg 12:739-744

NEW APPROACHES IN ELECTRICAL TREATMENT AND MANAGEMENT OF HEART FAILURE PATIENTS

What Have We Learned from Cardiac Resynchronization Trials?

F. Zanon, E. Baracca, C. Bilato, S. Aggio, P. Zonzin

Congestive heart failure (CHF) is a very frequent cardiovascular disease. Because of the large size of the affected population and the socioeconomic consequences, the management of chronic CHF is of great interest in clinical practice. Available therapeutic strategies based on medical therapy have evolved remarkably in recent years. Despite optimal medical management, however, many patients remain severely limited in their daily activities and only a minority of these subjects can receive cardiac transplantation. Currently there are no other verified treatments besides these medical and surgical alternatives.

A common feature in heart failure is lack of electromechanical synchronization between atrial and ventricular chambers, between ventricles, and among the different regions of the individual ventricle. In the last 10 years several attempts have been made to correct atrioventricular (AV) dyssynchrony by pacing, and more recently inter- and intraventricular resynchronization therapy has been tested to treat heart failure. Initially, small single-center observational studies suggested that pacing to shorten the PR interval alone might be of benefit in patients with severe heart failure [1, 2]. These results, however, were not confirmed in a randomized controlled trial using a crossover design with a 6-week treatment period [3]. Although this study failed to demonstrate a significant clinical improvement, it was too small to be conclusive and showed that only some patients with heart failure may benefit from this intervention. However, a precise identification of these individuals remains elusive.

More recently, different trials have tested the efficacy of cardiac resynchronization therapy (CRT) in patients with severe heart failure and increased AV delay or/and evidence of cardiac dyssynchrony as showed by a prolonged QRS interval [4-6].

The first short-term results of the PATH-CHF [7, 8] and the MUSTIC [9] studies were encouraging. PATH-CHF was planned as a single-blinded, ran-

Division of Cardiology, General Hospital, Rovigo, Italy

domized, controlled crossover trial of monoventricular versus biventricular cardiac resynchronization and investigated the effects on symptoms and exercise capacity. The left ventricular pacing system was implanted via thoracotomy and periods of CRT were alternated with 4 weeks of nonpaced washout. During CRT, patients' symptoms and exercise capacity improved significantly compared to baseline and the wash-out period. These observations strongly support the efficacy of CRT. However, the small sample size and the difficulties of the implantation technique are limitations on this study.

The MUSTIC program consists of two single-blinded crossover studies with 3 month treatment periods comparing CRT versus control. All patients (NYHA class III, EF ≤35%, QRS duration ≥150 ms) had a CRT device implanted (success rate: 93%) subcutaneously with pacing leads inserted transvenously in the right ventricle and in the coronary sinus for left ventricular pacing. Patients in atrial fibrillation (AF) were to be recruited only if they had a slow basal ventricular rate or after AV node ablation. In the patients with sinus rhythm (MUSTIC-SN), CRT resulted in a significant increase in the 6-min walking distance, a substantial increase in the peak exercise oxygen consumption, improvement of the quality-of-life score, and significantly fewer hospitalizations. Patients with AF (MUSTIC-AF) showed a similar although less significant trend. The MUSTIC study is the first properly designed trial on CRT and shows that CRT improves symptoms in patients with severe heart failure and left ventricular dyssynchrony. However, the program was unable to demonstrate whether CTR was safe or truly effective in reducing long-term morbidity and mortality, since neither of these end-points was investigated in the MUSTIC study.

The MIRACLE [10] trial is the first moderately large, medium-term (6 months) parallel group study. All patients (NYHA class III/IV, EF ≤35%, QRS duration ≥ 130 ms, left ventricular end-diastolic diameter >55 mm, optimized medical treatment) received a CRT device in a double-blind follow-up fashion, so that neither the investigator nor the patient was aware of who was receiving CRT. The study reported that CRT improved symptoms, quality of life, and exercise capacity while reducing left ventricular diameters and improving contractility. However, like the MUSTIC trial, this study was not designed to investigate potential benefit on morbidity and mortality.

A number of trials are ongoing in which patients have been randomized to CTR or control. The PAVE study is enrolling patients with AF who underwent AV node ablation and will provide important additional information to MUSTIC-AF. The VecToR study is designed to assess the effects of CRT on symptoms, ventricular function, and exercise capacity, but it will also test the effects of CRT on mortality.

Several trials are investigating the efficacy of CRT on patients who also require an intracardiac cardioverter defibrillator (ICD). The VENTAK-CHF and the CONTAK-CD [11] (thoracotomy and transvenous ICD respectively) programs will test whether CRT could also reduce short-term morbidity and mortality. Preliminary results show that the number of ICD interventions was significantly lower during CRT compared to the no-pacing period.

The ongoing multicenter trials COMPANION (in United States) and PACMAN (in Europe) will determine whether biventricular pacing with and without an ICD back-up will reduce overall mortality and hospitalization and will improve exercise performance in patients with severe heart failure. The results of these trials could determine a significant expansion of ICD indications in the future [12].

In conclusion, CRT may be a useful treatment for severe symptoms of heart failure that do not respond to conventional therapy. So far, CRT trials consistently suggest efficacy of CRT in improving symptoms, and amelioration of quality of life and cardiac function with an increase in exercise capacity has been generally observed. One single small study also suggests that resynchronization may reduce the density of premature ventricular beats, while other studies report that CRT decreases the incidence and/or the duration of hospital stay. Finally, in the next few years morbidity and mortality data are expected to definitively validate CRT as an important tool in the treatment of severe heart failure.

References

1. Hochleitner M, Hortnagl H, Fridrich L et al (1992) Long-term efficacy of physiologic dual-chamber pacing in the treatment of end stage idiopathic dilated cardiomyopathy. Am J Cardiol 70:1320-1325
2. Auricchio A, Sommariva L, Salo RW et al (1993) Improvement of cardiac function in patients with severe congestive heart failure and coronary artery disease by dual chamber pacing with shortened AV delay. Pacing Clin Electrophysiol 16:2034-2043
3. Gold MR, Feliciano Z, Gottlieb SS et al (1995) Dual-chamber pacing with a short atrioventricular delay in congestive heart failure: a randomized study. J Am Coll Cardiol 26:967-973
4. Cazeau S, Ritter P, Lazarus A et al (1996) Multisite pacing for end-stage heat failure: early experience. Pacing Clin Electrophysiol 19:1748-1757
5. Gras D, Mabo P, Tang T et al (1998) Multisite pacing as a supplemental treatment of congestive heart failure. Pacing Clin Electrophysiol 21:2249-2255
6. Daubert JC, Ritter P, Le Breton H et al (1998). Permanent left ventricular pacing with transvenous leads inserted into the coronary veins. Pacing Clin Electrophysiol 21:239-245
7. Auricchio A (1999) Effect of pacing chamber and atrioventricular delay on acute systolic function of paced patients with congestive heart failure. The Pacing Therapies for Congestive Heart Failure Study Group. The Guidant Congestive Heart Failure Research Group. Circulation 99:2993-3001
8. Auricchio A, Stellbrink C, Sack S et al (1999). The pacing therapies for congestive heart failure (PATH-CHF) study: rationale, design and endpoints of a prospective randomized multicenter study. Am J Cardiol 83:130D-135D
9. Cazeau S, Leclercq C, Lavergne T et al (2001) Multisite stimulation in Cardiomyopathies (MUSTIC) Study Investigators. Effects of multisite biventricular pacing in patients with heart failure and intraventricular conduction delay. N Engl J Med 344:873-880

10. Abraham WT (2000) Rationale and design of randomized clinical trial to assess the safety and efficacy of cardiac resynchronization therapy in patients with advanced heart failure: the Multicenter InSync Randomized Clinical Evaluation (MIRACLE). J Card Fail 6:369-380
11. Saxon LA, Boehmer JP, Hummel J et al (1999) Biventricular pacing in patients with congestive heart failure: two prospective randomized trials. The VIGOR CHF and VENTAK CHF Investigators. Am J Cardiol 83:120D-123D
12. Bristow MR, Feldman AM, Saxon LA (2000) Heart failure management using implantable devices for ventricular resynchronization: Comparison of Medical Therapy, Pacing and Defibrillation in Chronic Heart Failure (COMPANION) trial. J Card Fail 6:276-285

A Review of the SCD-HEFT, COMPANION, and CARE-HF Trials

D.S. Cannom

The past 10 years have provided a series of well-designed clinical trials to study the effect of the implantable cardioverter defibrillator (ICD) in patients at high risk of sudden death. These studies have been carried out on both sides of the Atlantic. Patient populations have been recruited both from post-event populations and from pre-event populations judged to be at high enough risk to warrant prophylactic ICD implantation. The results of both categories of trial have been remarkably similar. Interestingly, the primary prevention studies were both initiated first and have shown more positive impact of ICD implantation on survival than the secondary prevention trials.

A new number of randomized, prospective prophylactic ICD trials have demonstrated improved survival in well-defined ischemic cardiomyopathy populations. The MADIT I trial demonstrated a surprisingly effective role for the ICD in the coronary patient with a low ejection fraction (EF). Total mortality was reduced by 54% in coronary patients with an EF below 35% who were inducible (and nonsuppressed) in the electrophysiology laboratory and treated with an ICD [1]. Further analysis of these data demonstrated that ICD benefit in the MADIT I population was limited to a population with heart failure including those with an EF under 26%, left bundle branch block on EKG, and recently treated congestive heart failure (CHF) [2]. Subsequent data from the Multicenter Unsustained Tachycardia Trial (MUSTT), using a completely different trial design and a much larger population (2200 patients), confirmed the MADIT I data by clearly identifying the ICD as the reason for increased patient survival benefit in the inducible drug treatment arm of the trial [3].

The most recently completed prophylactic ICD trial is the MADIT II trial [4]. This trial was designed to extend the positive findings of MADIT I to a larger population of low-EF coronary artery disease patients. Eligible patients were those with coronary disease, prior infarction,and an EF equal to or under 30%. No additional marker of electrical instability (e.g., nonsustained VT or

Good Samaritan Hospital, Los Angeles, California, USA

arrhythmia inducibility) was required. Patients were randomized to receive either conventional therapy or an ICD. After 4 years, a total of 1232 patients were enrolled. Investigators employed aggressive background medical therapy. Beta-blocker use was 70% and ACE inhibitor use 70%. At a mean follow-up of 20 months the ICD provided an additional beneficial effect on survival. The mortality rate in the conventional therapy group was 19.8% and that in the ICD group 14.2%. These figures represent a hazard ratio for risk of death in the ICD arm of 0.69 (Fig. 1). Further analysis of the MADIT II data demonstrated that most of the benefit in this population was observed in the patients with a QRS duration greater than 120 ms: exactly one-half of patients in MADIT II had a wide QRS, and the risk reduction for this subset was 63% [5]. The combined data from MADIT I, MADIT II, and MUSTT demonstrate convincingly that the ICD can benefit low-EF patients with coronary disease.

There is one other major randomized clinical trial still underway which focuses more on a heart failure population for its enrollment. This is the SCD-HEFT trial and it has significant design features which are advantageous. It includes patients with both dilated and ischemic cardiomyopathies. Its treatment strategy employs a true placebo arm. The trial has enrolled 2500 patients and is now in a follow-up phase for at least 1 more year (from September 2002). The outcome of the trial depends to some extent on the actual risk of the dilated cardiomyopathy group. Recently published trials such as the CAT

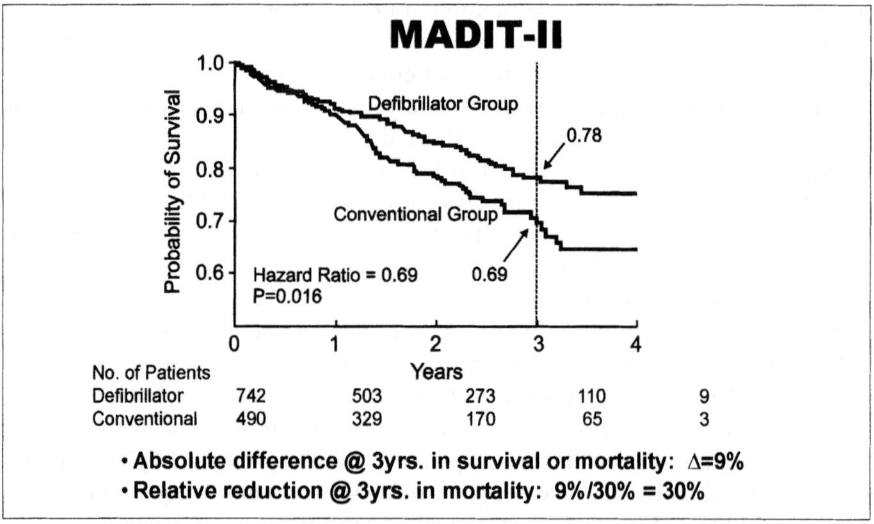

Fig. 1. Kaplan-Meier estimates of the probability of survival in the group assigned to receive an implantable cardioverter defibrillator (ICD) compared to the group assigned to receive conventional medical therapy, from the MADIT II study. The difference in survival between the two groups was significant. The mortality rate in the conventional therapy group is 19.8% and that in the ICD group 14.2% at 20 months. (From [4], reproduced with permission.)

trial have shown that the arrhythmic risk of the dilated cardiomyopathy population is lower than originally thought [6]. If dilated cardiomyopathy patients, who constitute one-half of the total number of the 2500 patients, have a low risk as in the CAT study, it will surely make it difficult for the ICD to show benefit in the ischemic population. The effect of amiodarone is also uncertain. Other trials employing amiodarone in heart failure patients have not shown a benefit for amiodarone (EMIAT, CAMIAT). The large number of enrolled patients in the SCD-HEFT trial will allow important substudies.

Finally, there are two trials underway, COMPANION and CARE-HF, which are studying the effect of the ICD with biventricular pacing. The ventricular resynchronization trials to date have shown improvement in functional indices - such as the second minute walk, CHF class, and quality of life - but have now shown a difference in total or cardiac mortality.

The COMPANION trial is designed to determine whether optimal pharmacological therapy (OPT) used with (1) ventricular resynchronizaion therapy (VRT) alone, or (2) VRT combined with an ICD, decreases mortality, alleviates cardiac symptoms, and improves function when compared with OPT alone (Fig. 2). The COMPANION trial is recruiting patients with New York Heart Association class III-IV heart failure, an admission for CHF within the 12 months prior to enrollment, and a PR interval greater than 150 ms and a QRS duration greater than 120 ms. Either ischemic or nonischemic patients may be

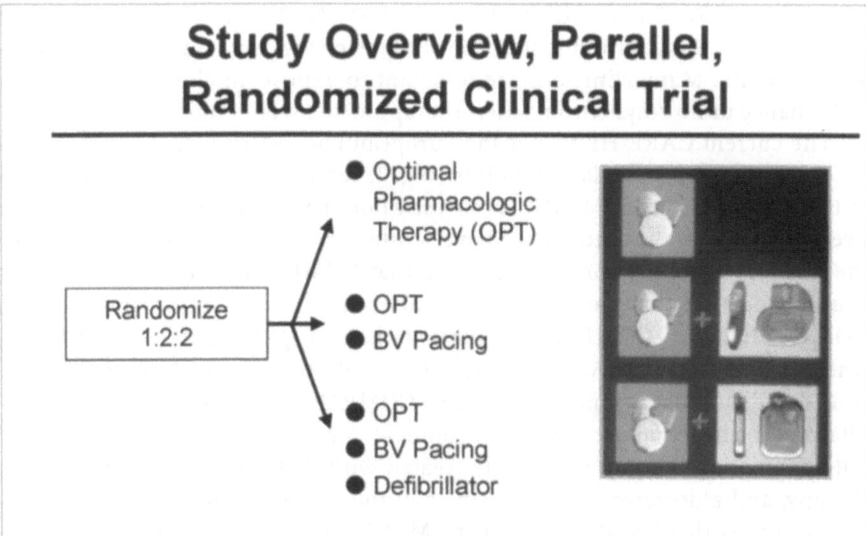

Fig. 2. Randomization scheme for the COMPANION trial. Patients are randomized to optimal pharmacological therapy alone, ventricular synchronization therapy alone, or ventricular synchronization therapy combined with an ICD. Enrollment has been handicapped by the reluctance of investigators to randomize a patient to pharmacological therapy alone. (From [7], reproduced with permission.)

enrolled. The primary endpoint is reduction of all-cause mortality and hospitalization for CHF. Secondary endpoints include reduction of cardiac morbidity, improvement of cardiac performance and quality of life, and increase in total survival [7].

A primary endpoint of the trial is total mortality. Significant attention is given to what constitutes appropriate medical therapy. All patients must be treated optimally for CHF for at least 1 month including a stable dose of beta-blocker for least 3 months before randomization. This is a very important consideration. As the MERIT trial has taught us, optimized medical therapy for NYHA class III-IV patients results in risk reductions, for both total mortality and sudden cardiac death, which are superior to those observed in MADIT II.

The enrollment goal is 2200 patients randomized. The primary endpoint of all-cause mortality and all-cause hospitalization assumes that the VRT device will result in a 25% reduction compared to a control annual rate of 40%.

The scientific appeal of this study is obvious and it has been supported enthusiastically by the heart failure community in the United States. The anticipated enrollment is 2200 patients, but patient recruitment has been slower than originally projected. Enrollment is now at 1500 patients (as of May 2002), and the hope is to complete enrollment by the end of 2002.

Many of the difficulties in enrollment relate not to trial design but to the reluctance of physicians to enroll patients when therapy is available outside of the trial. Enrollment in COMPANION suffered when a market-approved VRT device (Insync) was approved by the Food and Drug Administration (FDA) in September, 2001. Another difficulty for COMPANION was the publication of the MADIT II data. Enrollment in the study declined from 120 a month to 30-40 per month. Many clinicians are reluctant to expose an eligible patient to a 20% chance of no resynchronization therapy as the trial requires.

The current CARE-HF trial is the European trial which is looking at a similar population with similar endpoints (Fig. 3, Table 1). It is two-thirds enrolled at this time [8]. The COMPANION investigators have been emphatic about the need to complete the study. They have written to all investigative centers after the MADIT II publication to emphasize that COMPANION remains "ethically sound" and that there are significant differences in the intent and focus of COMPANION. All COMPANION patients have a QRS greater than 120 ms, whereas only half of MADIT II patients do. All etiologies of heart failure are considered, not just coronary disease. All COMPANION patients have been hospitalized for heart failure prior to enrollment. Most importantly, the COMPANION population is more adequately treated with ACE inhibition, beta-blocker therapy, and aldosterone antagonism than the MADIT population. Early estimates suggest that less than 15% of the MADIT II population would qualify for enrollment in COMPANION (Lorenzo DiCarlo, personal communication).

The fate of COMPANION remains uncertain. Certainly if a VRT-ICD mortality trial is not done now, it will never be done. The true role of VRT therapy in the treatment of the heart failure population depends upon the completion of a mortality trial. Whether the true benefit of this therapy is underestimated or overestimated is irrelevant. We are in an era now (similar to the early days of

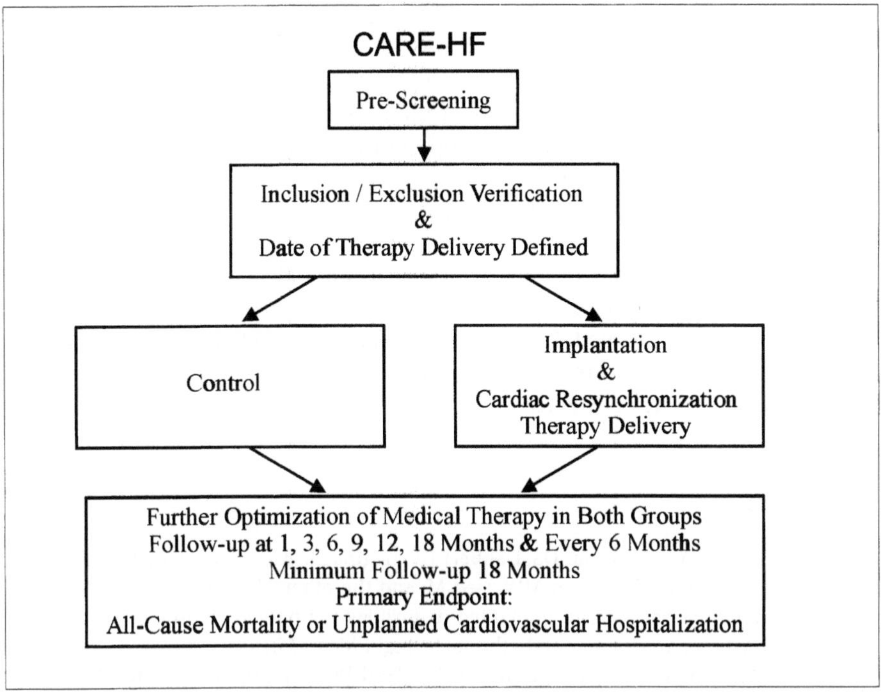

Fig. 3. CARE-HF randomization scheme. Enrollment criteria are very similar to the COMPANION trial (See Table 1). (From [8], reproduced with permission.)

Table 1. CARE-HF inclusion criteria

Chronic (>6 weeks) heart failure in the investigator's opinion
Symptom class NYHA III-IV
Stable (minimum 1 week) doses of diuretics (minimum 40 mg furosemide or equivalent)
Optimal drug treatment in the investigator's opinion
Sinus rhythm
Ventricular asynchrony as evidenced by QRS or echo:

1. QRS duration ≥ 150 ms as evidenced in at least two derivations of an ECG
2. QRS > 120 ms and at least 2 out of the following 3 echo criteria:
   - Aortic pre-ejection delay >140 ms, the interval between the onset ofthe QRS complex and the onset of aortic flow using pulsed wave Doppler
   - Interventricular mechanical delay ‘40 ms, the time difference between the onset of pulmonary ejection and aortic ejection, using pulsed wave Doppler
   - Delayed activation of the posterolateral left ventricular wall, defined as the maximal posterolateral wall inward movement, using M-mode or tissue Doppler echo, occurring later than the start of the left ventricular filling, using the transmitral Doppler flow signal.

Left ventricular ejection fraction ≤35%
LVEDD >30 mm

From [8]

ICD therapy in the 1990s) when only a mortality trial will do: of course, prospective randomized trials proved the VRT benefit was more than expected.

The results of the VRT-ICD trials are very important as a way to round out this era of important scientific study of the ICD. The fact that practice patterns in the United States have brought enrollment to a virtual standstill is unfortunate. Both the physician and patient community are now insisting that VRT devices be implanted with an ICD after wide dissemination of the results of the MADIT II study.

An enormous amount of data has been accumulated from clinical trials in the past 10-12 years. These data have had a major impact on patient management and ultimate survival. Even if the remaining important questions regarding the ICD in heart failure are not answered, this has been an extraordinary time for the advocates of device therapy.

References

1. Moss AJ, Hall WJ, Cannom DS, Daubert JP, Higgins SL, Klein H, Levine JH, Saksena S, Waldo AL, Wilber D, Brown MW, Heo M, and the other MADIT investigators (1996) Improved survival with an implanted defibrillator in patients with coronary disease at high risk for ventricular arrhythmia. N Engl J Med 335:1933-1940
2. Moss AJ, Fadi Y, Zareba W, Cannom DS, Hall WJ, for the Multicenter Automatic Defibrillator Implantation Trial Research Group (2001) Survival benefit with an implanted defibrillator in relation to mortality risk in chronic coronary heart disease. Am J Cardiol 88:516-520
3. Buxton AE, Lee KL, Fisher JD, Josephson ME, Prystowsky EN, Hafley G (1999) A randomized study of the prevention of sudden death in patients with coronary artery disease. Multicenter Unsustained Tachycardia Trial (MUSTT) Investigators. N Engl J Med 341:1882-1890
4. Moss AJ, Zareba W, Hall J, Klein H, Wilber DJ, Cannom DS, Daubert JP, Higgins SL, Brown MW, Andrews ML, for the MADIT-II Investigators (2002) Prophylactic implantation of a defibrillator in patients with myocardial infarction and reduced ejection fraction. N Engl J Med 346:877-883
5. Zareba W (2002) Presented at NASPE's 23rd Annual Scientific Sessions in San Diego on 11 May, 2002 in the Late Breaking Trial Session on MADIT II
6. Bansch D, Antz M, Boczor S, Volkner M, Tebbenjohanns J, Seidl K, Block M, Gietzen F, Berger J, Kuck KH, for the CAT investigators (2002) Primary prevention of sudden cardiac death in idiopathic dilated cardiomyopathy: the Cardiomyopathy Trial (CAT). Circulation 105:1453-1458
7. Bristow MR, Feldman AM, Saxon LA, for the COMPANION Steering Committee and COMPANION Clinical Investigators (2000) Heart failure management using implantable devices for ventricular resynchronization: comparison of medical therapy, pacing, and defibrillation in chronic heart failure (COMPANION) trial. J Card Fail 6:276-285
8. Cleland JGF, Daubert JC, Erdmann E, Freemantle N, Gras D, Kappenberger L, Klein W, Tavazzi L, on behalf of the CARE-HF study steering committee and investigators (2001) The CARE-HF study (Cardiac REsynchronisation in Heart Failure study): rationale, design and end-points. Eur J Heart Fail 3:481-489

Dual-Site Right Ventricular Pacing in Heart Failure Patients

L. Zamparelli, L. Cioffi, A. Di Costanzo, S. De Vivo, A. Settembre

It is known that monofocal pacing performed at the apical site of the right ventricle is not physiological. It induces an artificial left bundle block, evidenced by the widening of the evoked QRS complex. This pacing also has a deleterious effect on the patient's hemodynamics, introducing both systolic and diastolic dysfunction that, in most cases, induces an increase in functional mitral regurgitation.

The negative effects of inotropic asynchrony caused by monofocal ectopic ventricular activation are particularly in evidence in patients with severe dilated cardiomyopathy, in whom functional mitral regurgitation associated with a pathological left bundle block, with or without chronotropic incompetence, is very common [1-3]. Several reports have shown the advantages of left ventricular or biventricular pacing [4-7]. However, the inherent difficulties related to left ventricular access make this approach unsuitable in some cases.

Recently, Pachon Mateos et al. tried out a new endocardial, bifocal right ventricular pacing approach that requires simultaneous stimulation of the apex and of the upper portion of the interventricular septum. During that study, performed in patients with dilated cardiomyopathy associated with heart failure and functional mitral regurgitation, it was observed that bifocal pacing, compared to monofocal apical, caused a significant decrease in mitral regurgitation (better activation of papillary muscles) and a substantial narrowing of the evoked QRS complex (absence of induced left bundle block). Moreover, the kinetics of the apex-to-base contraction seemed to achieve better coordination [8].

The aim of our ongoing study is to assess whether DDD pacing with bifocal stimulation in the right ventricle, performed in patients with dilated cardiomyopathy (ejection fraction <40% and left ventricular diastolic diameter >65 mm), pathological QRS (> 120 ms), and chronotropic incompetence, leads to significant and durable benefits in terms of: electrophysiology (narrowing of the QRS complex), hemodynamics (increase of ejection fraction and

Department of Cardiac Pacing, Ospedale Monaldi, Naples, Italy decrease in mitral regurgitation), cardiac remodeling (reduction of left ventricular diastolic diameter), and quality of life (NYHA class improvement).

At present, nine patients (6 male, mean age 64.6±9.2 years) were included and completed the first year of follow-up. All had severe dilated cardiomyopathy (mean values: ejection fraction = 30.3±7.1%, left ventricular diastolic diameter = 69.8±3.3 mm, pulmonary arterial pressure = 56.0±4.1 mmHg), functional mitral regurgitation (mitral regurgitation index = 3+), and pacemaker indication due to left bundle block with AV block or sinus bradycardia (QRS duration = 148.2±5.7 ms). The mean NYHA functional class was 3.3±0.4. The etiologies were dilated cardiomyopathy of primitive origin in six patients and chronic ischemic cardiomyopahty in three patients.

All patients underwent permanent pacemaker implantation with two endocardial right ventricular leads. The first one (active fixation) was placed in the septal outflow tract of the pulmonary valve in seven patients and in the root area of the interventricular septum in two patients. The second one (passive fixation) was conventionally positioned at the apex of the right ventricle. An active fixation atrial lead was also implanted in accordance with the conventional endocardial technique. The pacemakers were: one Biotronik DDDR INOS^{2+} CLS, three Biotronik DDD Kairos D, one Biotronik DDD Actros D, one St. Jude DDDR Trilogy DR, and three St. Jude three-chamber DDDR Frontier 5510 pakemakers. The active fixation septal leads were: four Medtronic Capsure-FIX 5068, three St. Jude SDX 1488, one St. Jude 1055 K, and one Biotronik ELOX 53-BP leads.

The right ventricular bifocal stimulation was achieved using a Y adapter to "split" the ventricular output on two leads in six patients. In the remaining three patients the adapter was avoided by using a device with three chambers output (Frontier 5510). The electrical data collected during implantation and follow-up were within the normal range.

All patients were studied with electrocardiographic and two-dimensional echo-Doppler cardiogram at 3, 6, and 12 months after surgery. QRS complex duration, ejection fraction, pulmonary arterial pressure, mitral regurgitation index, and left ventricular diastolic diameter were assessed at each follow-up. The NYHA class was evaluated using a 6-min walking test (modified Bruce protocol). Table 1 summarizes the results achieved before implantation and during follow-up.

Monofocal pacing at the right ventricular apex induces a significant inotropic asynergy among the ventricular myocardial cells. The systole, the isometric contraction phase, and the mitral regurgitation time are extended. In consequence, the pulmonary venous system is additionally affected by the increase in mitral regurgitation and the reduced diastolic efficiency. These unphysiological conditions will contribute to generating or increasing a pulmonary hypertension and to progression of the heart failure.

The data collected in the limited group of patients who completed the first year of follow-up show that right ventricular bifocal stimulation induced obvious improvements in terms of:

Table 1. Electrophysiological and hemodynamic follow-up data (values ± SD)

	Before implantation	3-Month follow-up	6-Months follow-up	12-Month follow-up
QRS duration (ms)	148.2 ± 5.7	119.8 ± 12.9	107.6 ± 9.9	109.8 ± 10.5
Ejection fraction (%)	30.3 ± 7.1	36.9 ± 8.8	40.8 ± 8.9	39.7 ± 8.8
Pulmonary arterial pressure (mmHg)	56.0 ± 4.1	50.4 ± 5.8	45.7 ± 6.5	46.9 ± 5.6
Mitral regurgitaion index (+)	3.0 ± 0	2.1 ± 0.4	1.5 ± 0.4	1.6 ± 0.3
Left ventricular diastolic diameter (mm)	69.8 ± 3.3	65.1 ± 4.6	61.2 ± 3.8	62.4 ± 4.1
NYHA class	3.3 ± 0.4	2.8 ± 0.4	2.2 ± 0.4	2.1 ± 0.6

1. Electrophysiology: It avoided the left bundle block, narrowing the QRS duration (-19.1% at 3 months), and allowing a progressive electrical remodeling of the ventricles (additional -10.2% reduction of QRS duration in the following 3 months). Although the difference between data groups was not statistically significant, the trend to reduction in QRS duration was present in all patients. No significant changes were seen in the last 6 months of follow-up.
2. Hemodynamics: Ejection fraction increased (+21.8% during the first 3 months), with a constant trend (+10.6% in the following 3 months) and the increase was statistically significant ($p<0.05$). Pulmonary arterial pressure also decreased significantly ($p<0.05$; -10% at 3 months and -18.4% at 6 months). The mitral regurgitation index improved from 3+ before implantation to 1-2+ at 6 months with a trend to reduction detected in all patients, although the difference between groups of data was not statistically significant. No significant hemodynamic changes were observed in the last 6 months follow-up.
3. Anatomical remodeling: The left ventricular diastolic diameter decreases progressively (-6.7% at 3m), but constantly (-12.3% at 6m) during the first 6 months of pacing, and the reduction is statistically significative.
4. Quality of life: NYHA class decreased in all patients with a difference that was statistically significant within the 12 months of follow-up.

This preliminary study, although performed in a limited population, shows that in patients with severe dilated cardiomyopathy with functional mitral regurgitation and wide QRS, endocardial right ventricular bifocal stimulation performed in a context of DDD pacing induces, at least in the medium term, obvious beneficial effects on hemodynamics, left ventricular electrical and anatomical remodeling, and quality of life. These consequences of bifocal pacing seem to be due to more physiological activation of the papillary muscles, shortening of the systole (shorter mitral regurgitation time), and prolongation of the diastole (improvement of diastolic function).

It is too early to compare this new approach to the more widely used biventricular resynchronization therapy. However, given the easier implantation procedure, it may be considered an alternative when the coronary sinus approach is not viable and/or stable positioning of the left ventricular lead is impossible.

References

1. Xiao HB, Lee CH, Gibson DG (1991) Effect of left bundle branch block on diastolic function in dilated cardiomyopathy. Br Heart J 66:443-447
2. Hanna SR, Chung ES, Aurigemma G et al (2000) Worsening of mitral regurgitation secondary to ventricular pacing. J Heart Valve Dis 9:273-275
3. Cannan CR, Higano ST, Holmes DR Jr (1997) Pacemaker induced mitral regurgitation: an alternative form of pacemaker syndrome. Pacing Clin Electrophysiol 20(Pt. 1):735-738
4. Auricchio A, Stellbrink C, Block M et al 1999) Effect of pacing chamber and atrioventricular delay on acute systolic function of paced patients with congestive heart failure. The Pacing Therapies for Congestive Heart Failure Study Group. The Guidant Congestive Heart Failure Research Group. Circulation 99:2993-3001
5. Bakker PF, Meijburg H, Jonge N et al (1994) Beneficial effects of biventricular pacing in congestive heart failure. Pacing Clin Electrophysiol 17: 820 (abstract)
6. Cazeau S, Ritter P, Bakdach S et al (1994) Four chamber pacing in dilated cardiomyopathy. Pacing Clin Electrophysiol 17:1974-1979
7. Gras D, Mabo P, Tang T et al (1998) Multisite pacing as a supplemental treatment of congestive heart failure: preliminary results of the Medtronic Inc InSync Study. Pacing Clin Electrophysiol 21:2249-2255
8. Pachon Mateos JC, Albornoz RN, Pachon Mateos EI et al (2000) Right ventricular bifocal stimulation in dilated cardiomyopathy with heart failure. Europace 1[Suppl D]:210 (abstract)

Biventricular Pacing: A Simplified Technique For Transvenous Implantation

R. Cazzin[1], L. Sciarra[1], D. Milan[1], G. Paparella[1], T. Scalise[2]

Biventricular pacing in patients with advanced heart failure and intraventricular conduction delay has been associated with improvement in hemodynamics, functional class, and quality of life [1-3]. More information is needed about clinical and instrumental identification of responders and the long-term follow-up of these patients. Nevertheless, a positive response to biventricular pacing is expected when the electrical resynchronization is achieved [4].

The early leads available in the late 1990s for transvenous stimulation of the left ventricle through the coronary sinus were provided with an annular ring-tip electrode, and had a shaped configuration with a small diameter. Cannulation of the coronary sinus with preshaped guiding sheaths permitted the introduction of the lead through the sheath, and enabled coronary sinus angiography as well.

Improved technological support and the increasing experience of operators significantly reduced the rate of the unsuccessful procedures. Nevertheless, delivery of the therapy in an effective and minimally invasive way still presents some technical and methodological challenges.

Two kinds of leads are currently most popular for transvenous access to the coronary sinus. The "over-the-wire" system includes a tined electrode with a central lumen and an open tip for a wire-guided fixation. Other systems available are characterized by preshaped lead terminations that are available in many kinds of shapes and configurations to facilitate passive fixation in the collateral veins.

The implant success rate for the over-the-wire system [5] has been reported to be up to 83%, with an implantation procedure lasting from 1 to 8 h (mean 169 min) depending on the operator's experience. A large number of dislocations of the electrodes were reported in the first experience, then the rate dropped to 2%. The recent data of the Miracle study [6], which included 228 patients in the pacing arm, evidenced a rate of 8% of unsuccessful implants

[1]U. O. Cardiologia, Ospedale di Portogruaro, Portogruaro (VE), [2]Biotronik-Seda, Trezzano (MI), Italy

and a 2.6% rate of major complications (coronary sinus dissection, infections, shock, and two deaths). The mean implantation duration was 2.7 h, and lead displacements were reported in 3.8% of cases. In other experiences [7], lead displacement was observed in 11% of the patients even at the end of a relatively long learning period. Implantation success with these techniques strongly depends on the learning curve of the operators and the number of implants performed per year at the pacing center. Mean fluoroscopy times for this procedure are reported to be about 45 min [7, 8] even in the implantation centers with better experience; in many cases mean fluoroscopy time is significantly longer.

From the analysis of the literature therefore, it is evident that methodological aspects such as the difficulty of cannulating the coronary sinus and placing the lead in the collateral veins, the long X-ray expositive and total implantation times, and the stability of the lead are still problems to be further clarified. Moreover, patients in whom biventricular pacing is indicated are frequently hemodynamically unstable and liable to experience exacerbation of congestive heart failure and other major complications.

Methods

Recently we evaluated a novel implantation system for biventricular pacing with a new lead model, Corox LVS (Biotronik, Germany). The Corox LVS (Fig. 1) is a silicon-insulated, unipolar lead with a passive soft silicon tip (8.5 mm long, 3 F thick) to improve the self-guiding characteristic. An annular ring electrode with an iridium fractal surface structure just proximal to the soft

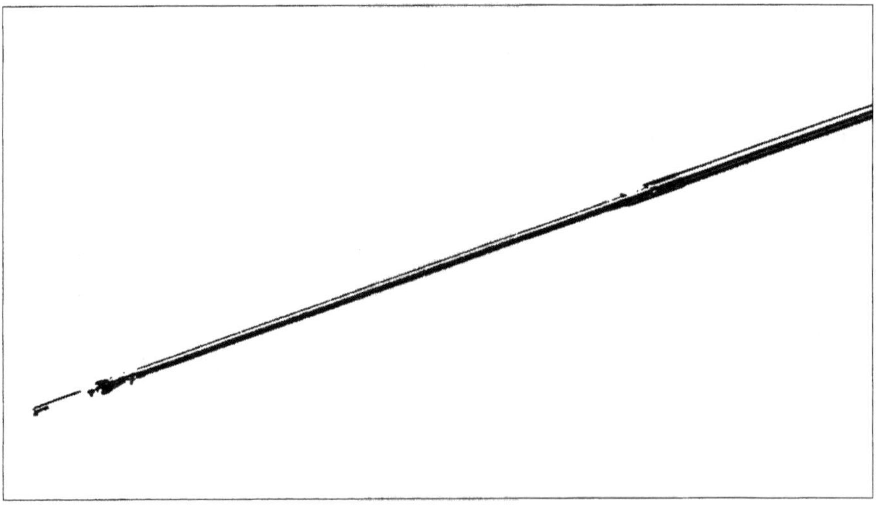

Fig. 1. Detail of the distal part of the Corox LVS lead

passive tip performs the stimulation. Then, the silicon beyond the ring electrode assumes a screw-like thread design for fixation of the lead into a coronary vein. The distal part of the lead has a 4.35 F diameter and ends at 8.5 cm from the tip, where a coaxial outer coil, up to the connector, provides a stiffer support that allows good maneuverability, increasing the lead body up to 6.6 F.

The aim of our study was to assess the feasibility of implantation with this novel device. From May 2001 to August 2002, 19 consecutive patients (17 male; mean age 75±6 years) underwent biventricular pacing in our center by means of the Corox LVS lead and were enrolled in the study. All the patients had severe heart failure (1 patient NYHA class II-III, 12 patients NYHA class III, and 6 patients NYHA class IV) despite maximal medical therapy. To be selected for implantation the patient had to have an ejection fraction of 35% or less with a dilated left ventricle. The electrocardiographic pattern required was a left bundle branch block, with an intrinsic QRS duration greater than 140 ms. In six patients the procedure was an upgrading from conventional to biventricular pacing. In such patients the symptoms of heart failure were reasonably related to the left asynchrony induced by the right stimulation, with an electrocardiographic pattern of a left-branch-block-like wide QRS. The presence of left ventricular asynchrony was diagnosed by means of echocardiography. Five patients were in atrial fibrillation and two of these underwent ablation of the atrioventricular node as well.

Two operators performed the implantation procedures with the patients under local anesthesia. Patients were premedicated with atropine and received antibiotic prophylaxis. For the lead placement the left subclavian vein and, whenever possible, the left cephalic vein were used. In one upgrading procedure, neither the left cephalic nor the subclavian approach was possible, so a right jugular vein approach was used. In the first six patients a preformed sheath catheter (Scout model, Biotronik, Germany), available in two preformed curves was used for coronary sinus cannulation. When necessary, the coronary sinus cannulation was facilitated by means of an electrophysiologic Josephson fixed-curve or steerable-curve catheter. The stable coronary sinus catheterization obtained with the sheath allowed a selective retrograde occlusive venogram to be performed by means of a Swan-Ganz catheter and the lead to be placed in the preferred branch. To simplify the procedure and to reduce both implantation and fluoroscopy times, in the last 13 patients we tried to approach the coronary sinus directly with the Corox LVS lead.

After the placement of the right ventricular lead we manually preformed the stylet in order to place the tip of the lead toward the interatrial septum, and then, with twisting movements, the coronary sinus could be cannulated. The definitive position of the Corox LVS lead was established according to pacing and sensing parameters. When an anterior or anterolateral branch was reached, we decided to move the lead toward a lateral, posterolateral or posterior branch. When the definitive position was achieved, the lead was rotated three times clockwise, keeping the stylet fixed, to allow better stabilization of the screw-like thread in the vein (Fig. 2).

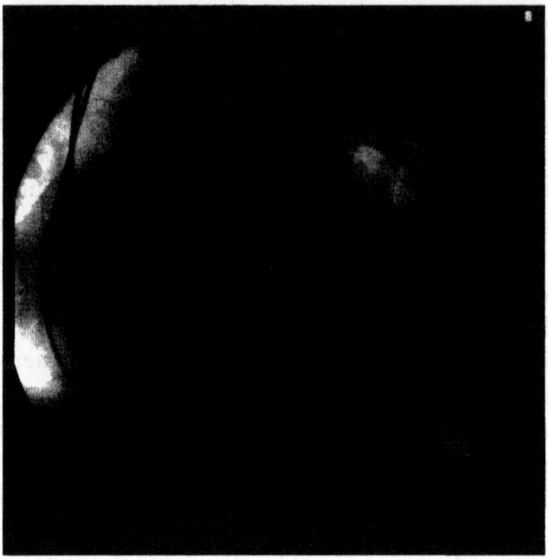

Fig. 2. Fluoroscopic image in the anteroposterior projection after placement of the right ventricular and left ventricular leads

Results

Eighteen procedures were successfully performed. In one patient (5.3%) we did not cannulate the coronary sinus either with the direct approach or with the sheath or with a steerable electrophysiologic catheter. The mean implantation time (skin to skin time) was 103±45 min. Mean X-ray expositive time was 20±9 min. The Corox LVS lead was placed in a posterolateral branch in seven patients, in a posterior branch in one patients, and in a lateral branch in ten patients. In the absence of the venogram, the collateral branch was identified by means of fluoroscopic projections of the heart. Mean threshold value at implantation was 1.2±1.0 V. No significant increments of the thresholds were observed during the follow-up (mean duration 80±50 days). In one patient (5.3%) we observed an early displacement of the lead that was successfully repositioned the day after. No significant complications were observed during the follow-up. In one patient local stimulation of the intercostal muscles was observed and solved by adjustment of the pacing parameters. Two patients did not benefit from ventricular resynchronization (nonresponders). In 16 patients an improvement in the functional NYHA class was observed. All the patients showed significant reduction of the QRS duration in biventricular pacing.

In our experience the implantation of the Corox LVS lead for biventricular pacing appeared to be feasible and safe. The fluoroscopy exposure and total implantation times were quite low. The approach to the coronary sinus, either with the Scout sheath or directly with the lead, was successful. Actually, we prefer to approach the coronary sinus directly with the lead. This technique seems to significantly simplify the procedure with a success rate at least comparable to other systems and without loosing the chance to pace an effective site of the left ventricle, in spite of the absence of a guiding venogram of the coronary sinus. The rate of unsuccessful procedures (only one case) appeared to be relatively low. Further investigations are required to confirm our data in a larger population.

References

1. Leclercq C, Cazeau S, Le Breton H, Ritter P et al (1998) Acute hemodynamic effects of biventricular DDD pacing in patients with end stage heart failure. J Am Coll Cardiol 32:1825-1831
2. Kass DA, Chen CH, Curry C et al (1999) Improved left ventricular mechanism from acute VDD pacing in patients with dilated cardiomyopathy and ventricular conduction delay. Circulation 99:1567-1573
3. Breithard OA, Stellbrink C, Franke A et al (2000) Echocardiographic evidence of hemodynamic and clinical improvement in patients paced for heart failure. Am J Cardiol 86:K133-K137
4. Cazeau S, Leclercq C, Lavergne T et al (2001) Multisite Stimulation in Cardiomyopathies (MUSTIC) study investigation: effects of multisite biventricular pacing in patients with heart failure and interventricular conduction delay. N Engl J Med 12:873-880
5. Purerfellner H, Nesser HJ, Winter S et al (2000) Transvenous ventricular lead implantation with the EASYTRAK lead system: the European experience. Am J Cardiol 86:K157-K164
6. William T, Abraham MD, Wetsby G et al (2002) Cardiac resynchronization in chronic heart failure. N Engl J Med 24:1845-1853
7. Alonso C, Leclercq C, Revault d'Allonnes F et al (2001) Six years experience of transvenous left ventricular lead implantation for permanent biventricular pacing in patients with advanced heart failure: technical aspects. Heart 86:405-410
8. Emile G, Daoud MD, Steven J et al (2002) Implantation technique and chronic lead parameters of biventricular pacing dual-chamber defibrillators. J Cardiovasc Electrophysiol 10:964-970

Optimization of Resynchronization Therapy by Intracardiac Ventricular Impedance

M. Bocchiardo[1], D. Caponi[1], P. Di Donna[1], M. Scaglione[1], G. Corgniati[1], M. Alciati[1], S. Miceli[1], L. Libero[2], C. Militello[3], R. Audoglio[3], F. Gaita[1]

Introduction

Cardiac resynchronization through biventricular pacing has proved to be an effective therapy in patients with severe heart failure (HF) with interventricular conduction disorders [1-7]. Nevertheless, about 25% of selected HF patients do not respond to synchronous biventricular pacing. The optimization of therapy in terms of pacing site(s) and interventricular delay is still under discussion.

At present, cardiac resynchronization therapy (CRT) optimization requires echographic measurements that consume time and resources. An automatic algorithm for CRT optimization implemented in a multisite pacemaker or in the programmer would improve patient quality of life and reduce follow-up costs. Intracardiac impedance is inversely proportional to blood volume in the cardiac chambers [8, 9]. This physiologic signal can be measured in vivo (Fig. 1) and might be a useful tool for CRT monitoring.

The aim of this study was to verify whether intracardiac ventricular impedance measured by a pacemaker might be used to optimize CRT.

Materials and Methods

Patients

Ten patients with HF (9 male, 1 female, age 71±6 years) were included in this study. The origin of the underlying cardiomyopathy was idiopathic (*n*=8) or ischemic (*n*=2). All patients had drug-refractory chronic HF (8 were in NHYA class III, 2 in class IV), left bundle branch block (mean QRS width 178 ± 36), ejection fraction below 35% (mean 22.7±3.1%) and chronic atrial fibrillation. All patients gave their informed, written consent to the procedures.

[1]Cardiology Division, Civil Hospital, Asti; [2]University Clinic, S. G. Battista Hospital, Turin, Italy; [3]Biotronik GmbH, Erlangen, Germany

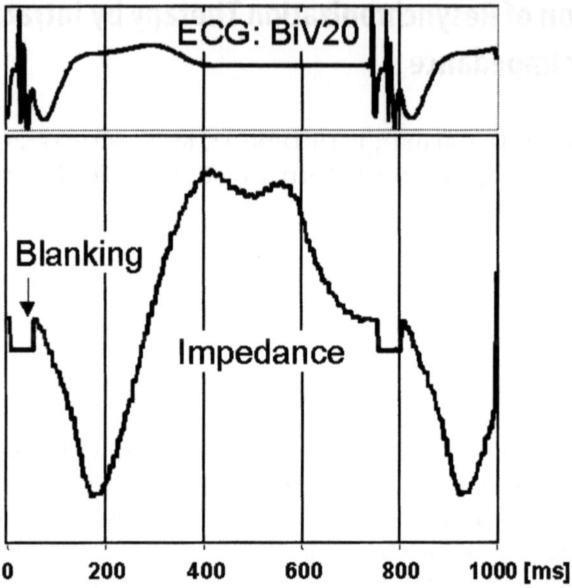

Fig. 1. Intracardiac impedance measured by the $Inos^{2+}$ CLS pacemaker during biventricular pacing with 20 ms interventricular delay

Device

All patients were implanted with an $Inos^{2+}$ CLS dual chamber pacemaker. All of them received a unipolar left ventricular (LV) lead through the coronary sinus and a passive fixation right ventricular lead. The LV lead was connected to the atrial channel of the pacemaker.

The pacemaker implements a closed loop system for rate adaptation based on intracardiac impedance analysis. In the standard operating mode, the intracardiac impedance signal is measured by injecting sub-threshold current pulses (200 μA, 30.5 μs) between pacemaker case and ventricular tip electrode and detecting the corresponding voltage at the same electrode pair. Dedicated research software can be downloaded to the device through the programmer. This allows one to select the electrodes involved in the impedance measurement, to increase the sampling rate to 128 Hz, and to enable beat-by-beat impedance and pacemaker flag transmission via telemetry.

Study Protocol

At baseline, drug therapy is optimized to minimize atrioventricular (AV) conduction. At implantation, the device is programmed in DDD mode and the AV delay is set at the minimum programmable value (20 ms). These parameters are kept throughout the study period. At 1 month follow-up, if the pacing percentage is still below 95%, the AV node is ablated.

At follow-ups (discharge, 1, 3, 6, and 12 months), pulmonary to aortic opening delay, mitral regurgitation area, and aortic and pulmonary velocity-time integrals are assessed by Doppler echocardiography during biventricular pacing at 20 and 40 ms interventricular delay, LV and RV pacing, and intrinsic activity when present. Based on the hemodynamic benefit assessed by echocardiography, the physician ranked the pacing modalities.

During the echocardiography procedures the intracardiac impedance was measured by the pacemaker using five consecutive electrode setups for current injection and voltage detection (Table 1). Impedance signal, pacemaker markers, and flags were downloaded via telemetry and stored in a laptop for post analysis.

Table 1. Electrode setups used for intracardiac impedance measurement

Impedance measurement configuration	Current injection	Voltage detection
Bipolar 1	Case–RV tip	Case–RV tip
Bipolar 2	Case–LV tip	Case–LV tip
Tripolar	LV tip–RV ring	LV tip–RV tip
Quadripolar	Case–RV ring	LV tip–RV tip

Data Analysis

The intracardiac impedance was averaged in a 50- to 300-ms window after LV events and digitally low-pass-filtered at 10 Hz in order to remove noise. Parameters calculated on the resulting impedance waveforms (Fig. 2) were correlated to the pacing modalities rank assigned by the physician.

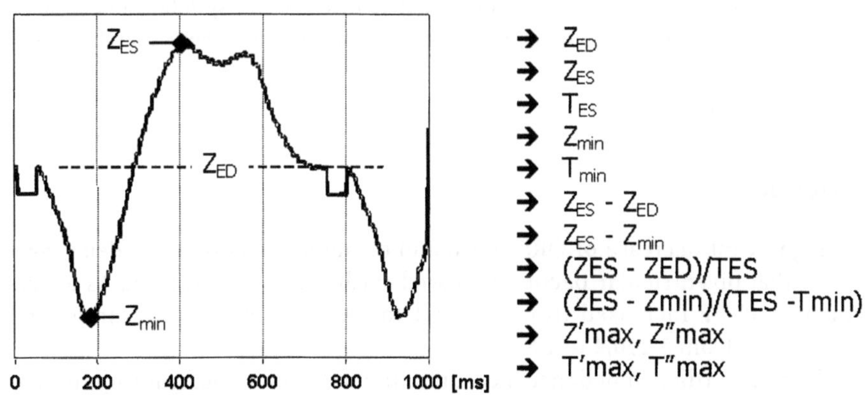

Fig. 2. Impedance-calculated parameters. Z_{ES}: maximum; Z_{ED}: baseline; Z_{min}: minimum; T_{ES}: LV event to Z_{ES} interval; T_{min}: LV event to Z_{min} interval; Z'_{max}, Z''_{max}: maximum of the 1st and 2nd derivative; T'_{max}, T''_{max}: LV event to Z'_{max}, Z''_{max} interval

Clinical variables were analyzed with the independent Student's *t*-test for paired data. A p value below 0.05 was considered statistically significant.

Results

With biventricular pacing, QRS width shortened to 158±35 ms. During a mean follow-up period of 7.8 months, 33 follow-ups were performed. The clinical results are summarized in Table 2.

In 32 out of 33 follow-ups, the pacing mode with the best rank assigned by the physician based on echocardiographic measurements was the same as the one showing the highest maximum of the second derivative (Z''_{max}) of the impedance measured in quadripolar configuration. When ranking the pacing mode based on Z''_{max}, the physician vs impedance rank correlation was 0.74 ($p<0.001$).

Table 2. Clinical results

	Baseline	Last follow-up	Δ[a]	p
NYHA class	3.2±0.4	1.8±0.6	−1.4	<0.001
LVEF (%)	22.7±3.1	30.9±7.1	8.2	<0.001
Mitral regurgitation area[b]	6.34±4.17	4.17±3.28	−2.17	0.07
Pulmonary to aortic delay (ms)	48.8±18.7	10.0±11.5	−38.0	<0.05
Aortic VTI	23.0±7.9	23.6±7.1	0.6	NS
Pulmonary VTI	15.0±3.0	13.4±4.1	1.57	<0.05
LVEDD	67.0±8.7	64.3±9.6	2.7	NS
LVSED	57.5±10.1	53.9±9.9	3.6	NS

VTI, velocity time integral; LVEDD, LVESD, left ventricular end-systolic and end-diastolic diameter; [a] Difference between last follow-up and baseline; [b] Four-chamber apical view

Discussion

The significant decrease of QRS width and of pulmonary-to-aortic delay confirmed that biventricular pacing improved cardiac synchronization. As a consequence, LVEF increased from 22.7±3.1 to 30.9±7.1. NYHA class improved significantly from 3.2±0.4 to 1.8±0.6.

The intracardiac impedance measured in quadripolar configuration is proportional to the blood volume in the LV. Consequently, Z''_{max} is proportional to blood acceleration and therefore to LV contractility. This rationale might explaining the predictive value of Z''_{max} in terms of LV function.

Conclusions

Preliminary results of this pilot study show that a CRT optimization algorithm based on intracardiac impedance monitoring is feasible and can be implemented in a pacemaker or in the programmer. A larger number of patients and further hemodynamic measurements are necessary to confirm that this simple and fast intracardiac impedance monitoring could take the place of echocardiography in the evaluation of CRT benefits.

References

1. Blanc JJ, Etienne Y, Gilard M et al (1997) Evaluation of different ventricular pacing sites in patients with severe heart failure. Circulation 96:3273-3277
2. Auricchio A, Stellbrink C, Block M et al (1999) Effect of pacing chamber and atrioventricular delay on acute systolic function of paced patients with congestive heart failure. Circulation 99:2993-3001
3. Gras D, Mabo P, Tang T et al (1998) Multisite pacing as a supplemental treatment of congestive heart failure: preliminary results of the Medtronic InSync Study. Pacing Clin Electrophysiol 21[Pt II]:2249-2255
4. Cazeau S, Leclercq C, Lavergne T et al (2001) Effects of multisite biventricular pacing in patients with heart failure and intraventricular conduction delay. N Engl J Med 344:873-880
5. Porciani MC, Puglisi A, Colella A et al (2000) Echocardiographic evaluation of the effects of biventricular pacing: the InSync Italian Registry. Eur Heart J Suppl 2[Suppl J]:J23-J30
6. Breithardt OA, Stellbrink C, Franke A et al (2000) Echocardiographic evidence of hemodynamic and clinical improvement in patients paced for heart failure. Am J Cardiol 86(9 Suppl 1):K133-K137
7. Zardini M, Tritto M, Gargiggia G et al (2000) The InSync Italian Registry: analysis of clinical outcome and considerations on the selection of candidates for left ventricular resynchronization. Eur Heart J Suppl 2[Suppl J]: J16-J22
8. Osswald S, Cron T, Gradel C et al (2000) Closed-loop stimulation using intracardiac impedance as a sensor principle: correlation of right ventricular dP/dtmax and intracardiac impedance during dobutamine stress test. Pacing Clin Electrophysiol 23:1502-1508
9. Bernhard J, Lippert M, Ströbel JP et al (1996) Physiological rate-adaptive pacing using closed-loop contractility control. Biomed Tech 41[Suppl 2]:13-15

Benefits of Closed Loop Stimulation in Resynchronization Therapy

A. Ravazzi, P. Diotallevi, G. De Marchi, E. Gostoli, F. Provera

Closed loop stimulation (CLS) is the algorithm implemented in the INOS^{2+} (Biotronik, Germany) pacemaker to perform rate modulation in dual or single chamber pacing. CLS is driven by a "virtual sensor" that detects the variations in intracardiac impedance during the systolic phase of right ventricular contraction [1, 2].

The sensor is the distal electrode tip of the ventricular pacing lead and the volume in which the impedance is measured is, in first approximation, a small sphere with the tip at the center in which blood and myocardium are included. During ventricular contraction the blood-to-myocardium ratio changes with a speed of variation that is proportional to the speed of the contraction, then to the duration of the shortening of the myocardial contractile element. During clinical investigations it was found that the intracardiac impedance and the dP/dt correlate well ($R > 0.90$). In essence the CLS sensor detects a hemodynamic parameter that is related to a large number of intrinsic and extrinsic factors such as ventricular preload and afterload, myofibril contractility, and contraction rate, all influencing cardiac performance [3, 4].

Cardiac performance is the resultant of a whole, physically ended and complete, that keeps its equilibrium constant thanks to a closed loop configuration with negative feedback. When the value of one element of this closed loop system (e.g. pre- or afterload, contractility, or chronotropy) changes, all the other elements change their value proportionally in order to maintain a constant equilibrium in the system as a whole.

The pacing algorithm based on the closed loop concept allows constant and automatic monitoring of variations in cardiac performance and modifies the hemodynamic equilibrium of the cardiac contraction controlling rate and atrioventricular (AV) synchrony [5, 6].

Division of Cardiology, Ospedale SS. Antonio e Biagio, Alessandria, Italy

Ventricular Filling

The amount of ventricular filling is a significant factor that influences myofibril contractility. When the ratio between the initial length of the myocardial fiber and the developed strength varies, the speed of shortening of the contractile element changes. In consequence, heart rate and afterload should alter to maintain the equilibrium of the system (cardiac output). This means that the CLS system is capable of measuring variations in ventricular filling via changes in contractility. In experimental clinical studies it was demonstrated that measuring intracardiac impedance in conditions of AV sequential pacing it is possible to calculate the optimal AV delay, in both basal and dynamic conditions, in any pathophysiological condition of the patient [7].

Contractility

This physiological parameter is not directly measured by the CLS system and no objective information about the intrinsic quality of the myocardial fiber is supplied by the device. However, the course of intracardiac impedance and its changes over the time are in strong correlation to the variations in contractility. Therefore, the signal driving the CLS is, in good approximation, an effective hemodynamic indicator of cardiac performance.

Obviously, CLS pacing does not influence myocardial contractility directly, but it modulates two parameters, rate and ventricular filling (through the AV delay), that act directly on contractility. In patients in whom myocardial contractility is preserved, but chronotropic competence is lost, the hemodynamic performance can be optimized by CLS pacing in any contingent situation. On the other hand, if the strength of muscular fibers is deficient (as in the case of congestive heart failure), the CLS pacing system can improve the contractile profile, inducing changes in rate and ventricular filling.

From the clinical point of view this means that in the first case a smaller amount of energy is spent by the myocardial cells, and in the second the cardiac performance is optimized at the best level allowed by the compromised contractile function [8].

Cardiac Capture

Additional information that can be obtained by measuring intracardiac impedance variations relates to the efficacy of the pacing stimulus delivered by the pacemaker. A clinical investigation has demonstrated that, by monitoring the impedance during an early time window immediately after the pacing stimulus, it is possible to detect a "dip" in the impedance course, caused by the opening of the cellular sodium channels. This dip is not present when the stimulus does not induce a cardiac evoked response. Unlike the case of the ventricular evoked response, this method is expected to perform in any of the paced cardiac chambers [9].

If such an algorithm is implemented in an implantable device, continuous control of cardiac capture and optimal dosage of the pulse energy in each paced site will be easily achieved. The advantages offered by this solution are:
- Increased patient safety and optimization of resynchronization therapy
- Substantial saving in battery energy, especially in dual and triple chamber devices
- Limitation of the electromechanical noxa caused by the intensity of the stimulus in the myocardial cell

The concept on which the CLS stimulation is based has introduced and will in the near future continue to introduce several advances in conventional pacing and ventricular resynchronization therapies:
1. Physiological stimulation, adapting the heart rate to metabolic needs not only during exercise, but also during unconscious stress conditions, and respecting the pathophysiological conditions of the patient as well. This is the main clinical application of the system at present.
2. Continuous optimization of the AV delay through the analysis of impedance variations during automatic scanning of the AV delay, in both basal and dynamic conditions. The improvement is represented by beat-to-beat optimization of ventricular filling.
3. Myocardial capture control and minimization of pacing energy. Although the advantage connected to the saving in battery energy is self-evident, almost nothing is known about the long-term response of myocardial cell performance when the electromechanical stress of pacing is reduced. It is expected that constant monitoring of intracardiac impedance will provide some answers in this matter as well.
4. Improvement of cardiac performance. At present, this aspect has not been completely evaluated in all its clinical applications, even though it is the most obvious from the theoretical point of view. The potential benefits represented by continuous monitoring of cardiac performance on the basis of intracardiac impedance are several and significant, starting from the evolution of the natural history of cardiac contractility, both in normal and deficient conditions, and ending with long-term, real-time monitoring of the effects of pharmacological therapy and/or mechanical synchronization therapy using models of sequential biventricular pacing.

Combining all the above advances in a three chamber resynchronization device will substantially improve the benefits of biventricular stimulation and enable an accurate, easy, and noninvasive monitoring of therapy.

In conclusion, the CLS concept based on intracardiac impedance offers several fascinating applications at various stages of pacing or resynchronization therapy. During device implantation and the postsurgical acute phase, it may allow optimization of the modality and parameters of cardiac resynchronization and early detection of "nonresponding" patients. In the chronic phase it will combine continuous hemodynamic monitoring with the therapeutic efficacy of a self-regulating, automatic pacing system that constantly optimizes the profile of the cardiac contraction despite evolving pathology.

References

1. Zecchi P, Bellocci F, Ravazzi AP et al (2000) Closed loop stimulation: a new philosophy of pacing. Prog Biomed Res 5:126-131
2. Ravazzi AP, Zecchi P, Bellocci F et al (2000) Physiologic rate response of closed-loop stimulation. Results of the VICRA validation study. Pacing Clin Electrophysiol 23(Pt. 2):725 (abstract)
3. Ravazzi AP, Carosio G, Diotallevi P et al (2000) Clinical assessment of the correlation between right ventricular impedance and left ventricular contractility. Prog Biomed Res 5:478-481
4. Ravazzi AP, Carosio G, Diotallevi P et al (2001) Right ventricular impedance and myocardial contractility. Clinical correlation assessment during left heart catheterization. Pacing Clin Electrophysiol 24(Pt. 2):685 (abstract)
5. Orazi S, Ravazzi AP, Diotallevi P et al (2001) Closed loop stimulation versus peak endocardial acceleration. Clinical evaluation of two contractility based pacing systems. Europace 2[Suppl A]:A11 (abstract)
6. Occhetta E, Vassanelli C, Ravazzi AP et al (2000) Myocardial contractility guided dual chamber rate-responsive pacing: toward a closed-loop stimulation. In: Santini M (ed) Progress in clinical pacing 2000. CEPI-AIM Group, Rome, pp 268-277
7. Ravazzi AP, Diotallevi P, Provera MF et al (2001) A-V delay optimization according to the right ventricular intracardiac impedance. Prog Biomed Res 6:409-412
8. Ravazzi AP, Carosio G, Diotallevi P et al (2001) Effetti della modulazione del ritmo sull'emodinamica. Prog Biomed Res (Italian edition) 2:36-40
9. Ravazzi AP, Diotallevi P, Provera MF et al (2001) AV delay optimization using ventricular intracardiac impedance. Europace 2 [Suppl C]:C26 (abstract)

Clinical Issues in the Ventricular Synchronization Therapy of Heart Failure

C. Borasteros

Introduction

Population ageing, the high prevalence of hypertension, obesity and diabetes and especially the very high incidence of ischaemic heart disease, make advanced chronic heart failure (HF) an epidemic and extremely serious public health problem in the developed world. Spain, a country with a relatively low incidence of ischaemic heart disease, has about 40,000 new cases of myocardial infarction annually.

The Framingham heart study [1] reported an improvement in the mortality rate of patients suffering from HF between 1990–1999, in comparison to the period of 1950–1969. Between 1950–1969, male mortality occurring within 30 days, 1 year or 5 years of HF was 12%, 30% and 70% respectively, while in the period of 1990–1999 it was reduced to 11%, 28% and 59%. The observed 10% reduction in mortality within 5 years coincides with the extensive use of angiotensin converting enzyme inhibitors (ACEI) and beta-blockers (BB) in the treatment of HF. However, a 60% mortality rate within 5 years of HF is still a significant number, and is a higher rate than in many cancers. The quality of life in these patients is poor, where they are often disabled and have multiple hospital admissions.

The most ambitious investigational treatment of HF today includes cellular therapy, genetic therapy and angiogenesis. However, these options are still a long way from widespread clinical application. A more modest and limited contribution to a considerable group of patients (those with moderate to severe systolic dysfunction, advanced functional class and intraventricular conduction delay) is the therapy of ventricular resynchronization with biventricular stimulation. This has been shown in a short period of time not only to improve the quality of life, functional class of the disease and exercise capacity, but also to reduce hospital admissions (MUSTIC, PATH-CHF, MIRACLE, CONTAK CD Studies) and mortality (COMPANION study).

Service of Cardiology, SACYL, Avila, Spain

Recent updating in the ACC/AHA/NASPE 2002 guidelines for the implantation of cardiac pacemakers and antiarrhythmic devices [2] includes cardiac resynchronization(CR) therapy as a II a indication with level of evidence A for patients with dilated cardiomyopathy in functional class III/IV, not responding to medical treatment, with QRS >= 130 ms, left ventricle diastolic diameter >= 55 mm, and ejection fraction (EF) <= 35%.

Frequently, at the moment of their publication, guidelines are not yet updated to the results of new studies, so that a QRS durations of 130 ms could be reduced to 120 ms, and the functional class III/IV to class II/III, as will be discussed later.

In patients with advanced systolic dysfunction, intraventricular conduction delay occurs between 20% and 50% of the cases, depending on the cut-off point of the QRS, be it 120 ms, 130 ms or 150 ms. Moreover, the width of the QRS correlates with EF and mortality [3]. Cianfrocca et al. reported that a QRS of 115 ±18 ms was associated with an EF < 25%, whilst a QRS of 105 ± 21 ms was related with higher EF. A QRS of 119 ± 25 ms was recorded in patients who died, versus 105 ± 22 ms in the survivors. Strong evidence supports the independent contribution of intraventricular conduction delay to mortality rate in HF. Gothipaty et al. [4] evaluated 3654 ECGs in the VEST study, following up the patients for a year after treatment. The independent predictors of mortality were: age, creatinine, EF, heart rate and QRS duration. Patients with a wide QRS showed a five-fold increase in mortality in comparison to those with a narrow QRS.

Silvet et al. [5] followed up 2263 patients with an EF <40% for 1007 consecutive days. Where the QRS ≥110 ms, the mortality rate within 6 years of HF was 66%, versus 40% with a QRS <110 ms (P<0.0001). Patients with an EF <30% and a QRS >110 ms had a mortality rate of up to 75%, whilst if the EF was higher than 30% and the QRS <110 ms, mortality rates were only 30%.

The mortality rate for patients suffering from HF with a wide QRS may double in relation to those with a narrow QRS, mortality being directly proportional to QRS width and further increasing as the EF falls.

The hemodynamic consequences of left bundle branch block (LBBB) are well known: desynchronization between right ventricle, septum and left ventricle (LV) with overlapping systole and diastole; shortening of the left ventricle filling time; reduction of the EF; uncoupling of the septum and the LV free wall and worsening of mitral insufficiency (MI). The hemodynamic alteration in systole and diastole increases as the QRS widens and provides the basis for the correlation between the QRS width and parameters like EF, oxygen consumption and functional class in the patient with HF. In addition, the QRS width is a useful prognostic marker in regards to mortality. It is a vicious circle, with the altered hemodynamics causing further deterioration of the heart.

The hypothesis that is widely accepted today, is that pacemaker-based resynchronization therapy (RT) coordinates both ventricles each other and the septum with the free wall, optimizes the filling time and reduces MI, without increasing myocardium oxygen consumption, but, on the contrary, reducing it, as shown by Nelson et al. [6].

Several randomized studies have shown the functional improvement and the reduction of hospital admissions of patients receiving RT. Recent data from the COMPANION study have shown for the first time a significant reduction of mortality in patients with HF treated with RT .

Therefore, pacing-induced RT is a therapeutic option that clinical cardiologists must include in their treatment of patients with HF, systolic dysfunction and left bundle branch block (LBBB) and not consider it as an "exotic" resource confined to sophisticated groups of investigators.

The more interesting clinical issues to discuss are:

1. In which patient should a pacemaker be indicated for CR?
2. Which are the most significant parameters to follow up?
3. How to deal with the patient with moderate to severe mitral insufficiency (MI)?
4. In which patient is it necessary to choose a defibrillator-resynchronizer?

Clinical Indications

According to the present indications from the AHA/ACC/NASPE guidelines, the functional class of patients for RT must be III/IV. Class IV implies a very advanced state of cardiac disease, though many cardiologists following up patients with HF have seen impressive results with RT, with an improvement from class IV to class II and removal of the patient from the transplant waiting list. Furthermore, current data suggest that a deceleration in the progress of HF, a regression of remodelling and a reduction in mortality rate can also occur. Taken with the results from clinical trials of patients with class II cardiac disease, these data have lead clinicians to consider treating with RT patients in functional class II/III/IV, instead of class III/IV only, in the presence of an EF <35%, LV dilatation, a wide QRS with LBBB, and echocardiographic evidence of cardiac desynchronization.

The CONTAK-CD study [7] randomized 581 patients with functional class II to IV, a QRS >120 ms and risk of sudden death, with indication for an implantable cardiac defibrillator (ICD). The presence of an ICD could affect itself patients' mortality, but HF evolution under RT can still be evaluated. The ICD was programmed double-blind for 6 months of resynchronization versus no resynchronization. Patients under RT showed improvement in the classical follow up parameters, e.g., the 6 minute walk test (35 m increase), the oxygen consumption (VO_2 0.9 ml/Kg/m) or the Minnesota survey (16%). However, if we consider events resulting from further heart deterioration, like death, hospital admissions for HF, the need for other medical intervention and malignant arrhythmia, resynchronized patients showed a 21% reduction in the progression of the disease. Furthermore, LV diameters were reduced suggesting a regression of remodelling. After 6 months of treatment, 80% of resynchronized patients were in NYHA class I or II.

The analysis of ECG data from the " VIGOR Congestive Heart Failure" study [8], proves that resynchronization is associated with a reduction of atrial volume, LV telesystolic and telediastolic diameters and an improvement of systolic function. Patients under the VIGOR study were in class III/IV at the start, but the criteria of the QRS width was set at 120 ms only. The improvement became stable from the twelfth week of treatment.

The MIRACLE study [9] from Medtronic, analyzed a higher number of patients and a had longer follow up programme (298 for 12 months) than either the VIGOR or MUSTIC studies. This study also found a regression of ventricular remodelling in echocardiographic parameters, including a reduction of LV mass. This confirms in mid-term clinical evaluation the data of acute studies, i.e. an increase in mechanical efficiency of the heart linked to a reduction in energy cost. In addition, resynchronization resulted in a very significant reduction of MI (P=0.003). One year after treatment, the improvement in functional class, 6 minute walk test, quality of life, and the decrease in the number of hospital admissions (50% reduction) were confirmed, with a tendency of a reduction in mortality rate that did not reach statistical significance.

If these data are added to those from the COMPANION study (discussed below), enough arguments can be derived in favour of including patients in functional class II/III/IV, with a QRS ≥120 ms and moderate to severe systolic dysfunction, for pacing RT.

Follow Up

The follow up may be focused on simple clinical parameters, functional class being the most important one. Between 70%–80% of patients improve by at least one class and 30% by two classes, although 15%-20% do not improve and 5% get worse.

As a consequence, the quality of life is clearly improved and there is generally no need to apply the Minnesota score. In our opinion, a relevant clinical evidence is the increase in systolic pressure, which reaches 10–20 mm Hg in patients sensitive to resynchronization. It is then possible either to increase the doses of ACEI and BB, or to start the drug treatment if the patient could not tolerate it previously. This may have a significant impact on mortality reduction.

Of course, more sophisticated parameters can be included in the follow up, like assessment of norepinephrine or BNP levels, 6 minute walk test, or $V0_2$ consumption under stress test. However, we do not consider this essential in the clinical routine.

The echocardiogram is an excellent follow up tool to evaluate the efficiency of resynchronization, the improvement of atrial and ventricular volumes and systolic parameters, as well as the reduction of MI.

The AV interval must be programmed empirically on the basis of the obtained results. The proposed techniques and methods to optimize it, such as Ritter's formula, are controversial, and may even lead to contradictory effects.

Mitral Insufficiency

The mitral valvular apparatus and its closing mechanics during systole is altered in dilated cardiomyopathy, and this becomes more evident in the presence of LBBB. Just to point out the complexity of the mechanism leading to MI in dilated cardiomyopathy, it is important to remind that anatomic and functional alterations could involve: the valvular ring perimeter; the anchorage of anterior and posterior valvular leaflets; the proportions and dynamics of fibrous and muscular portions of cardiac trygonous forming the ring; the LV internal perimeter; the distance between the septum and the anterior and posterior papillary muscles; the distance between both papillary muscles and lastly, the extension and movement of the interventricular septum. In LBBB, abnormal and asynchronous contraction of the LV and the papillary muscles impairs the mitral valve apparatus to an even greater extent.

Currently we know that MI in dilated cardiomyopathy is not due to a ring dilatation secondary to LV dilatation. In fact, the severity of ventricular dilatation is not correlated with that of the ring and does not determine the occurrence of MI.

The posterior trygonous of the mitral ring is muscular and MI in these patients often involves this area of the valve. What does the surgeon do when performing a mitral anuloplasty? In simple terms, he moves the posterior wall of the ring towards the anterior valve (partial anuloplasty), or brings both valves together, shifting the muscular posterior wall and the fibrous anterior wall towards each other (total anuloplasty of G.Duran).

Resynchronization would imply a "functional anuloplasty". The early activation of the muscular area of the valvular trygonous, along with the resynchronization of the septum and papillary muscles, restores the "mitral sphincter" at the systole onset and reduces MI. Studies with real time ECHO-3D can confirm in vivo what 3D digitalization had previously shown in anatomic preparations of the isolated heart [10].

The differences observed in patients' response depending on the stimulation site in the LV, probably come more from induced changes in the activation sequence septum-posterior wall (close to the mitral ring-papillary muscles) than from global changes in the sequence septum-apex-anterior free wall. Interesting data on higher effectiveness of stimulation close to the atrio-ventricular ring in a postero-lateral position have been shown by Andrea Puglisi and colleagues.

Resynchronization and ICD: For whom?

The MADIT II study represents a significant change in the prophylactic indication of ICD [11], since ICD implantation is related exclusively to a low EF and not to the presence of arrhythmia in a wide range of patients (ischaemic heart disease and EF≤ 30%). Indeed, EF is well known as an excellent marker of mortality, but not of functional class or quality of life.

The MADIT II study proved a 31% reduction in the mortality of patients undergoing ICD implantation. The electrocardiographic substudy done by W. Zareba (Rochester, NY) and presented in the 23rd NASPE Meeting (San Diego) is extremely interesting. The multivariate analysis of the 364 patients treated by conventional therapy without an ICD, shows that a QRS width of >120 ms is an independent predictor of death. Furthermore, it is the only electrocardiographic parameter that predicts ICD shock for VT/VF in the randomized group with an ICD.

In patients with an ICD and a QRS >120 ms, the reduction in mortality was 63%, compared to those treated by conventional therapy (36% and 53% mortality within 2 and 3 years of HF with conventional therapy, versus 14% and 21% with an ICD, respectively).

Therefore, the results of the MADIT II study suggest that patients with an EF <30% and a QRS >120 ms can take the highest benefit from an ICD. If their functional class is II or more, ventricular diameters are increased, and/or moderate to severe MI occurs, we think there is no reason to refuse the implantation of an ICD capable of RT. Data on the mortality rate after 12 months from the implantation of the IncSync ICD will be provided by MEDTRONIC, as requested by the FDA. Together with the evaluation at 3 years that the company must carry out, these data will contribute to clarify the indications for a resynchronizing PM-ICD.

While the ICD indication depends on the EF, the indicators to the choice of a resynchronizing PM should be the functional class and the QRS width. In ischemic patients, the association of low EF with a wide QRS defines the group receiving higher benefit from a resynchronizing PM-ICD, and with highest mortality and worst functional class under conventional therapy.

Mortality is an issue already documented in the COMPANION study with solid and reliable data. The advances of the study have been reported by Dr. Bristow (University of Colorado Health Sciences Center, Denver) in a conference patronized by the Guidant Corporation. However, the final publication has not been produced so far.

The COMPANION study includes 1600 patients randomized under three teatments: optimal medical therapy; resynchronization alone or ICD-resynchronization. The inclusion criteria are: moderate to severe HF, QRS >120 ms with PR >150 ms and hospital admission for HF in the last year. End points are total mortality and hospital admissions.

In the two groups treated with RT, a 20% reduction in total mortality and number of hospital admissions was observed, in comparison to the group treated with optimal medical treatment. Moreover, the group with ICD-resynchronization showed a 40% reduction in the total mortality. The reduction in mortality in the resynchronization group was about one half of that noticed in the ICD-resynchronization group.

Conclusions

1. The cardiologist must consider resynchronization with a biventricular pacemaker in those patients suffering from moderate to severe HF, systolic dysfunction (EF <35%) and a QRS >120 ms with a LBBB pattern. Resynchronization is even more important if the above symptoms are accompanied by MI, whenever the patient does not respond to the best medical treatment (relapses to class III from II and always in class III/IV). It is proved beyond any reasonable doubt that RT can induce an improvement in the quality of life and a reduction in hospital admissions, along with strong evidence in favour of a diminution in mortality.
2. The follow up of these patients is easy, based on the clinical evaluation and the echocardiogram. A therapy with ACEI and BB may frequently be started if these drugs were not tolerated beforehand, or the doses can be increased.
3. The patients with a MADIT I or II indication of ICD, a QRS >120 ms and HF symptoms, are reasonable candidates for ICD-resynchronization.
4. In the group with LBBB and MI, the indication for RT is particularly attractive and can be summarized as "electric anuloplasty".

References

1. Levy D, Kenchaiah S, Larson MG et al (2002) Long- term trends in the incidence of and survival with heart failure. N Engl J Med 347:1397-1402
2. ACC/AHA/NASPE 2002. Guideline update for implantation of cardiac pacemakers and antiarrhythmia devices: summary article. Circulation, 106:2145-2161
3. Cianfrocca C et al (1992) Resting and ambulatory ECG predictors of mode of death in dilated cardiomyopathy. J Electrocardiol 25(5):295-303
4. Gothhipaty et al (1999) The resting ECG provides a sensitive and inexpensive marker of prognosis in patients with chronic congestive heart failure. JACC 33(2):A145 (Abstract 847-4)
5. Silvet H et al (1999) Increased QRS duration reduced survival in patients with left ventricular dysfunction: results from a cohort of 2263 patients. JACC 33(2):A145 (Abstract 847-5)
6. Nelson et al (2000) Left ventricular or biventricular pacing improves cardiac function at diminished energy cost in patients with dilated cardiomyopathy and left bundle branch block. Circulation 102:3053-3059
7. Guidant Corporation's CONTAK CD Trial. 22nd Annual Scientific Sessions of the North American Society of Pacing and Electrophysiology. Boston

8. Saxon LA, de Marco T, Schaefer J et al (2002) Effects of long-term biventricular stimulation for resynchronization on echocardiographic measures of remodeling. Circulation 105:1304-1310
9. Abraham WT, Ficher WG, Smiyh AL et al (2002) Cardiac resynchronization in chronic heart failure. NEJM 346:1845-1853
10. Ciappina Huch A, Biscegli Jatere F, Pinho Moreira LF et al (2002) Ventricular remodeling and mitral valve modifications in dilated cardiomyopathy: New insight from anatomic study. J Thotac Cardiovasc Surg 124:1216-1224
11. Moss AJ, Zeraba W, Hall J et al (2002) Prophylactic implantation of a defibrillator in patients with myocardial infarction and reduced ejection fraction. NEJM 346:877-83

New Advances in Biventricular Pacing: Improving Ventricular Sensing Function

F. Dorticós[1], P. Mazzone[2], R. Zayas[1], M.A. Quiñones[1], J. Castro[1], F. Di Gregorio[3]

Introduction

Several studies and increasing clinical experience suggest that interventricular resychronization can play an important role in the therapy of congestive heart failure (CHF) that is refractory to standard drug treatment. A remarkable percentage of CHF patients present with a delay in interventricular conduction and often with an ECG pattern of left bundle branch block (LBBB). The delayed left ventricular activation has detrimental effects on diastolic ventricular filling, with E wave and A wave overlapping, and can result in functional mitral regurgitation [1, 2]. In addition, desynchronization of myocardial contraction in the right and left ventricles (RV, LV) impairs the pump function, reducing the stroke volume (SV), and increasing the physical stress to the heart [3, 4].

Ventricular resynchronization can be achieved by simultaneous electrical stimulation of the two ventricles. To this purpose, specific biventricular (biV) pacemakers have been developed, as well as pacing leads suitable to be inserted into the coronary sinus in order to pace the LV from a cardiac vein. Several technical problems have progressively been solved, making biV pacing increasingly safe and effective [5]. Nevertheless, new advances in the implantable material are still requested to further improve LV lead positioning at implantation and stability during the follow-up.

The Optimal LV Pacing Site

The choice of the optimal pacing site in LV is a compromise of different considerations including physical accessibility, stability of the lead in situ, pacing threshold and sensing performance, and the effects of biV stimulation on the

[1]Instituto de Cardiología y Cirugía Cardiovascular, Habana, Cuba; [2]Cardiology Department, San Raffaele University Hospital, Milan; [3]Medico Clinical Research, Rubano (PD), Italy

QRS complex. Although the correlation between electrophysiological effects and actual clinical benefit of biV pacing is still a matter of debate, in principle the LV lead should be positioned where LV stimulation entails the maximum QRS shortening. This is generally obtained by pacing the basal region from a posterolateral vein [6].

Different techniques are available to drive the LV lead to a convenient pacing site, all with both advantages and disadvantages. However, in our experience, driving the LV lead along a coronary angioplasty guide-wire is the first-choice procedure. This approach ensures a high success rate in LV implantation, with the main limitation that, so far, the only available leads have been unipolar.

LV Sensing Specificity

Unipolar LV pacing is usually effective, although in some cases it can induce diaphragm or pectoralis muscle stimulation. The bipolar option may be more important in the prevention of sensing problems, which could be a critical issue in biV pacing. Sometimes, high ventricular sensitivity is required to ensure precise and timely detection of intrinsic activity, including ectopic beats generated in the LV. On the other hand, a high sensitivity increases the risk of oversensing, potentially resulting from environmental electromagnetic interferences, myopotentials, and atrial cross-talk. The latter should be a special concern, since far-field potentials generated in the left atrium could be sensed by a unipolar system in the LV, especially if the electrode is positioned in proximity to the coronary sinus. In contrast, bipolar sensing would allow better far-field rejection, greatly increasing LV sensing specificity.

New Tools in Biventricular Pacing

A new biV pacing system is currently under clinical evaluation in our center. It consists of the Ejection-P pacemaker and the Lifeline CS 750 LV lead (Medico, Padua, Italy). The pacing lead is bipolar and is designed to be positioned along a coronary angioplasty guide-wire (Table 1). The pacemaker is a DDD-R device which provides parallel biV pacing. It allows fine regulation of rate-adaptive AV delay, which is essential for biV pacing optimization, and high flexibility in individual pacing rate control, thanks to the special "dual-slope" rate-responsive system. A full series of pacing modes are available, including ventricular-triggered dual-chamber and single-chamber modes (DDT, VDT, VVT). Ventricular-triggered pacing also ensures biV stimulation in the event of intrinsic conduction, allowing free AV delay management on the basis of purely hemodynamic considerations.

Three Ejection-P pacemakers have been implanted: one with a unipolar lead in the LV (Corox LV, Biotronik, Germany) and two with the Lifeline CS 750 bipolar lead. All patients were affected by CHF of ischemic etiology with LBBB. The

Table 1. Technical specifications of Lifeline CS 750 bipolar lead

Suggested introducer	9 Fr
Total length	78 cm
Sheath diameter	1.7 mm
Inner lumen	0.45 mm
Insulation	Bio-compatible silicone
Electrodes (proximal / distal)	
Shape	Ring / ring
Diameter	1.9 / 1.9 mm
Surface	18 / 9 mm^2
Inter-electrode distance	20 mm
Material	Platinum-coated microporous titanium

implantation of the new Lifeline leads was performed quickly and without problems, with acute LV pacing thresholds of 0.7 V–0.5 ms and 0.8 V–0.5 ms. BiV pacing thresholds on discharge are reported in Table 2. The energy required for biV stimulation was about 50% lower in bipolar than in unipolar pacing. An example of threshold analysis by the implanted pacemaker is shown in Fig. 1. The QRS pattern and duration in VDD pacing can be compared under biV stimulation (energy above threshold), RV stimulation (energy between RV and biV threshold), and intrinsic conduction (total loss of ventricular capture).

In these patients, switching from unipolar to bipolar configuration did not substantially affect ventricular sensing, which was reliable in both sensing polarities even at the highest sensitivity. The permanent pacing mode was DDT, since two patients showed intrinsic conduction with PR interval in the normal range and AV delay shortening might have reduced the hemodynamic efficiency. In these cases, biV pacing was inhibited in DDD, while in DDT mode ventricular spikes were properly delivered and the resynchronization therapy was fully effective (Fig. 2).

Table 2. BiV pacing threshold on discharge

	Patient 1		Patient 2	
	Unipolar	Bipolar	Unipolar	Bipolar
V	2.5	2.5	1.25	1.25
ms	0.31	0.18	0.5	0.31
Impedance (Ω)	350	400	400	550
Energy (μJ)	5.5	2.8	1.9	0.8

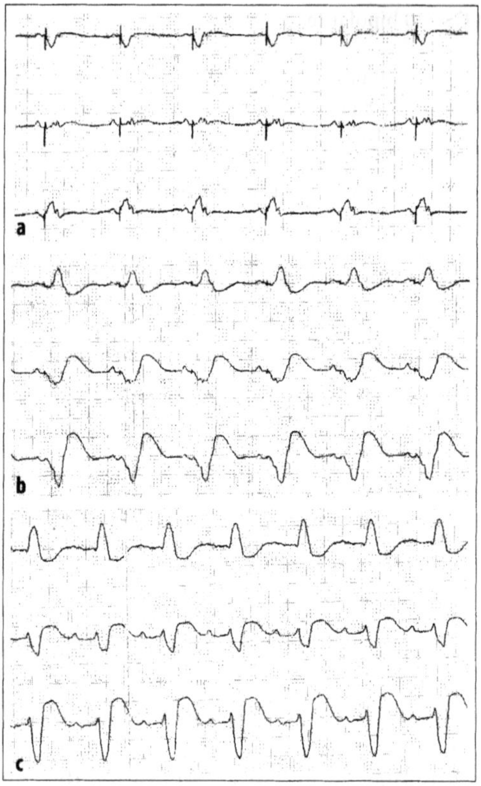

Fig. 1a-c. Threshold analysis with the implanted pacemaker (patient 2). **a** biV capture; **b** capture in RV only; **c** total loss of capture, resulting in intrinsic conduction with first-degree AV block and LBBB

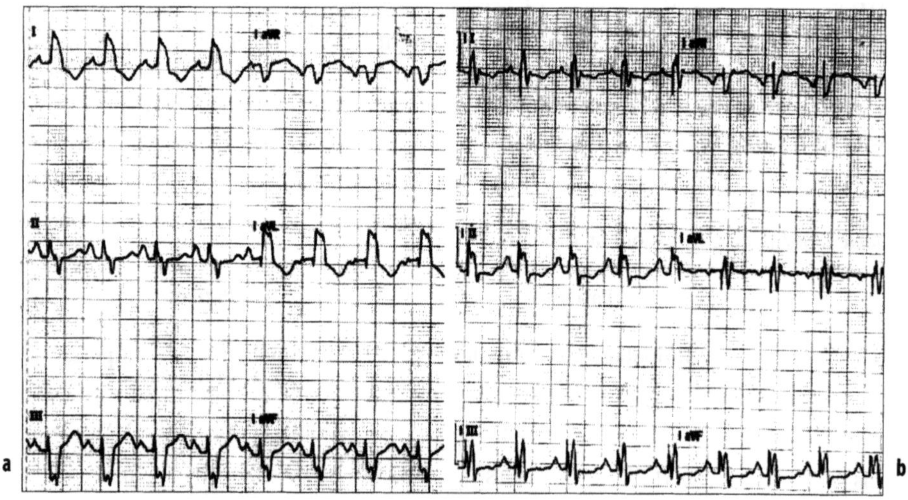

Fig. 2a,b. Patient 3. **a** DDD pacing mode, resulting in ventricular pacing inhibition due to intrinsic conduction with LBBB pattern. **b** DDT pacing mode with the same AV delay allowed regular biV pacing, resulting in marked QRS narrowing

At present, the longest follow-up is 12 months. A remarkable improvement in hemodynamic parameters and the patient's clinical condition was observed (Table 3). Pacing threshold and sensing performance remained quite stable over the period.

Table 3. Effects of ventricular resynchronization therapy (patient 1)

	Pre-implantation	1 month follow-up	12 month follow-up
QRS duration (ms)	202	180	170
SV (ml)	46	93	82
CO (l/min)	1.6	3.2	4
EF (%)	15	25	28
NYHA class	III	II	I
6-min walk (m)	390	545	500

Conclusions

A bipolar LV pacing lead to be positioned with a coronary angioplasty guidewire combines the advantages of high sensing specificity, reduced pacing threshold, and a quick and effective implantation procedure. In the presence of intrinsic conduction, the DDT pacing mode is the most advisable solution to prevent inhibition of ventricular pacing and loss of ventricular synchronization. Our experience with the Ejection pacing system is quite positive, both in terms of technical reliability and clinical results in treatment of CHF.

References

1. Schnittger I, Appleton CP, Hatle LK et al (1988) Diastolic mitral and tricuspid regurgitation by Doppler echocardiography in patients with atrioventricular block: new insight into the mechanism of atrioventricular valve closure. J Am Coll Cardiol 11:83-88
2. Auricchio A, Stellbrink C, Block M et al (1999) The effect of pacing chamber and atrio-ventricular delay on acute systolic function of paced patients with congestive heart failure. Circulation 99:2993-3001
3. Grines CL, Bashore TM, Boudoulas H et al (1989) Functional abnormalities in isolated left bundle branch block. The effect of interventricular asynchrony. Circulation 79:845-853
4. Xiao HB, Brecker SJD, Gibson DG (1992) Effects of abnormal activation on the time course of the left ventricular pressure pulse in dilated cardiomyopathy. Br Heart J 68:403-407

5. Curnis A, Mascioli G, Bontempi L et al (2002) Biventricular pacing: criteria for easier implantation procedure. In: Adornato E (ed) Progress on diagnosis and treatment of cardiac arrhythmias. Edizioni Luigi Pozza, Rome, pp 181-186
6. Pappone C, Rosanio S, Gulletta S et al (2000) Technological lead innovations and best sites for left ventricular pacing in patients with heart failure. In: Adornato E (ed) Cardiac arrhythmias: how to improve the reality in the third millennium? Edizioni Luigi Pozza, Rome, pp 369-375

Role of "Single Shock" ICD for Primary Prevention of Sudden Death in Heart Failure Patients

J. Brachmann

Introduction

When implantable cardioverter defibrillators (ICDs) were first introduced, ICD therapy was offered only to those patients who already had experienced an episode of ventricular fibrillation (VF). The dilemma of this approach in the particular field of ICD therapy, however, is that only a few per cent of patients survive their first VF episode. In other words, only a few thousand out of the 400 000 annual victims of sudden cardiac death in the USA have the chance to be treated with an ICD [1, 2]. However, if patients at an elevated risk were identified *before* they have their first VF episode and were implanted with an ICD prophylactically, the incidence of sudden cardiac death could be reduced.

Trials on the Use of ICD Therapy for Primary Prevention of Sudden Cardiac Death

In the early 1990s the first four controlled randomized trials for investigation of the use of ICD therapy in primary prevention of sudden cardiac death were initiated. MADIT I was able to clearly demonstrate a relative reduction in mortality of 42% after 4 years of follow-up. These results were eventually confirmed by the MUSTT trial 3 years later [3]. However, the CABG Patch trial failed to demonstrate a benefit from prophylactic ICD therapy in patients after coronary artery bypass graft surgery who were identified on the basis of a left ventricular ejection fraction (LVEF) below 0.36 and an abnormal signal-averaged electrocardiogram [4]. The Cardiomyopathy Trial (CAT), which investigated patients with idiopathic dilated cardiomyopathy and LVEF below 0.3, was terminated early because the all-cause mortality at 1 year did not reach the expected 30% in the control group [5].

Department of Cardiology, Klinikum Coburg, University of Würzburg, Coburg, Germany

The direct effect of MADIT I and MUSTT on ICD implantation numbers was not overwhelming since these two trials addressed a highly selected patient population. Neither did MADIT I or MUSTT affect the further development of ICD functionality: in 1997, Higgins et al. addressed the question whether MADIT I patients should be provided with ICDs with a reduced functionality and concluded that the answer was a clear no [6]. Only in 2001, did Zipes for the first time discussed this issue scientifically in his well-known *Circulation* editorial entitled "Implantable Cardioverter-Defibrillator: A Volkswagen or a Rolls Royce: How Much Will We Pay To Save A Life?" [7].

Just a few months later, in November 2001, after 2 years of follow-up the MADIT II trial demonstrated a reduction in mortality by 31% in patients with previous myocardial infarction and LVEF below 0.3 [8]. MADIT II could lead to an increase in the number of patients eligible for ICD therapy by as much as 100%. The positive outcome of the trial has stimulated intensive discussion of the socioeconomic impact of drastically increased patient numbers.

Concept of a Special Device for Prophylactic ICD Therapy

In the following, Zipes' idea of a special device for prophylactic implantation is further elaborated. These patients have never had a VT episode, and most of them never will have one: in MADIT II, the probability for receiving therapy for VT/VF within 3 years was 34%, and the probability of first appropriate shock for VF was 10% at 4 years [9]. Thus, the capacity for treatment delivery may be reduced, whereas the service time should be as long as possible. Patients without a history of arrhythmias will not need most of the functionality of modern ICDs. Their device should be as simple and robust as possible to make follow-up as easy and fast as possible. More precisely, a prophylactic ICD will certainly have to provide shock therapy, VVI pacing, and a VT episode Holter memory, but sophisticated antitachycardic or preventive pacing functions, for instance, may not be required.

After an episode of sustained VT/VF has occurred, in a patient, not primary but now secondary prevention is indicated. One would therefore expect this patient to use the device in the same way as those who had an indication for secondary prevention in the first place. Thus, it may be argued that the prophylactic ICD should then be replaced with a "standard" ICD. In other words, the capacity of such a device must ensure the safe and effective treatment of a single episode of VT/VF - a "single shock" device. Obviously, the capacity of a prophylactic ICD has to be somewhat greater, since ineffective or inappropriate therapies cannot be excluded completely.

Clinical Implications of a Prophylactic ICD

Assuming that a prophylactic ICD as defined above were to exist, how might it b-ehave in clinical practice? What is the mean episode-free survival of ICD patients? AVID reports that VT/VF occurred more frequently in patients whose index arrhythmia was VT than in those with VF [10]. The respective cumulative probabilities were 68% and 39% at 1 year of follow-up, 81% and 53% at 2 years, and 85% and 69% at 3 years. CIDS revealed a cumulative risk for receiving an ICD shock of 65.4% at 4 years [11]. For MADIT I, Higgins et al. report a cumulative probability for therapy release of more than 70% at 3 years of follow-up [6]. In MADIT II, the cumulative probability for receiving a therapy due to VT/VF was 34% at 3 years of follow-up [9].

There are several implications to be drawn from these figures. First, in all trials, a substantial portion of patients who receive an ICD after survived VF or sustained VT have no second episode at all. Second, a history of VT is associated with a higher incidence of therapy delivery than a history of VF. Third, in MADIT II, where inducibility was not required, the probability of receiving therapy was about 50% lower than in AVID, CIDS, or MADIT I. Its value is indeed in a range where a prophylactic ICD as described above becomes a reasonable alternative to standard devices.

To further analyze this issue, we retrospectively analyzed two ICD databases - our own clinical database and the database of the regulatory studies of one of the device manufactures (Biotronik GmbH & Co., Berlin). Our own ICD database includes 145 patients whose clinical characteristics are summarized in Table 1. We investigated the group of 43 patients (30%) who had no history of sustained VT/VF. Two of these patients had ICDs implanted for primary prevention, in the remaining 41 patients VT/VF was inducible during electrophysiological testing. The mean duration of follow-up in this patient group was 18.7±13.6 months (range: 0.1-53.2 months). During these 1.5 years on average

Table 1. Clinical characteristics of ICD patients in the Klinikum Coburg and Biotronik databases

	Coburg database	Biotronik database
Number of patients	43	400
Mean age (years)	65 ± 13	63 ± 11
Male sex (%)	82	83
Cardiac disease (%)		
Coronary artery disease	67	69
Myocardial infarction	61	35
Dilated cardiomyopathy	24	22
HOCM / RV dysplasia	-	4
Idiopathic	4	1
Other	4	4
Left ventricular ejection fraction	0.35 ± 0.14	0.34 ± 0.13
NYHA functional class	2.22 ± 0.79	2.1 ± 0.7

HOCM/RV, hypertrophic obstructive cardiomyopathy, right ventricle

of follow-up, 37% of the patients had at least one episode of sustained VT or VF. Inappropriate shocks occurred in four patients (9%) due to supraventricular tachycardias (n=2) or ventricular oversensing.

The Biotronik database included 400 patients. For details of the clinical characteristics see Table 1. Again, the analysis focused on the patients without a history of VT/VF (n=27; 6.8%). These patients were followed up for 10.9±6.4 months (range: 0.1-23.5 months). Six patients (22%) had an episode of VT or VF, and in four patients (15%) inappropriate detections were observed.

Conclusions

The potential of ICD therapy is that it could save up to 1000 lives per million population who die each year of sudden cardiac death. In the beginning, the application of ICD therapy was limited because we did not know how to identify the patients, and even today we can only identify a small fraction of them. Nevertheless, our health care system does not provide an ICD for all patients where there is general evidence that their lives could be saved by the device. In order to reach an implantation rate that is justified by the scientific evidence, it has been suggested that the cost of the devices be reduced, the health care budget for ICD therapy increased, and a special device offered to patients who have no history of sustained VT/VF. The functionality of such a device should be limited to detecting the first episode of life-threatening tachyarrhythmia in formerly asymptomatic patients and treating it through defibrillation. The device should then be replaced by a standard ICD. An analysis of the published literature on primary prevention trials and of two other databases provided evidence for the clinical validity of this new approach to ICD therapy. This analysis further reveals that there are two large patient groups who are expected to benefit from the proposed device for prophylactic ICD therapy: the post-myocardial infarction population and the heart failure population.

References

1. Engelstein ED, Zipes DP (1998) Sudden cardiac death. In: Alexander RW, Schlant RC, Fuster V (eds) The heart, arteries and veins. McGraw-Hill, New York, pp 1081-1112
2. Myerburg RJ, Castellanos A (1997) Cardiac arrest and sudden death. In: Braunwald E (ed) Heart disease: a textbook of cardiovascular medicine. WB Saunders, Philadelphia, pp 742-779
3. Buxton AE, Lee KL, Fisher JD et al (1999) A randomized study of the prevention of sudden death in patients with coronary artery disease. Multicenter Unsustained Tachycardia Trial investigators. N Engl J Med 341:1882-1890
4. Bigger JT Jr (1997) Prophylactic use of implanted cardiac defibrillators in patients at high risk for ventricular arrhythmias after coronary-artery bypass graft surgery. Coronary Artery Bypass Graft (CABG) Patch trial investigators. N Engl J Med 337:1569-1575

5. Bansch D, Antz M, Boczor S et al (2002) Primary prevention of sudden cardiac death in idiopathic dilated cardiomyopathy: the Cardiomyopathy Trial (CAT). Circulation 105:1453-1458
6. Higgins SL, Klein H, Nisam S (1997) Which device should "MADIT protocol" patients receive? Multicenter Automatic Defibrillator Implantation Trial. Am J Cardiol 79:31-35
7. Zipes DP (2001) Implantable cardioverter-defibrillator: a Volkswagen or a Rolls Royce: how much will we pay to save a life? Circulation 103:1372-1374
8. Moss AJ, Zareba W, Hall WJ et al (2002) Prophylactic implantation of a defibrillator in patients with myocardial infarction and reduced ejection fraction. N Engl J Med 346:877-883
9. MADIT II. FDA Premarket Approval Application: summary of safety and effectiveness. 2; P910077/S037 and P960040/S026. http://www.fda.gov/cdrh/pma/pmajul02.html
10. Anonymous (1997) A comparison of antiarrhythmic-drug therapy with implantable defibrillators in patients resuscitated from near-fatal ventricular arrhythmias. The Antiarrhythmics Versus Implantable Defibrillators (AVID) Investigators. N Engl J Med 337:1576-1583
11. Connolly SJ, Gent M, Roberts RS et al (2000) Canadian implantable defibrillator study (CIDS): a randomized trial of the implantable cardioverter defibrillator against amiodarone. Circulation 101:1297-1302

Subject Index

MIX
Papier aus verantwortungsvollen Quellen
Paper from responsible sources
FSC® C105338

If you have any concerns about our products,
you can contact us on
ProductSafety@springernature.com

In case Publisher is established outside the EU,
the EU authorized representative is:
Springer Nature Customer Service Center GmbH
Europaplatz 3, 69115 Heidelberg, Germany

Printed by Libri Plureos GmbH
in Hamburg, Germany